INSTRUCTOR'S RESOURCE MANUAL FOR

Being a Nursing Assistant

Lisa Friedman, MS, RN

Rose B. Schniedman, CNA, MSEd, BSN, RN

Susan S. Lambert, MAEd

Barbara R. Wander, BSN, RN

INSTRUCTOR'S RESOURCE MANUAL FOR

BEING A NURSING ASSISTANT

NINTH EDITION

FRANCIE WOLGIN

American Hospital Association

PEARSON Prentice Hall

HEALTH RESEARCH & EDUCATIONAL TRUST
In Partnership with AHA

Upper Saddle River, New Jersey

Notice: The procedures described in this textbook are based on consultation with nursing authorities. The author and publisher have taken care to make certain that these procedures reflect currently accepted clinical practice; however, they cannot be considered absolute recommendations.

The material in this textbook contains the most current information available at the time of publication. However, federal, state and local guidelines concerning clinical practices, including without limitation, those governing infection control and universal precautions, change rapidly. The reader should note, therefore, that new regulations may require changes in some procedures.

It is the responsibility of the reader to familiarize himself or herself with the policies and procedures set by federal, state and local agencies, as well as the institution or agency where the reader is employed. The authors and the publishers of this textbook, and the supplements written to accompany it, disclaim any liability, loss or risk resulting directly or indirectly from the suggested procedures and theory, from any undetected errors, or from the reader's misunderstanding of the text. It is the reader's responsibility to stay informed of any new changes or recommendations made by any federal, state and local agency as well as by his or her employing health care institution or agency.

Publisher: Julie Levin Alexander
Assistant to the Publisher: Regina Bruno
Editor-in-Chief: Maura Connor
Executive Editor: Barbara Krawiec
Assistant Editor: Sladjana Repic
Managing Development Editor: Marilyn Meserve
Development Editor: Maureen Muncaster
Editorial Assistant: Jennifer Dwyer
Director of Production and Manufacturing: Bruce Johnson
Managing Production Editor: Patrick Walsh
Production Liaison: Mary C. Treacy
Production Editor: John Probst, The GTS Companies/York, PA Campus
Manufacturing Manager: Ilene Sanford
Manufacturing Buyer: Pat Brown
Design Director: Cheryl Asherman
Senior Design Coordinator: Maria Guglielmo Walsh
Senior Marketing Manager: Nicole Benson
Marketing Coordinator: Janet Ryerson
Channel Marketing Manager: Rachele Strober
Composition: The GTS Companies/York, PA Campus
Cover Printer: Coral Graphics
Printer/Binder: Banta Harrisonburg

Pearson Education LTD.
Pearson Education Singapore, Pte. Ltd
Pearson Education, Canada, Ltd
Pearson Education—Japan
Pearson Education Australia PTY, Limited
Pearson Education North Asia Ltd
Pearson Educación de Mexico, S.A. de C.V.
Pearson Education Malaysia, Pte. Ltd
Pearson Education, Upper Saddle River, New Jersey

PEARSON
Prentice Hall

10 9 8
ISBN 0-13-177990-7

Contents

To the Instructor

This Instructor's Resource Manual is intended to help you use the *Being a Nursing Assistant* textbook to train students to become nursing assistants. The preparation of nonprofessional personnel to be effective and efficient members of the health care team is the responsibility of the instructor. It is usually the nursing assistant who has the most direct, prolonged contact with patients in the process of providing care for their basic daily needs. Be determined to improve the level of patient care beginning with your new class. You have, within your grasp, the means to effect constructive and positive change.

This Instructor's Resource Manual is written to assist you in the development of methods and means to transfer the content and fundamental skills from *Being a Nursing Assistant,* Ninth Edition, plus your knowledge and experience, to your students.

This manual can assist you in maximizing the use of your time and energy with increased benefits from your efforts. It is to this end that this manual has been prepared.

The needs, abilities, and characteristics of your students will require individualized instructional techniques. The able learner will require additional challenge in related in-depth study. Slow learners must be encouraged to expand their total effort.

When possible, use theater-style seating for lecture/discussion or film presentation. Use small-group clusters for team problem solving. Arrange a circle group for procedure instruction requiring close observation, and separated seating for quizzes and tests.

Assess time constraints within which you will have to work. Demonstration of a procedure will take twice the usual completion time, due to explanations and attention to key points.

To evaluate the level of comprehension, employ testing after each chapter followed by review of subject matter. You may wish to use the Instructor's Resource CD-Rom and the Companion Website online study guide to assist you in testing and assessment.

Provide each student with a copy of the textbook, *Being a Nursing Assistant,* Ninth Edition (ISBN 0-13-182873-8), by Francie Wolgin, and the *Workbook for Being a Nursing Assistant,* Ninth Edition (ISBN 0-13-177986-9), by Pulliam, Schniedman, Lambert, Wander.

SUGGESTED TEACHING STRATEGIES

- Provide opportunities for group participation
- Provide discussion opportunities to exchange points of view
- Continually diagnose the nature of students' learning deficiencies
- Use examples and/or case studies
- Provide participants with opportunities for independent study
- Provide lectures on subject matter
- Encourage students to take notes
- Provide tutoring
- Provide audiovisual presentations to reinforce lessons

To Present Theory

- Lecture—instructor, guest speaker, audiovisual presentation, movies, slides, overheads, charts, and posters
- Panel of authorities
- Resource materials

To Present Concept

- Discussion
- Small groups
- Role play
- Dramatization
- Handouts/workbook assignments

To Broaden Concept

- Field trips
- Clinical observation
- Peer-panel presentation and/or experts

To Present Skills

- Demonstration
- Observation
- Audiovisual presentation

To Develop Skills

- Return demonstration
- Laboratory practice with supervision
- Clinical practice with supervision
- At home practice

To Evaluate

- Written—worksheets, puzzles, quizzes, tests, exams, key questions
- Verbal—questioning, games
- Performance—procedure skill
- Evaluation should occur continually throughout the training period
- Evaluation should be based on the objectives identified for the content being tested
- Performance of skills must be observed to assure proper execution of procedures
- Establish a policy concerning the score necessary to complete/pass a procedure; when a score is unacceptable, the student should be given the time to practice and then repeat the procedure for evaluation
- Provide immediate review following evaluation

To Meet OSHA Standards, Continually Stress Standard/Universal Precautions

Nursing assistants will adhere to the following precautions when delivering care to all patients. This will decrease the risk of transmission of disease when the infection status of the patient is unknown.

- Gloves must be worn when contact with blood or body fluids (urine, feces, emesis, etc.) is likely, for example, when taking a rectal temperature.
- Gowns or aprons must be worn during procedures or situations when there will be exposure to body fluids, blood, draining wounds, or mucous membranes.
- Mask and protective eyewear or face shield must be worn during procedures that are likely to generate droplets of body fluids or blood or when the patient is coughing excessively.
- Gloves are to be worn when collecting all specimens to prevent contamination from body specimen fluids or blood.
- Handwashing: Hands must be washed before gloving and after gloves are removed. Hands and other skin surfaces must be washed immediately and thoroughly if contaminated with body fluids or blood and after all patient care activities.
- Nursing assistants who have open cuts, sores, or dermatitis on their hands must wear gloves for all patient contact.

This Instructor's Resource Manual can assist you in utilizing your time and energy with increased benefits from your efforts. It is to this end that this manual has been prepared. May you always enjoy your opportunity to teach and to share your knowledge and experience for the benefit of others.

PREPARATION FOR STATE AND/OR NATIONAL CERTIFICATION

The successful end of a nursing assistant course will be the completion by students of all requirements for state and/or national certification. Instructors should have a very clear understanding of these requirements.

Most of the state and national exams use the multiple-choice format. There are definite keys to successfully passing multiple-choice examinations. In a multiple-choice question or problem, the question or problem is called a stem. Four or five alternatives follow the stem and include the correct answer and the wrong ones, or distracters. The student must separate the correct, or most correct, answer from the distracters. The student should know that the stem deserves as much attention as the distracters. Discovering what the stem *is asking for* leads one in the right direction to finding the correct answer. It is important to thoroughly read and understand what the stem *is asking or looking for* before selecting an answer. Careless mistakes made on examinations are most often the result of not taking the time to read the question, or stem, of the question completely.

One of the best ways to prepare students for taking certification exams is to make multiple-choice examinations a part of the course from the very beginning. Doing so will sharpen students' test-taking skills and will prepare them for the format they are most likely to see.

Each chapter in this Instructor's Resource Manual contains a multiple-choice exercise to build student familiarity with the format. In addition, the Instructor's Resource CD-Rom allows you to easily prepare multiple-choice tests custom tailored to your students' needs.

If multiple-choice testing reveals some deficiencies in student understanding of chapter material, you might use the textbook end-of-chapter material for additional reinforcement, review, and practice. The Chapter Review provides fill-in-the-blank, multiple-choice, and critical thinking formats for reviewing chapter content.

INSTRUCTIONAL MEDIA

Companion Website: www.prenhall.com/wolgin

The interactive Companion Website, which is tied chapter-by-chapter to the text, gives students an online study guide that provides immediate feedback, helps bolster their self-confidence and provides links to interesting and relevant sites on the World Wide Web. The Companion Website also enables instructors to create a customized syllabus.

Free Student CD-Rom

Helps students master key terminology with an audio glossary. Includes test questions and videos.

Instructor's Resource CD-Rom

Includes a test bank, animations, and PowerPoints for classroom presentation.

Care Provider Skills Video Series

Allows students to see how procedures are actually performed. Videos are available individually or in a ten-video set.

Focus on Professionalism Video

Teaches students how to develop a professional image by demonstrating what professionalism is—and isn't.

1

The Health Care System

CHAPTER OVERVIEW

I. **The Health Care Environment**
   A. Health Care Reimbursement
   B. Medicare and Medicaid
   C. Diagnosis-Related Groups
   D. Managed Care
   E. HIPAA

II. **Health Care Delivery Sites**

III. **The Patient/Health Care Team**
   A. Organization of the Health Care Team
   B. Patient-focused Care

IV. **The Nursing Assistant: Part of the Team**
   A. Relationship of Nurse and NA/PCT

Instructor Notes

Instructor Notes

OBJECTIVES

When the students have completed this chapter, they will be able to:

- Explain the purpose and organization of the health care delivery system.
- Explain how managed care influences the health care delivery system.
- Describe the effects of DRGs on the American health care system.
- Describe five ways of organizing the patient care services/nursing health care team.
- Identify the members of the patient care services/nursing health care team.
- Explain the purpose and function of a multidisciplinary team approach to patient care.
- Explain the difference between the qualifications of the registered nurse and the licensed practical nurse, and between the jobs of the patient/nursing assistant and the unit clerk/secretary.

KEY TERMS

Diagnosis: Finding out what kind of disease or medical condition a patient has; diagnosis is always made by a physician

Diagnosis-related Groups (DRGs): Diagnostically related groups of patients; a DRG includes patients whose diagnoses are related, usually by body system or broad disease type, such as heart disease

Functional Nursing: A method of organizing the health care team in which the head nurse assigns and directs all patient care responsibilities for the nursing staff; this is sometimes called direct assignment

Health Care Institution (Facility): Hospital, hospice, nursing home, convalescent home, or clinic where health care services are provided both on an inpatient and outpatient basis

Health Insurance Portability and Accountability (HIPAA): Federal regulation governing the privacy of medical records and encouraging electronic transactions.

Hospice: An extended, or long-term, care facility that provides health care services to terminally ill patients and their families

Hospital: A short-term, or emergency, care facility that provides health care services to patients

Immediate Supervisor: An individual responsible for providing direction, critiquing performance, and giving feedback related to that performance

Multidisciplinary Team: A team of professionals and nonprofessionals from different disciplines that plans, makes decisions, and implements the delivery of patient care that is focused, or centered, on the patient's needs rather than any particular discipline's (department's) needs

Nurse: A person educated and trained to provide health care for people and to help physicians and surgeons; nurses are licensed as registered nurses (RNs) and licensed practical nurses (LPNs)

Nurse Manager: The RN leader responsible for the care delivery, personnel supervision, and operating budget of a unit, area, or facility

Instructor Notes

Nursing Assistant: A person who helps the registered nurse to care for patients; nursing assistants work in hospitals, long-term care or other health care facilities, or in the patient's home

Patient-focused Care: A care delivery model in which multidisciplinary teams plan, make decisions, and deliver care with the patient's needs as a focus rather than the needs or convenience of various departments or caregivers

Primary Nursing: A patient-oriented method of organizing the health care team in which the professional registered nurses are responsible for the total nursing care of the patient

Preferred provider organization (PPOs): An organization that contracts with an employer to provide health care and physicians' services to employees at a discounted rate

Task Oriented: Nursing care that is arranged according to what must be done

Team Leader: The nurse responsible for one area of a nursing unit, including patient care assignments

Team Nursing: A task-oriented method of organizing the health care team in which the team leader gives patient care assignments to each team member

CORE STUDENT ASSIGNMENTS

Students should:

- Read this chapter in their textbook, *Being a Nursing Assistant.*
- Underline any words or sentences they do not understand. Write down any questions they have.
- Complete the Chapter Review in their textbook.
- Read the Time Management Tip for this chapter and think about how they might use this tip in their work.
- Complete the Nursing Assistant in Action exercise.

OPTIONAL STUDENT ASSIGNMENTS

Students should:

- Complete all workbook assignments for this chapter in their copy of *Workbook for Being a Nursing Assistant.*
- Use the CD/CD-Rom disk enclosed with their textbook to hear the pronunciation of the key terms in the chapter.
- Watch the "Studying/Reading about Your Field" and the "Learning from Your Coworkers" sections of the "Focus on Professionalism" video from the Care Provider Skills series.
- Use the Website address **(www.prenhall.com/wolgin)** to access the free, interactive Companion Website created for this textbook. Get hints, instant feedback, and textbook references to chapter-related multiple-choice questions. Read and react to the Nursing Assistant in Action exercise. Link to other interesting sites.

Instructor Notes

METHODOLOGY AND SUGGESTED ACTIVITIES

I. Lecture/Discussion

- Answer any questions the students may have.
- Discuss the key terms and related abbreviations. Repeat them out loud and practice using them in sentences.
- Discuss the Time Management Tip for this chapter.
- Discuss the Nursing Assistant in Action exercise.
- Discuss the Critical Thinking points for this chapter.
- Discuss personal safety and protection. Emphasize the importance of following Universal Precautions. Stress the need to wear protective equipment.
- Tour a major hospital, a long-term care facility, and/or a home care agency.
- Draw a chart on the board as you discuss the organization of the health care team.
- Advise the students to contact community college admissions offices to get information on LPN and RN training programs, or invite an admissions director to be a guest speaker for your class.
- Enhance your lecture as you explain the levels of nursing by education required, job responsibilities, employment opportunities, and probable salary at each level.
- Review DRGs and managed care. Give examples from your institution.
- Review ways that medical information can be protected under HIPAA. Review common accidental disclosures that can be avoided.
- Compare and contrast the different ways to deliver nursing care.

II. Role Play/Lab

- Show the videos for this chapter. Discuss the different kinds and levels of nurses in the profession. Discuss the different ways that people learn, from formal education and from each other, and the importance of working as a team for optimal patient care.
- Have the students practice being the nurse and being the nursing assistant in different situations that require giving and receiving delegation.
- Have the group brainstorm how they might resolve nurse/nurse assistant conflict scenarios.
- Have students role play situations where confidentiality is an issue. Discuss precautions the students should take to be in compliance with HIPPA.

III. Evaluation

- Review the answers to the Chapter Review with students.
- Review the answers to the workbook exercises with students.
- Review the students' understanding of the Time Management Tip.
- To evaluate student comprehension, give a quiz.
- To evaluate student skills, administer the competency checklist.
- Have the students visit the interactive Companion Website and take the quiz.

ANSWERS TO CHAPTER REVIEW

Instructor Notes

FILL IN THE BLANK

Read each sentence and fill in the blank line with a word that completes the sentence. (Note: Hyphenated words get one line.)

1. The ___team___ ___leader___ is the nurse responsible for one area of a nursing unit.
2. An ___organizational___ ___chart___ is a chart that shows the chain of command within an institution.
3. An extended care facility that takes care of terminal patients is called a ___hospice___.
4. ___Managed___ ___care___ is a type of insurance that is based on prepayments, negotiated contracts, and agreements for prior service authorization.
5. Patient-focused care is a ___care___ ___delivery___ model for assigning care to patients.

MULTIPLE CHOICE

Choose the best answer for each question or statement.

1. Which of the following is not a function of a health care delivery system?
   A. Provide care for the ill and injured
   B. Prevent disease
   (C.) Provide free care to the indigent
   D. Provide facilities for the education of health care workers
2. A physician's determination of a patient's condition or disease is called a:
   A. hospice.
   B. referral.
   (C.) diagnosis.
   D. HIPAA code.
3. Which of the following is not a health care delivery site?
   A. Birthing center
   (B.) Fitness center
   C. Skilled nursing facility
   D. Community care home
4. Which of the following is not a care delivery model?
   A. Primary nursing
   (B.) Quad care
   C. Team nursing
   D. Partners in practice

Instructor Notes

5. HIPAA's primary concern is
   A. streamlining payments for health care.
   B. fighting obesity.
   C. regulating hip replacements.
   (D.) protecting patient privacy and treatment information.

6. Nursing assistants who work in nursing homes must complete
   (A.) competency evaluation programs.
   B. college.
   C. training programs.
   D. written tests.

CRITICAL THINKING

CUSTOMER SERVICE

Encourage students to reflect and share their thoughts and experiences. Respect their privacy and confidentiality. Share your own viewpoints with the students.

CULTURAL CARE

Encourage students to reflect and share their thoughts and experiences. Respect their privacy and confidentiality. Share your own viewpoints with the students.

COOPERATION WITHIN THE TEAM

Encourage students to reflect and share their thoughts and experiences. Respect their privacy and confidentiality. Share your own viewpoints with the students.

NURSING ASSISTANT IN ACTION

You will be working with a group of people you do not know. You report to the unit and a team member approaches you saying, "Oh you must be the new guy. I was told to show you around."

What Is Your Response/Action?

Introduce yourself and express your interest in learning. Ask questions about the plan of the day and the organization of tasks and duties. Watch for not only what is being done, but also how it is being performed for the patients.

1

Answers to Workbook Exercises

The following exercises will assist you to apply what you have read in Chapter 1, "The Health Care System." For each exercise, read the objective and use information you have read in Chapter 1 to answer the questions, complete the sentences, or label the diagrams.

EXERCISE 1-1

Objective: To recognize and correctly spell words related to the health care system.

Directions: Unscramble the words in the Word List at the left. Then circle these same words in the Word Search at the right.

Word List

1. RDG ______ *DRG*
2. AANMDGE RAEC ______ *MANAGED CARE*
3. AETM ______ *TEAM*
4. IMRPRYA ______ *PRIMARY*
5. AKST ______ *TASK*
6. SPRUEVRIOS ______ *SUPERVISOR*
7. TAIPNET OCFSDUE ______ *PATIENT FOCUSED*
8. SRGIETEEDR ESRUN ______ *REGISTERED NURSE*
9. AIPHA ______ *HIPAA*

Word Search

L	E	S	I	T	K	X	S	H	K	L	F	Q	Y	K
P	S	B	Q	A	W	Z	F	W	U	D	G	C	P	Z
A	R	U	O	V	B	U	D	I	O	P	N	I	W	X
T	U	T	A	G	S	C	R	H	A	R	G	N	E	Y
I	N	E	I	L	Y	E	A	C	Q	I	B	Y	O	T
E	D	A	B	F	T	I	G	F	N	M	S	K	L	U
N	E	M	A	N	A	G	E	D	C	A	R	E	I	K
T	R	A	B	E	S	O	N	R	U	R	D	P	G	Q
F	E	H	I	M	K	J	A	G	N	Y	S	E	M	X
O	T	K	D	T	R	H	K	D	B	L	C	J	E	R
C	S	R	O	S	I	V	R	E	P	U	S	S	N	I
U	I	G	F	G	X	I	M	P	A	Y	T	O	H	O
S	G	L	B	I	C	P	E	R	O	I	A	C	J	U
E	E	W	M	O	V	O	T	Y	M	U	V	T	X	D
D	R	N	C	P	S	A	W	J	H	I	P	A	A	Z
C	B	V	A	E	F	Z	X	A	W	Q	B	M	X	A
Y	R	T	B	D	L	K	U	O	J	P	N	Z	G	W
Z	I	K	O	E	B	Z	H	Z	E	C	V	J	C	H
X	F	M	Q	R	L	T	Y	H	A	Y	K	I	S	E

EXERCISE 1-2

Objective: To apply what you have learned about the health care system and the nursing assistant.

Directions: Circle the letter next to the statement that best completes the sentence or describes the sentence as true or false. If the sentence is false, draw a line through the incorrect part of the sentence and write the correction on the blank line.

1. Factors directly affecting the health care system are all of the following *except*
   A. government legislation.
   B. an aging population.
   C. managed care.
   (D.) floral deliveries.
2. The nursing assistant in his role is able to directly contribute to the health care system if he can effectively participate in
   A. culturally sensitive care.
   B. the team approach.
   C. cost-effective quality care.
   (D.) all of the above.
3. It is important to understand the organizational structure of the facility you work at because
   (A.) knowing this will help you to be more successful in your role.
   B. it might be asked on a test.
   C. you will get paid more for knowing this.
   D. you want to impress your friends.
4. At the center of the multidisciplinary team approach is the
   A. nurse.
   B. nursing assistant.
   C. doctor.
   (D.) patient.
5. Patient-focused care means that the patient's needs are considered ~~last~~ when planning individualized care.
   A. True
   (B.) False
   Correct Answer: *first*
6. Preventing disease is an important aspect of the ________ system.
   A. postal
   B. digestive
   C. infective
   (D.) health care

7. Because the health care system is continually changing, the successful nursing assistant will be looking for opportunities to

A. work fewer hours.
(B.) learn new skills to keep up with these changes.
C. remain the same, because it always worked in the past.
D. do her best to resist change.

8. Which of the following is not a type of insurance?

A. managed care
(B.) HIPAA
C. PPO
D. Blue Cross

9. DRG stands for

A. divisional regulated growth.
B. diagnostic rules and groups.
(C.) diagnosis-related groups.
D. diagonally related growth.

10. To be effective, health care must go beyond the care provided in the hospital to consider the health needs of the community.

(A.) True
B. False
Correct Answer: ______________________________

11. CPT–4 stands for

A. Cost-Preventive Treatment–4th edition.
B. Currently Posted Trials–4th edition.
C. Collective Procedural Terminology–4th edition.
(D.) Current Procedural Terminology–4th edition.

12. The goal of quality care is to improve the individual's health status as much as possible.

(A.) True
B. False
Correct Answer: ______________________________

13. The goal of managed care is to balance quality care, cost, and access.

(A.) True
B. False
Correct Answer: ______________________________

14. Health care financing refers to __________ , who pay for hospital visits, clinic visits, prescription medications, home care visits, hospice care, and other health care services.

A. insurance companies
B. managed care entities
C. individuals
(D.) all of the above

15. Health care delivery refers to ________, who provide health care services to patients.

A. nursing assistants, doctors, nurses, and therapists
B. hospitals, clinics, and surgical centers
C. rehabilitation centers, hospices, and home care agencies
(D.) all of the above

16. There are several different kinds of nursing care team structures, but a common element is

(A.) a nurse accountable for the patient's nursing care.
B. a nursing assistant as part of the team.
C. fee-for-service payment.
D. a doctor performing nursing tasks.

17. The nursing assistant will need to focus on providing all of the following *except*

A. privacy.
B. culturally specific care.
C. customer service.
(D.) financial advice.

18. No matter what team the nursing assistant works on, the most important element of his success is

A. to discuss his assignments with the patient.
(B.) to discuss his assignment and any questions he may have with his immediate supervisor.
C. to discuss everything with the team.
D. to discuss the patients he cares for with his friends.

19. Based on the ________, nursing assistants must complete an approved training program before working in skilled nursing facilities and nursing homes.

(A.) Omnibus Budget Reconciliation Act (OBRA) of 1987
B. direction of the Skilled Nursing Act
C. American Nursing Home Authority
D. TEFRA of 1982

EXERCISE 1-3

Objective: To apply what you have learned about organizational structures and the nursing assistant's "chain of command."

Directions: Label the blank spaces on the organizational chart in Figure 1-1. Place the words from the Word List below in the proper order on the diagram.

Word List

Board of Directors	Staff Nurses	Director of Nurses
VP of Operations	LPNs	Nursing Assistants
Nurse Managers	President	

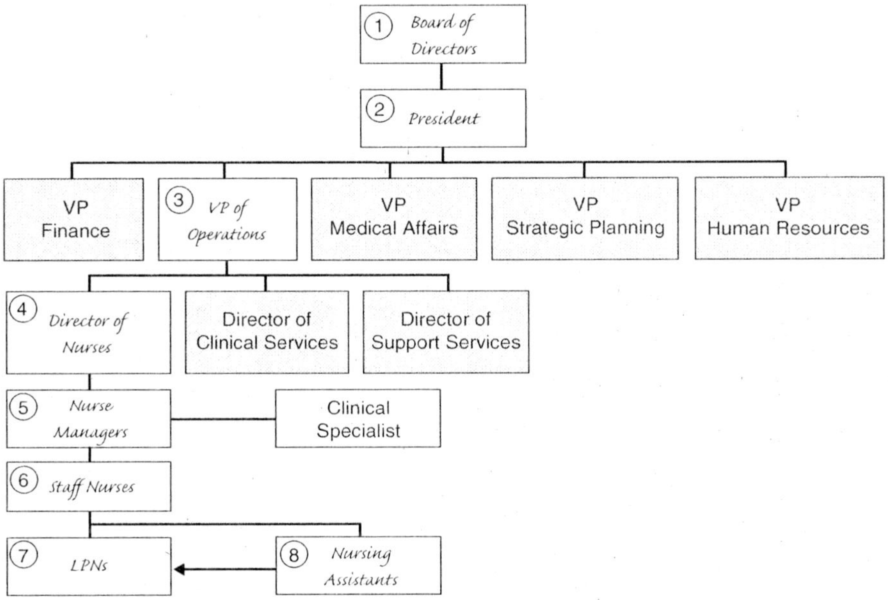

FIGURE 1-1

EXERCISE 1-4

Objective: To apply what you have learned about the multidisciplinary patient care team.

Directions: Label the multidisciplinary patient care team diagram in Figure 1-2 with the correct words from the Word List below. Choose from the list only those who are part of this team.

Word List

Clergy	Veterinarian	Physician	Speech Therapist
Patient	Family	Social Worker	Coach
Manicurist	Engineer	Pilot	Registered Nurse
Dentist	Beautician	Nursing Assistant	Patient Care Technician
Pharmacist			

FIGURE 1-2

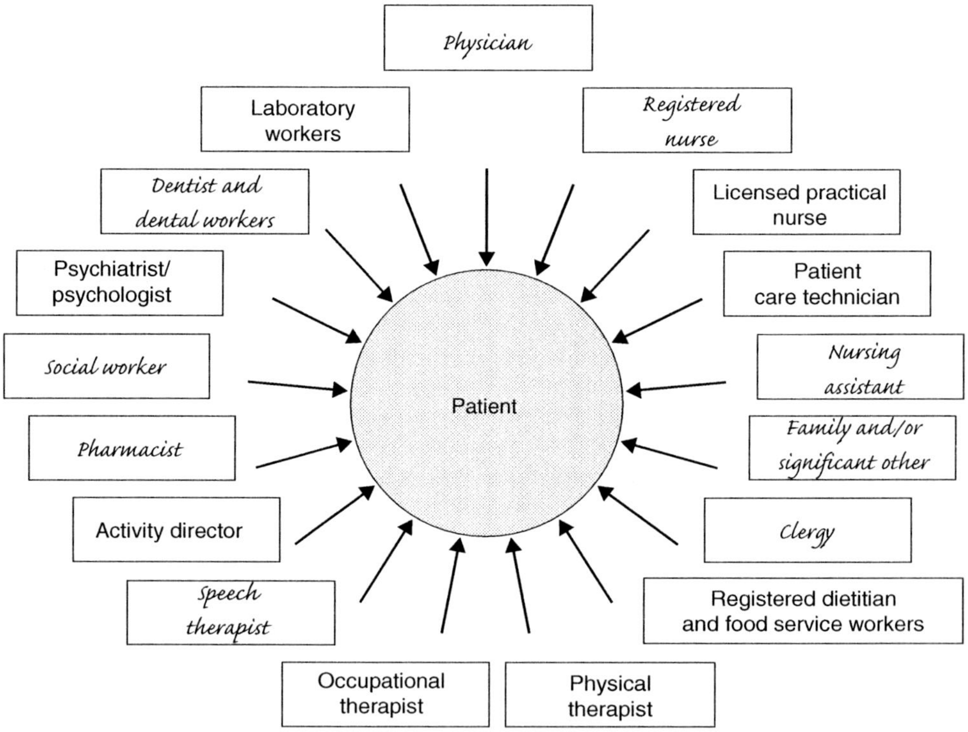

EXERCISE 1-5

Objective: To recognize the definitions of words related to the health care system.

Directions: Place the letter of the correct definition next to the matching word(s) from the Word List.

Word List

I 1. nurse
E 2. hospice
A 3. diagnosis
B 4. DRGs
H 5. multidisciplinary team
C 6. functional nursing
D 7. health care institution
G 8. immediate supervisor
F 9. hospital
N 10. managed care
Q 11. team nursing
P 12. team leader
O 13. task oriented
K 14. nurse manager
M 15. primary nursing
J 16. nursing assistant
L 17. patient-focused care
R 18. preferred provider organization

Definitions

A. A physician's determination of a patient's disease or condition
B. Diagnostically related groups of patients
C. A method of organizing the health care team in which the head nurse assigns and directs all patient care responsibilities for the nursing staff
D. Hospital, hospice, nursing home, convalescent home, or clinic where health care services are provided both on an inpatient and outpatient basis
E. An extended, or long-term, care facility that provides health care services to terminally ill patients and their families
F. A short-term, or emergency, care facility that provides health care services to patients
G. An individual responsible for providing direction, critiquing performance, and giving feedback related to that performance
H. A team of professionals and nonprofessionals from different disciplines that plans and implements patient-focused care
I. A person educated and trained to provide health care for people, working with physicians and other health care team members; licensed as RNs and LPNs
J. A person who helps the registered nurse to care for patients
K. The RN leader responsible for the care delivery, personnel supervision, and operating budget of a unit, area, or facility

L. A care delivery model in which multidisciplinary teams plan and implement care based on the patient's individual needs

M. A patient-oriented method of organizing the health care team in which the professional registered nurses are responsible and accountable for the entire nursing care of the patient

N. Care provided under a wide variety of prepayment agreements, negotiated contracts and discounts, agreements for prior service authorization or approval, and performance audits

O. Nursing care that is arranged according to what must be done

P. The nurse responsible for one area of a nursing unit, including patient care assignments

Q. A task-oriented method of organizing the health care team in which the team leader gives patient care assignments to each team member

R. A company that provides health care and physician services to members for a discounted price as long as they use services within the plan

2

Your Role as a Nursing Assistant

CHAPTER OVERVIEW

Instructor Notes

I. The Nursing Assistant: An Important Caregiver
- A. Role of the Nursing Assistant
- B. Duties and Functions of the Nursing Assistant

II. Personal Qualities
- A. Personal Hygiene and Appearance

III. Organizing Your Work
- A. Time Management
- B. Goal Setting
- C. Stress Reduction

IV. Ethical Behavior

V. Legal Aspects of Patient Care
- A. The Patient's Bill of Rights
- B. Incidents

Instructor Notes

OBJECTIVES

When the students have completed this chapter, they will be able to:

- Display qualities that are desirable in a good patient/nursing assistant.
- Identify duties and role functions of nursing assistants.
- Practice good personal hygiene.
- Organize their work efficiently.
- Behave ethically.
- Keep confidences to themselves.
- Work accurately.
- Be dependable.
- Follow rules and instructions.
- Develop cooperative staff relationships.
- Show respect for patients' rights.
- Explain how laws affect them and the patients they care for.
- Report incidents.

KEY TERMS

Accountable: To be answerable for one's behavior; legally or ethically responsible for the care of another

Accuracy: The quality of being exact or correct; exact conformity to truth and rules; free from errors or defects

Competency: A demonstrable skill or ability

Cooperation: Working or acting together; uniting to produce an effect or to share an activity for mutual benefit

Dependability: A quality shown by coming to work every day on time and doing what is asked at the proper time and in the proper way

Ethical Behavior: To keep promises and do what you should do; to act in accordance with the rules or standards for right conduct or practice

Hazard: A source of danger; a possible cause of an accident

Hygiene: The science that deals with the preservation of health; when used to describe an object or a person, it means clean and sanitary

Incident: An unforeseen event that occurs without intent

Informed Consent: A voluntary act by which a conscious and mentally competent person gives permission for someone else to do something for him

Interpersonal Skills: Skills used in interacting with other persons, such as courtesy; good interpersonal skills enable people to interact or work together in a productive and satisfying manner

Malpractice: Negligence when applied to the performance of a professional

Negligence: The commission of an act or failure to perform an act, where the respective performance or nonperformance deviates from the act that should have been done by a reasonably prudent person under the same or similar conditions

Stress: A physical, mental, or emotional tension or strain triggered by a stimulus that requires some response or type of adjustment

Instructor Notes

CORE STUDENT ASSIGNMENTS

Students should:

- Read this chapter in their textbook, *Being a Nursing Assistant.*
- Underline any words or sentences they do not understand. Write down any questions they have.
- Complete the Chapter Review in their textbook.
- Read the Time Management Tip for this chapter and think about how they might use this tip in their work.
- Complete the Nursing Assistant in Action exercise.

OPTIONAL STUDENT ASSIGNMENTS

Students should:

- Complete all workbook assignments for this chapter in their copy of *Workbook for Being a Nursing Assistant.*
- Use the CD/CD-Rom disk enclosed with their textbook to hear the pronunciation of the key terms in the chapter.
- Watch the "Studying/Reading about Your Field" and the "Learning from Your Coworkers" sections of the "Focus on Professionalism" video from the Care Provider Skills series.
- Use the Website address **(www.prenhall.com/wolgin)** to access the free, interactive Companion Website created for this textbook. Get hints, instant feedback, and textbook references to chapter-related multiple-choice questions. Read and react to the Nursing Assistant in Action exercise. Link to other interesting sites.

METHODOLOGY AND SUGGESTED ACTIVITIES

I. Lecture/Discussion

- Answer any questions the students may have.
- Discuss the key terms and related abbreviations. Repeat them out loud and practice using them in sentences.
- Discuss the Time Management Tip for this chapter.
- Discuss the Nursing Assistant in Action exercise.
- Discuss the Critical Thinking points for this chapter.
- Emphasize the rules to follow.
- Give examples of the policies on lateness and absenteeism from a few health care institutions where your former students are employed.
- Give examples of possible mistakes and what to do when they happen.
- Invite a lawyer to be a guest speaker.
- Discuss how different cultures' practices have an effect on students' thoughts on ethics.

Instructor Notes

II. Role Play/Lab

- Show the videos for this chapter. Discuss what kinds of behavior make you feel well cared for and respected when you are receiving health care. Discuss the issues of patient rights and, especially, the patient's right to refuse care. Relate these themes to various cultures.
- Have the students role play factors that increase or decrease friendliness or stress in the workplace.
- Explain qualities that make a well-rounded nursing assistant. To demonstrate, draw a large circle and divide it into pie-shaped sections. Have the students fill in each slice with a quality.
- Invite a few former students to return as an informal panel to describe their jobs. Have your students prepare questions in advance.
- To *dramatize* the importance of proper grooming, you may wish to ask one student to dress up as a living example of what not to do. For example, she should wear a black slip an inch too long under her uniform, too much jewelry, dirty tennis shoes, and a bright scarf around her hair. Expand on this with further explanations and examples.

III. Evaluation

- Review the answers to the Chapter Review with students.
- Review the answers to the workbook exercises with students.
- Review the students' understanding of the Time Management Tip.
- To evaluate student comprehension, give a quiz.
- To evaluate student skills, administer the competency checklist.
- Have the students visit the interactive Companion Website and take the quiz.

ANSWERS TO CHAPTER REVIEW

FILL IN THE BLANK

Read each sentence and fill in the blank line with a word that completes the sentence. (Note: Hyphenated words get one line.)

1. When you are legally or ethically responsible for the care of another, you are said to be ___accountable___.
2. Working or acting together for mutual benefit is called ___cooperation___.
3. Good ___hygiene___ includes good personal cleanliness and appearance.
4. You demonstrate good ___time___ ___management___ when you plan, prioritize, and organize your work in order to get it done in a given time period.
5. ___Ethical___ behavior includes keeping promises, doing what you should do, and acting in accordance with the rules and standards for right conduct and practice.

Instructor Notes

MULTIPLE CHOICE

Choose the best answer for each question or statement.

1. Positive traits in a nursing assistant are all of the following *except*
- A. being trustworthy.
- B. enjoying working with others.
- (C.) liking things only a certain way.
- D. liking to learn new things.

2. The code of ethics includes which of the following standards?
- A. Carrying out faithfully the instructions you are given
- B. Respecting the right of all patients to beliefs that are different from yours
- C. Letting the patient know it is your pleasure to do your job
- (D.) All of the above

3. Do not discuss patient information with
- A. other patients.
- B. relatives and friends of the patient.
- C. your family.
- (D.) All of the above.

4. Doing something or not doing something when a reasonably prudent nursing assistance would have done it under the same conditions is called
- (A.) negligence.
- B. invasion of privacy.
- C. accountability.
- D. battery.

5. Because an incident is an unforeseen event that occurs without intent,
- A. it does not need to be reported.
- B. it only needs to be reported if the patient is harmed.
- (C.) failure to report it could lead to losing your job.
- D. there is no liability for it.

CRITICAL THINKING

CUSTOMER SERVICE

Encourage students to reflect and share their thoughts and experiences. Respect their privacy and confidentiality. Share your own viewpoints with the students.

CULTURAL CARE

Encourage students to reflect and share their thoughts and experiences. Respect their privacy and confidentiality. Share your own viewpoints with the students.

COOPERATION WITHIN THE TEAM

Encourage students to reflect and share their thoughts and experiences. Respect their privacy and confidentiality. Share your own viewpoints with the students.

Instructor Notes

NURSING ASSISTANT IN ACTION

You are in the elevator at work along with two doctors and three visitors. The doctors start a conversation about one of the patients you are assigned to care for today. You notice the visitors paying attention to the doctors' conversation about treatment options for Mr. Chu, your patient.

What Is Your Response/Action?

Sometimes caregivers get so wrapped up in their conversations that they do not see others who should not hear what they are saying. A good thing to do in this situation is to politely interrupt the physicians to remind them of the visitors' presence without being rude. You could say something like "Excuse me, be alert"; this is a familiar signal to watch what you are saying. Or "Excuse me, doctors, we have visitors with us." If that does not work, you could divert the visitors' attention away from the physicians by starting a conversation with them.

2

Answers to Workbook Exercises

The following exercises will assist you to apply what you have read in Chapter 2, "Your Role as a Nursing Assistant." For each exercise, read the objective and use information you have read in Chapter 2 to answer the questions, complete the sentences, or label the diagrams.

EXERCISE 2-1

Objective: To apply what you have learned about personal hygiene and appearance.

Directions: Look carefully at the pictures in Figure 2-1. Choose the number of the sentence on the Personal Hygiene List that indicates the correct personal grooming rule you need to practice on a daily basis. Label the item in Figure 2-1 with the correctly matching number.

Personal Hygiene List

1. Dress properly and neatly. Follow the dress code of the health care institution where you work.
2. Use good personal hygiene, bathing or showering daily.
3. Keep your mouth and teeth clean and in good condition.
4. Keep your hair clean and neatly combed. Long hair should be braided, pulled back, or pinned up.
5. Keep your nails short and clean. Wear only clear nail polish, if any.
6. Wear no or very little makeup.
7. Try to be completely free of odor. Do not use heavy perfume, scented sprays, or heavy shaving lotion. Use an unscented deodorant.
8. Get plenty of sleep. Be alert when you come to work.
9. Keep your body fit; do daily exercises.
10. Wear your name tag where patients can see it.
11. Wear comfortable, low-heeled, enclosed shoes with nonskid soles and heels.
12. Keep your shoes polished and the laces clean.
13. Repair rips and hems and replace missing buttons on your clothing.

14. Eat a well-balanced diet every day.
15. Always wear your name pin and institutional badge.
16. Always wear a wristwatch with a second hand.
17. Always carry a pen and a pad of paper.

Figure 2-1

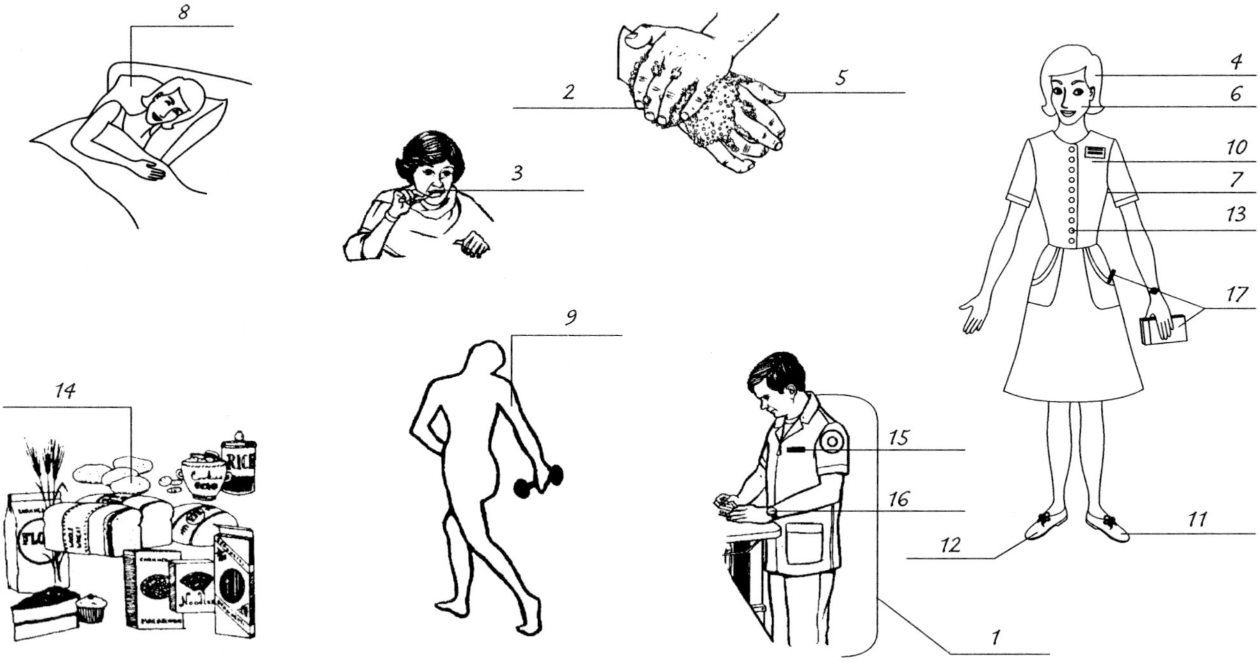

EXERCISE 2-2

Objective: To be able to recognize important concepts of work organization, ethics, work rules, staff relationships, and the legal requirements of patient care.

Directions: Place the correct letters next to the closest matching phrase. There may be more than one correct answer.

WO = work organization WR = work rules
LR = legal requirements SR = staff relationships
E = ethics

_LR_ **1.** The Patient's Bill of Rights

_WR_ **2.** Never discuss your personal problems with patients.

_WR_ **3.** Do not waste or destroy supplies or equipment.

_E_ **4.** Check the patient's ID bracelet for accuracy.

_WO_ **5.** Prioritize your work.

_LR_ **6.** Understand how the law affects you and your patient.

_E_ **7.** Dependability means more than coming to work on time every day.

E 8. Work to be a good team member.

WR 9. Be ready to adjust quickly to new situations.

LR 10. Know the laws of your particular state.

LR 11. Civil rights must be guaranteed to all citizens.

LR 12. Good Samaritan laws protect you if you act in good faith during emergencies.

WR 13. Patient confidentiality must be protected.

LR 14. Standards of care are based on laws, administrative policy, and guidelines.

WO 15. Report all complaints from patients and visitors to the immediate supervisor.

SR 16. Volunteer to assist coworkers when you can.

E 17. Respect the right of all patients to have beliefs and opinions that are different from yours.

WO 18. New needs and unexpected situations may arise, requiring you to adjust your priorities.

WR 19. Perform only procedures that you have been educated to do.

WO 20. Make a written list of your assignments. Review or change the list as you prioritize your work, and check off each item as it is completed.

EXERCISE 2-3

Objective: To apply principles of ethical behavior to challenging situations in which you may be involved.

Directions: Next to each Practice Description, write the number of the correct response.

Practice Description

C 1. A patient offers you a tip.

E 2. A patient inquires about another patient across the hall.

D 3. The patient's ID bracelet is on the bedside stand.

B 4. You discover that Mrs. Chang, who is on a low-salt diet, has eaten all of her lunch from a regular diet tray, which you gave her earlier by mistake.

A 5. You have a headache, and nothing seems to be going the way it should today.

Response

A. Refrain from sharing your personal problems as you provide care for others.

B. You notify your immediate supervisor at once.

C. You say, "No, thank you," and pleasantly explain that it is against written policy to accept.

D. You follow the policy of your institution to place the ID bracelet on the patient's wrist for safety.

E. You give no information about the patient, but you do explain the institution's policy on confidentiality.

EXERCISE 2-4

Objective: To apply what you have learned about your role as a nursing assistant.

Directions: Circle the letter next to the statement that best completes the sentence or describes the sentence as true or false. If the sentence is false, draw a line through the incorrect part of the sentence and write the correction on the blank line.

1. Making false or damaging statements about another person is
(A.) known as defamation of character.
B. known as a good standard of care.
C. a breach of duty.
D. a way to strengthen a relationship.

2. Patients have the right to refuse care, ~~even if they are not conscious.~~
A. True
(B.) False
Correct Answer: *if they are conscious and mentally alert.*

3. Leaving your patients without permission or without notifying the immediate supervisor is
A. acceptable if you are sick.
B. acceptable at the end of your shift, even if no other caregiver has arrived to take your place.
(C.) known as abandonment.
D. important to you.

4. If a nursing assistant leaves a weak, unstable patient alone in the bathroom and the patient is seriously injured,
A. the nursing assistant is guilty of malpractice.
B. there is no breach of duty.
C. the nursing assistant is protected under the Good Samaritan Act.
(D.) the nursing assistant may be charged with negligence.

5. Putting a patient in a restraining device without a written doctor's order is known as
A. invasion of privacy.
B. liability.
(C.) false imprisonment.
D. a prudent practice.

6. A person can give written instructions in advance that life-support systems shall not be used in the event that they are ~~sick~~.
A. True
(B.) False
Correct Answer: *near death*

7. Voluntary acts by which a conscious and mentally competent person gives permission for someone else to do something for him is known as ~~a civil law~~.

A. True

(B.) False

Correct Answer: *informed consent.*

8. A quality shown by coming to work every day on time and doing what is asked at the proper time and in the proper way is known as

A. good hygiene.

B. malpractice.

C. liability.

(D.) dependability.

9. When professionals, such as registered nurses, are negligent, they can be charged with

A. the patient's hospital bill.

B. an advance directive.

C. impersonating a Good Samaritan.

(D.) malpractice.

10. The document from the American Hospital Association describing the basic rights to which a patient is entitled is known as

A. the Good Samaritan Act.

B. the Hospital Bill of Rights.

C. a living will.

(D.) the Patient's Bill of Rights.

Communication Skills

3

CHAPTER OVERVIEW

Instructor Notes

I. Communication Skills
- A. Verbal Communication (Communicating through Words)
- B. Written Communication
- C. Nonverbal Communication and Body Language
- D. Barriers to Effective Communication

II. Aids to Effective Communication and Relating to People
- A. Relationships with Patients
- B. Communicating with Patients
- C. Communicating with the Pediatric Patient
  1. Importance of the Child's Family
- D. Communicating with Older Adults
- E. Communicating with Family and Visitors
- F. Communicating with Sensory-Impaired, Blind, or Deaf Patients
- G. Communicating with Non-English-Speaking Patients
- H. Communicating with Other Staff Members
- I. Answering the Patient Call Signal
- J. Using the Telephone
- K. Reporting Incidents
- L. Complaints and Grievance Procedures

III. Observing the Patient

IV. Methods of Observation
- A. Objective Observations: Signs
- B. Subjective Observations: Symptoms
- C. Observation of an Infant or Child

V. Reporting and Recording Observations
- A. Subjective and Objective Reporting
- B. Forms and Records Used in Documentation
- C. Computerization of Medical Records
- D. Computer Documentation
- E. Basic Parts, or Components, of a Computer

Instructor Notes

F. Hardware
G. Software
H. Network
I. Confidentiality
J. Medical Terminology

OBJECTIVES

When the students have completed this chapter, they will be able to:

- Demonstrate a courteous and professional manner toward patients, family, visitors, and coworkers.
- Keep their emotions under control while on the job.
- Deal with patients and visitors in an empathetic and tactful manner.
- Show interest and concern about the patient's welfare.
- Communicate effectively with pediatric patients and their parents.
- Use communication skills effectively when relating to patients and their visitors.
- List seven barriers to effective communication.
- Answer the patient's call light signal promptly.
- Meet the patient's physical and psychological needs.
- Teach a patient with a visual or hearing impairment how to use the call light.
- Take complete and accurate telephone messages.
- Use their senses of sight, touch, hearing, and smell to observe their patients.
- List the behaviors to observe in a patient.
- List the behaviors to report when they are observed in infants or children.
- Differentiate between objective and subjective reporting.
- Report observations promptly, accurately, and objectively.
- Identify the basic parts and functions of a computer used to document and communicate patient information.

KEY TERMS

Body Language: Communication through hand movements (gestures), facial expressions, body movements, and touch

Boot Up: To start up the computer

Central Processing Unit (CPU): The "computer brain" where information is stored or directed to appropriate pathways

Communication: The exchange of thoughts, messages, or ideas by speech, signals, gestures, or writing between two or more people

Courtesy: Being polite and considerate

Cursor: Flashing bar, or symbol, that indicates where the next character is to be placed or location on the computer screen

Cyanosis: When the skin looks blue or gray, especially on the lips, nailbeds, and under the fingernails; in a black patient, it may appear as a darkening of color. This occurs when there is not enough oxygen in the blood

Instructor Notes

Data: Information that a user enters into a computer

Edema: Abnormal swelling of a part of the body caused by fluid collecting in that area; usually the swelling is in the ankles, legs, hands, or abdomen

Empathy: The ability to put yourself in another's place and to see things as they see them

Feedback: Response of the receiver to the sender's message; the response, or feedback, lets the sender know if the message is acknowledged and clearly understood

Hardware: The actual physical equipment that is used by a computer to process data

Keyboard: An input device similar to a typewriter keyboard; has additional keys that allow the user to make selections to direct computer activity

Light Pen: A hand-held device shaped like a pen that has an electronic sensor for making selections on a computer screen

Log On: To sign on to the computer using a password or personal identification number

Memory: The capacity of the computer to store data

Monitor: A screen, similar to a television screen, that allows the user to see input and output

Mouse: A pointing and selecting device to input data; a small tabletop electronic pointing device used to make selections on a computer screen

Network: Several computers that are connected or wired together, having access to central computer programs; can interface to obtain information; located at different workstations

Objective Observations: Signs that can be observed and reported exactly as they are seen

Objective Reporting: Reporting exactly what you observe

Observation: Gathering information about the patient by noticing any change

Password: A word or phrase that identifies a person and allows access to or entry to a program or record

Pediatric Patient: Any patient under the age of 16 years

Personal Identification Number (PIN): Password

Printer: An output device for creating a hard copy

Prompt: A reminder that the user must take some action so further processing of the data can continue

Retrieval: To recall data stored in computer memory

Screen: A portion of data that is displayed at one time within the confined area of the computer monitor

Secretions: The substances that flow out of or are produced by glandular organs; the process of producing this substance; for example: sweat, bile, lymph, saliva, or urine

Instructor Notes

Software: Set or sets of instructions that direct computer operations; computer programs

Subjective Observations: Symptoms that can be felt and described only by the patient himself, such as pain, nausea, dizziness, ringing in the ears, and headache

Subjective Reporting: Giving your opinion about what you have observed; the nursing assistant should never use subjective reporting

Tact: Doing or saying the right thing at the right time

Terminal: A computer monitor that allows the computer operator to see input and output on a screen

CORE STUDENT ASSIGNMENTS

Students should:

- Read this chapter in their textbook, *Being a Nursing Assistant.*
- Underline any words or sentences they do not understand. Write down any questions they have.
- Complete the Chapter Review in their textbook.
- Read the Time Management Tip for this chapter and think about how they might use this tip in their work.
- Complete the Nursing Assistant in Action exercise.

OPTIONAL STUDENT ASSIGNMENTS

Students should:

- Complete all workbook assignments for this chapter in their copy of *Workbook for Being a Nursing Assistant.*
- Use the CD/CD-Rom disk enclosed with their textbook to hear the pronunciation of the key terms in the chapter.
- Watch the "Age-Specific Competencies" video from the Care Provider Skills series.
- Use the Website address **(www.prenhall.com/wolgin)** to access the free, interactive Companion Website created for this textbook. Get hints, instant feedback, and textbook references to chapter-related multiple-choice questions. Read and react to the Nursing Assistant in Action exercise. Link to other interesting sites.

METHODOLOGY AND SUGGESTED ACTIVITIES

I. Lecture/Discussion

- Answer any questions the students may have.
- Discuss the key terms and related abbreviations. Repeat them out loud and practice using them in sentences.
- Discuss the Time Management Tip for this chapter.
- Discuss the Nursing Assistant in Action exercise.

Instructor Notes

- Discuss the Critical Thinking points for this chapter.
- Discuss the computer documentation that occurs in your institution.
- Ask the students how they act when sick and how they like to be treated.
- Ask the students if any of their relatives or friends were born in another country. If so, let them describe a few of their customs or beliefs. These examples should help the students realize how difficult the hospital situation is for a patient who has difficulty communicating because of language or cultural differences.
- Have the students think of other situations that might arise. For example, ask them how they would ask for the bedpan if they were patients who did not speak English.
- Nonverbal communication is especially important with children. A friendly smile and a gentle touch will help. Nursing assistants should treat children in ways that are appropriate to the children's ages.
- The nursing assistant should make visitors feel welcome. Discuss how different cultures are made to feel welcome.
- Being a good listener is important in all interactions.
- Discuss what to do when a patient signals frequently and makes many trivial requests. Include some probable reasons for this type of behavior and how it affects personnel. What can be done to cope with the problem?
- Discuss caring for blind individuals. Find out from them how to best set up their living areas.

II. Role Play/Lab

- Show the videos for this chapter. Discuss with the students how their care differs based on the age of the patient. Using the same nursing assistant/patient scenario, have students role play a scenario with the patient being different ages. Discuss the verbal and nonverbal differences that the caregiver made in caring for the patient.
- Have the students practice using your institution's computer system as they document patient care scenarios.
- Role play conversations between the nursing assistant and the patient of a different culture. Have the nursing assistant practice setting the patient at ease.
- Practice entering a patient's room to give care. Be sure the students identify the patient by name, introduce themselves, and explain what they are going to do.
- Being a good listener is always helpful when establishing positive relationships. Role play scenarios where poor listening is seen.
- Role play distraction techniques to help most children stop crying after the parent is gone.
- Role play phone calls. Give messages but omit a necessary point and request a return call. For example, don't identify yourself, omit your phone number, or neglect to say whom you were calling. See if the students request the information.

III. Evaluation

- Review the answers to the Chapter Review with students.
- Review the answers to the workbook exercises with students.

Instructor Notes

- Review the students' understanding of the Time Management Tip.
- To evaluate student comprehension, give a quiz.
- To evaluate student skills, administer the competency checklist.
- Have the students visit the interactive Companion Website and take the quiz.

ANSWERS TO CHAPTER REVIEW

FILL IN THE BLANK

Read each sentence and fill in the blank line with a word that complete the sentence. (Note: Hyphenated words get one line.)

1. Signs that can be observed and reported exactly as they are seen are called __objective__ __observations__.
2. __Body__ __language__ is a type of communication through movements (gestures), facial expressions, body movements, and touch.
3. For the pediatric patient, __family__ is extremely important in helping calm the fears of the patient.
4. It is very important to answer the __call__ __light__ when the patient signals so that she can receive help without delay.
5. __Computers__ are an electronic medical record that makes it easy for institutions to record and store information for retrieval or recall.

MULTIPLE CHOICE

Choose the best answer for each question or statement.

1. Communication
   (A.) may be written.
   B. may be spoken.
   C. is an exchange of information with others.
   D. All of the above.
2. Which of the following is not a key element of communication?
   A. The sender must obtain the receiver's attention, and make sure the message is understood.
   (B.) The sender must speak loudly.
   C. The receiver must listen carefully and respond appropriately.
   D. The message must be organized, simple, and clear.

Instructor Notes

3. The patient's medical record is an example of
   A. verbal communication.
   (B.) written communication.
   C. nonverbal communication.
   D. body language.
4. To maintain patient confidentiality, you should do all of the following *except*
   (A.) discuss one patient's problems with another patient.
   B. keep confidences.
   C. keep out of earshot of others when discussing a patient's concerns.
   D. only discuss the patient's problems with your supervisor.
5. Which of the following guidelines does not promote good communication?
   A. Showing an interest in the patient
   (B.) Speaking loudly at all times
   C. Using good manners
   D. Using language the patient can understand

CRITICAL THINKING

CUSTOMER SERVICE

Encourage students to reflect and share their thoughts and experiences. Respect their privacy and confidentiality. Share your own viewpoints with the students.

CULTURAL CARE

Encourage students to reflect and share their thoughts and experiences. Respect their privacy and confidentiality. Share your own viewpoints with the students.

COOPERATION WITHIN THE TEAM

Encourage students to reflect and share their thoughts and experiences. Respect their privacy and confidentiality. Share your own viewpoints with the students.

NURSING ASSISTANT IN ACTION

You are working as a CNA in a long-term care facility assisting a group of residents during their dinner. You overhear a confused resident, Mrs. Loud, rebuffing a newly admitted tablemate, Mrs. Brauns, who just introduced herself. Mrs. Loud says, "I have told you a thousand times what my name is so do not ask me again! I will not tell you again what my name is!" Mrs. Brauns now is in tears.

What Is Your Response/Action?

Remind Mrs. Loud that Mrs. Brauns is a new resident. Re-orient her to time and place. If possible separate the two residents. Apologize to Ms. Brauns and reassure her that it is not her fault. Help her to get acquainted with other residents.

Instructor Notes

Answers to Workbook Exercises

3

The following exercises will assist you to apply what you have read in Chapter 3, "Communication Skills." For each exercise, read the objective and use information you have read in Chapter 3 to answer the questions, complete the sentences, or label the diagrams.

EXERCISE 3-1

Objective: To recognize and correctly spell words related to communication skills.

Directions: Unscramble the words in the Word List at the left. Then circle the same words in the Word Search at the right.

Word List

1. BSJUTCEVEI ______ SUBJECTIVE
2. OJECBVETI ______ OBJECTIVE
3. YOBD GNAULGAE ______ BODY LANGUAGE
4. EPROTR ______ REPORT
5. SERBVOE ______ OBSERVE
6. SEDRCBIE ______ DESCRIBE
7. VRNOBNALE ______ NONVERBAL
8. RITTNWE ______ WRITTEN
9. REMOPWCT ______ COMPUTER

Word Search

N	O	N	V	E	R	B	A	L	L	O	T	D	N	A
J	H	I	P	Q	T	Z	M	V	E	R	P	Q	G	D
N	T	L	O	X	V	N	G	R	O	E	R	E	H	E
M	L	W	A	K	B	U	E	F	V	J	G	C	B	S
P	G	D	U	V	D	T	L	I	N	A	H	I	E	C
B	R	W	C	W	U	F	T	S	U	P	R	C	M	R
S	X	I	E	P	R	C	G	G	P	E	D	O	B	I
Q	B	O	M	X	E	S	N	X	P	B	N	L	I	B
F	Q	O	L	J	X	A	Q	O	B	S	E	R	V	E
M	C	Q	B	A	L	J	R	C	S	A	D	J	D	C
C	L	U	R	Y	S	T	E	N	U	T	Q	E	A	O
E	S	T	D	E	G	M	N	W	R	I	T	T	E	N
H	O	O	Z	A	I	Y	J	N	R	B	D	A	F	F
I	B	S	O	B	J	E	C	T	I	V	E	K	G	E
K	R	L	C	U	Y	K	X	Y	V	M	G	Y	N	O

EXERCISE 3-2

Objective: To apply what you have learned about methods of observation.

Directions: Read the following riddles carefully before writing the correct answer on the blank line.

1. If the patient complained about spots and flashes, what area of his body is involved, and what sense would you be interested in observing? *Hint:* It isn't the skin or the sense of touch.
   eyes; sight
2. This could be an important sign of internal bleeding. *Hint:* It resembles something used to brew a morning beverage.
   emesis that looks like coffee grounds
3. What would you suspect if the patient you were conversing with yesterday now only nods and smiles at everything you say? *Hint:* You will often find this in the patient's bedside table drawer.
   The patient is not wearing his hearing aid.

EXERCISE 3-3

Objective: To recognize the definitions of words related to communication skills that the nursing assistant will use in patient care.

Directions: Place the letter of the correct definition next to the matching word(s) from the Word List.

Word List

- *P* 1. tact
- *J* 2. observation
- *N* 3. subjective observation
- *O* 4. subjective reporting
- *F* 5. edema
- *C* 6. communication
- *H* 7. objective observations
- *B* 8. body language
- *D* 9. courtesy
- *M* 10. secretions
- *E* 11. cyanosis
- *G* 12. empathy
- *I* 13. objective reporting
- *K* 14. pediatric patient
- *L* 15. feedback
- *A* 16. cliché

Definitions

A. A familiar phrase used without thinking about what one is saying
B. Communication through hand movements (gestures), facial expressions, body movements, and touch
C. The exchange of thoughts, messages, or ideas by speech, signals, gestures, or writing between two or more people

D. Being polite and considerate
E. When the skin looks blue or gray, especially on the lips, nailbeds, and under the fingernails; in a black patient, it may appear as a darkening of color: This occurs when there is not enough oxygen in the blood.
F. Abnormal swelling of a part of the body caused by fluid collecting in that area; usually the swelling is in the ankles, legs, hands, or abdomen
G. The ability to put yourself in another's place and to see things as they see them
H. Signs that can be observed and reported exactly as they are seen
I. Reporting exactly what you observe
J. Gathering information about the patient by noticing any change
K. Any patient under the age of 16 years
L. Response of the receiver to the sender's message; the response lets the sender know if the message is acknowledged and clearly understood
M. The substances that flow out of or are produced by glandular organs; the process of producing this substance; for example: sweat, bile, lymph, saliva, or urine
N. Symptoms that can be felt and described only by the patient himself, such as pain, nausea, dizziness, ringing in the ears, and headache
O. Giving your opinion about what you have observed; the nursing assistant should never use subjective reporting
P. Doing or saying the right and polite thing at the right time

EXERCISE 3-4

Objective: To demonstrate appropriate responses to changes in the patient's condition.

Directions: Read the situation description and then circle the appropriate response.

1. You have been taking care of Mrs. Jones, 101-A bed, for the past 2 days. Mrs. Jones has been able to get out of bed and brush her teeth in the bathroom; however, today she says to you, "I will brush my teeth later. I don't feel so good today. I am going to stay in bed. Don't bring me any breakfast." What would you say?

A. "Stay in bed and later you can get out and brush."
(B.) "Are you comfortable? Would you like another blanket? I will be back in half an hour to see how you are feeling." The nursing assistant then goes to the nurse or immediate supervisor to report this change in the patient's condition.
C. "If you don't brush for one day, it will not hurt you."
D. "When you give in to feeling sick, you will become very sick."

2. Mr. Murray, the patient in room 209-C bed, had four bowel movements in the past 2 hours. The last time he wasn't able to wait for the bedpan and soiled the bed. Yesterday, he had one bowel movement the entire day. After you have cleaned the patient and changed his bed, what would you do?
   A. Continue to clean up Mr. Murray as needed.
   (B.) Report this to your nurse or immediate supervisor; this is a definite change in the patient's condition.
   C. Tell the patient he is awful for messing up the bed.
   D. Tell the doctor that the patient has moved his bowels in bed.

3. Mrs. Hernandez, the patient in room 103-A bed, is receiving a blood transfusion that has been running for the past hour. As you are making her bed, you notice that the color of the patient's face has changed. She now has very red cheeks. Mrs. Hernandez cannot speak English and you cannot converse with her. You then notice that Mrs. Hernandez is scratching her arms and legs and seems very agitated. What would you do?
   A. Tell the doctor that Mrs. Hernandez is scratching her arms and legs.
   B. Tell the patient's visitors to tell her to stop scratching.
   C. Use body language so that Mrs. Hernandez will understand and stop scratching.
   (D.) Use the emergency signal to call for help. Report on the intercom to the nurse or immediate supervisor that Mrs. Hernandez seems to be having a reaction to her treatment, and you need help with this patient.

4. A patient complains to you that his IV hurts. You look at the area on the patient's arm around the needle, and it appears red and swollen. What would you do?
   A. Nothing. As a nursing assistant, this is not your job.
   B. Tell the patient to mention it to the nurse next time she comes in.
   (C.) Report this immediately to your nurse or immediate supervisor. Although a nursing assistant does not regulate IVs, you still must be observant and report anything unusual.
   D. Tell the doctor.

5. Communication is basic to the mutual exchanges of messages that make a connection between the nursing assistant and the patient. What types of things would you do to show good communication skills?
   A. Show an interest in what the patient is saying.
   B. Speak in a pleasant tone.
   C. Use good manners, courtesy, emotional control, sympathy, empathy, and tact.
   (D.) All of the above.

6. Your patient appears to be very irritable. What would you do?
   A. Try to calm him down.
   B. Try to be an attentive, sympathetic listener.
   (C.) Report this excessive irritability to the nurse or immediate supervisor.
   D. Answer the patient in the same irritable manner.

7. Mrs. Smith is a preoperative patient. She is scheduled to go to the operating room in the morning. You notice that when the nurse or immediate supervisor is not around, Mrs. Smith drinks whiskey right from a bottle she keeps in her bedside table. What would you do?
   A. Tell the patient to stop drinking.
   (B.) Report this to your nurse or immediate supervisor right away.
   C. Tell Mrs. Smith's visitors that she is drinking.
   D. Tell the doctor that the patient is drinking.

8. Your patient has just been admitted to the health care institution. The doctor ordered oxygen by face mask for this patient. You notice that as soon as the nurse or immediate supervisor leaves the room, the patient takes the mask off. What would you do?
   A. Tell the doctor.
   (B.) Report this to the nurse or immediate supervisor right away.
   C. Tell another nursing assistant.
   D. Call the pharmacy.

9. Your patient is in the health care institution because of a diabetic condition. The doctor ordered a special therapeutic diet for her. You notice the patient eating a candy bar when she is alone. What would you do?
   A. Let her eat it; she really does not want to get well.
   B. Tell the patient she should not eat the candy without the nurse or immediate supervisor's permission.
   (C.) Report this incident to the nurse or immediate supervisor, who will tell you what to do.
   D. Ignore the whole thing.

10. Your objective is to report your observations. Which of the following best describes this process?
   A. Tell the nurse or immediate supervisor what you think is wrong with the patient.
   B. Tell the nurse or immediate supervisor to give the patient some pills.
   (C.) Tell the nurse or immediate supervisor exactly what you saw, smelled, or felt or what the patient said.
   D. Tell the nurse or immediate supervisor to observe the patient.

11. The nurse or immediate supervisor has given you instructions to report exactly what the patient eats at mealtime and not to give the patient anything between meals. However, during visiting hours, you notice that the patient is eating a hot dog that was brought in by a visitor. What would you do?
   A. Speak to the patient and take the food away immediately.
   B. Call the visitors outside the room and send them home.
   C. Tell the doctor.
   (D.) Report this to the nurse or immediate supervisor right away.

12. Your patient was fine this morning and was able to get out of bed and walk around his room. However, after lunch, you notice that the patient is lying very quietly in his bed, does not answer when you talk to him, and his face is very red. What would you do?

A. Shake the patient to wake him every 5 minutes for 1 hour.
B. Call the visitors in to see the patient.
C. Call the doctor.
(D.) Report this to the nurse or immediate supervisor right away; this is a change in the patient's condition.

EXERCISE 3-5

Objective: To demonstrate appropriate communication skills.

Directions: Circle the appropriate response to the following patient situations.

1. A patient rings his call bell at mealtime. The nursing assistant answers the signal and the patient angrily says, "What's wrong with this place? I have no fork and my coffee is cold!" The nursing assistant should respond by saying:

A. "I'll do something about it later."
(B.) "I'll get you a fork and hot coffee right now."
C. "The dietary department must have a lot of new help."
D. "Well, that's the way it is around here."

2. A patient signals by ringing the call bell every 15 to 20 minutes. The nursing assistant responds and notices that the patient is making a lot of small requests, such as "Please raise the window shade"; "Please lower the window shade"; "Please turn on the radio"; "Please turn my pillow." The nursing assistant should respond by

A. telling the patient politely not to ring so often.
B. deliberately delaying in answering the call signal or neglecting to answer it at all.
C. explaining to the patient that she has other work to do.
(D.) reporting to the immediate supervisor, asking what to do and how to handle the situation, and asking the nurse to visit the patient; something is obviously wrong.

3. Mrs. White, a nursing assistant, finished her assignment and is walking down the hall toward the nurses' lounge when another nursing assistant approaches her and says, "Please get Mrs. Smalling in 203-B back to bed for me now. Her doctor is on the nursing unit in another room and wants to examine her. Thank you, Mrs. White. I have to go and get the dressing cart for the nurse so the doctor can change my patient's bandages." The nursing assistant on her way to the lounge should respond by saying:

A. "That's not my job, because it is not my patient."
(B.) "I will do this right away. By the time you get to Mrs. Smalling's room, she will be in bed."
C. "I am going to complain to the nurse that you are always asking me to do your work."

D. "I am tired from my own assignment, and if this hospital wants me to do two jobs, let them pay me two salaries."

4. The nursing assistant has just been told by the nurse that walking to the linen closet five times during one patient's bed bath is bad technique, time consuming, and not acceptable. One trip should be made, and all the linen needed for one patient must be brought into the room at one time. The nursing assistant should respond by saying:

(A.) "Thank you for taking the time to teach me. I will try your suggestion now that I understand that what I have been doing is not acceptable."

B. "How dare you criticize me!"

C. "I went to school to learn how to be a nursing assistant, and you have no right to tell me how to do anything."

D. "You always manage to think of something else I do that you do not like; this is the fourth time this morning that you have told me that I am doing something wrong."

5. Miss Smith, a nursing assistant, is told to go to 201-A bed to give the patient, Mrs. Joseph, a message from her family. Miss Smith has never met this patient, and even though other staff members refer to all of the patients by room and bed number, she does not feel this is right. What would be the right way for Miss Smith to greet the patient?

A. "Are you 201-A bed? Your husband called. . . ."

(B.) "How do you do, Mrs. Joseph. I am Miss Smith, a nursing assistant. May I check your identification bracelet? Thank you. The nurse asked me to give you this message. . . ."

C. "Hi, your husband called. . . ."

D. "Hi, are you the diabetic patient? Well, I have a message for you. . . ."

EXERCISE 3-6

Objective: To apply what you have learned about good communication techniques.

Directions: Write the word *Do* or *Don't* next to each statement below as appropriate.

1. ___Don't___ use a shrill or loud voice, especially if the patient does not speak the same language as you do.

2. ___Do___ speak clearly and slowly, especially to patients with hearing impairments.

3. ___Don't___ speak in a harsh manner so that the patient will not bother you as often.

4. ___Don't___ use complex medical terms and abbreviations when talking with patients.

5. ___Do___ use age-specific communication styles.

6. ___Don't___ let the patient think you are too busy to listen, even if you are.

7. ___Do___ respect the patient's cultural preferences.

8. ___Do___ show an interest in what the patient is saying.

9. ___Don't___ use slang words or clichés.

10. ___Do___ speak using a pleasant tone of voice.

EXERCISE 3-7

Objective: To apply what you have learned about communication with patients, families, and your health care team members.

Directions: Circle the letter next to the statement that best completes the sentence or describes the sentence as true or false. If the sentence is false, draw a line through the incorrect part of the sentence and write the correction on the blank line.

1. Both verbal and nonverbal communication involve three important elements:
   A. a criticizer, a moderator, and an evaluator.
   B. a host, an audience, and a sponsor.
   C. a stretcher, a toner, and an exerciser.
   (D.) a sender, a receiver, and a message.

2. The sender must send a clear message.
   (A.) True
   B. False
   Correct Answer: ______________________

3. The receiver should ask for clarification if necessary.
   (A.) True
   B. False
   Correct Answer: ______________________

4. When working with patients, the message should be ~~unclear, complex, disorganized~~, and ~~complicated in order to challenge the listening skills of the receiver~~.
   A. True
   (B.) False
   Correct Answer: clear, organized, simple, and uncomplicated.

5. An example of good body language to use when providing care to a patient is to
   A. pause briefly to ask, "How are you?" and then leave quickly before the reply is completed.
   B. back slowly out of the room as you are talking.
   C. glance out the window often while speaking to the patient about his level of pain.
   (D.) look directly at the arm the patient is describing as painful.

6. A key to good communication is to be ____________ when you listen.
A. talking
(B.) nonjudgmental
C. ready to reply
D. opinionated

7. To distract the child when he is unhappy or fearful means to
A. discipline him for crying.
(B.) turn his attention to other things, such as a toy or book.
C. tell him to be happy.
D. contact the parents immediately.

8. Being sensitive to times when a patient may not want to talk means
A. you sing happy songs so he won't feel he has to talk to you.
(B.) you convey your support with positive body language instead of carrying on a conversation with him.
C. you encourage him to "talk things over" with you so he will feel better.
D. you should be offended that he does not talk to you.

9. Pediatric patients are sometimes grouped according to age because
A. children of different ages play well together.
(B.) children of different ages need different kinds of care.
C. children age differently.
D. children do better if grouped.

10. A smile can communicate many positive things to a child.
(A.) True
B. False
Correct Answer: ________________________________

11. Addressing adults in the manner they prefer, such as "Mrs. Smith" rather than "Grandma," shows that you respect them as people.
(A.) True
B. False
Correct Answer: ________________________________

12. For pediatric patients, all of the following are true *except*
A. family members need to be with their children.
B. most children first learn about the world from their families.
C. family members are normally concerned about the child.
(D.) the less serious the illness, the less they need their family.

13. If you suspect the child has been abused by the family,
A. ask them if they have stopped beating the child.
(B.) report your suspicions and any objective observations to your immediate supervisor at once.
C. call 911.
D. take the child away from them immediately.

14. It is helpful to make visitors feel welcome by making pleasant comments about

A. their appearance.
B. flowers or gifts they may give you.
(C.) flowers or gifts they may bring for the patient.
D. the new, shorter visiting hours.

15. When visitors bring food for the patient,

A. you must taste the food before the patient eats it.
B. ask if you may have some.
C. tell them it is not allowed.
(D.) find out if the nurse or doctor has approved this practice.

16. If your patient has a visual impairment, make sure you

(A.) have him demonstrate to you that he can use the call light.
B. leave the call light on the bedside table.
C. remind him to shut off the light.
D. All of the above.

17. Communicating with patients who have hearing or speaking impairments is helped by the use of a pad of paper and a pencil to communicate in writing.

(A.) True
B. False

Correct Answer: ______________________________

18. If your patient speaks a different language or needs sign language, your employer or institution must address that need.

(A.) True
B. False

Correct Answer: ______________________________

19. A(n) ______________ has pictures of the patient's equipment and is a tool to help you communicate with the patient.

A. story board
B. outboard
(C.) communication board
D. notice board

20. Incidents, such as a patient fall, should be reported to your immediate supervisor as soon as you

A. have time to do so after your break.
(B.) observe it or it is reported to you.
C. can after completing your daily assignment.
D. can after discussing it with the patient's family.

21. As a nursing assistant, you should be aware of the ________________ in your institution so that you can follow it when you or others have a complaint that must be resolved by your employer.
    (A.) grievance procedure
    B. problem road map
    C. critical pathway
    D. case management process

22. Computers are tools to assist in ________________________ information and getting work done.
    A. entering
    B. storing
    C. retrieving
    (D.) all of the above

23. Because all patient computer information deals with the private and personal care of the patient, it must be treated in a ________________ manner.
    A. public
    (B.) confidential
    C. humorous
    D. all of the above

4

Patients, Residents, and Clients

CHAPTER OVERVIEW

Instructor Notes

I. Understanding and Relating to Patients, Residents, and Clients

II. Customer-focused Care
   A. Seven Goals of Customer-focused Care

III. Cultural Differences and Diversity
   A. Transcultural Nursing

IV. Basic Human Needs
   A. Basic Physical and Psychological Needs
   B. Rest and Sleep
   C. Influences on Patient Behavior: Unmet Needs

V. Dealing with Difficult Behavior

VI. Physical Crisis Management

Instructor Notes

OBJECTIVES

When the students have completed this chapter, they will be able to:

- Describe seven goals of customer-focused care.
- Demonstrate an understanding of cultural differences among patients, residents, and clients.
- Provide service that meets the basic human needs of those who are in their care.
- Identify actions they can take to promote rest and sleep for their patients.
- Describe how unmet needs can influence patient behavior.
- Use methods to deal with disruptive behavior.

KEY TERMS

Client: An individual cared for by a home health agency or provider

Culture: The thoughts, beliefs, and values of a social group

Customer-focused Care: Care designed to meet the needs of patients, residents, and clients (customers)

Ethnic Diversity: The variety of races, religions, and cultures in the world

Need: A requirement for survival

Patient: An individual admitted to an inpatient or outpatient hospital, physician office, or clinic

Physical Crisis Management: Methods for dealing with a dangerous situation involving a patient, resident, or client

Resident: An individual cared for in a nursing home or other long-term/extended care facility

Service: Factors, such as attentiveness, quality of food, and cleanliness of environment, that affect the care and comfort of the individual receiving health care

CORE STUDENT ASSIGNMENTS

Students should:

- Read this chapter in their textbook, *Being a Nursing Assistant.*
- Underline any words or sentences they do not understand. Write down any questions they have.
- Complete the Chapter Review in their textbook.
- Read the Time Management Tip for this chapter and think about how they might use this tip in their work.
- Complete the Nursing Assistant in Action exercise.

OPTIONAL STUDENT ASSIGNMENTS

Instructor Notes

Students should:

- Complete all workbook assignments for this chapter in their copy of *Workbook for Being a Nursing Assistant.*
- Use the CD/CD-Rom disk enclosed with their textbook to hear the pronunciation of the key terms in the chapter.
- Watch the "Dealing with Dementia" video and the "Professionalism: Dealing with Anger" video from the Care Provider Skills series.
- Use the Website address **(www.prenhall.com/wolgin)** to access the free, interactive Companion Website created for this textbook. Get hints, instant feedback, and textbook references to chapter-related multiple-choice questions. Read and react to the Nursing Assistant in Action exercise. Link to other interesting sites.

METHODOLOGY AND SUGGESTED ACTIVITIES

I. Lecture/Discussion

- Answer any questions the students may have.
- Discuss the key terms and related abbreviations. Repeat them out loud and practice using them in sentences.
- Discuss the Time Management Tip for this chapter.
- Discuss the Nursing Assistant in Action exercise.
- Discuss the Critical Thinking points for this chapter.
- Discuss personal safety and protection. Emphasize the importance of following Universal Precautions. Stress the need to wear protective equipment.
- As you explain these patient rights, ask the students to pretend that they are patients and imagine how they would like to be treated.
- Ask the students if any of their relatives or friends were born in another country. If so, let them describe a few of their customs or traditions related to health care.
- Discuss the mission or philosophy of your institution or of those in which you are training. Discuss how this influences care.
- Discuss the definitions and ramifications of good customer service.
- Have the students discuss how they like to be treated as customers.
- Review the seven goals of customer-focused care.
- Discuss cultures and look for signs of diversity in your area. Give case examples of issues that affect care.
- Review the cross-cultural guidelines.
- Discuss and review sleep habits and factors that affect sleep; review the effects of aging in sleep.

II. Role Play/Lab

- Show the videos for this chapter. Discuss the difference between delirium and dementia. Practice using techniques for working with patients who are experiencing dementia. Discuss and role play working with angry patients, families, and coworkers.

Instructor Notes

- Have the students practice being upset patients and caregivers. Point out service and customer care guidelines in practice.
- Have the students practice caring for people of other cultures.
- Have the students examine their own cultural values related to health, illness, and care.
- Have the students keep a sleep diary for a week. Review the diaries in class.

III. Evaluation

- Review the answers to the Chapter Review with students.
- Review the answers to the workbook exercises with students.
- Review the students' understanding of the Time Management Tip.
- To evaluate student comprehension, give a quiz.
- To evaluate student skills, administer the competency checklist.
- Have the students visit the interactive Companion Website and take the quiz.

ANSWERS TO CHAPTER REVIEW

FILL IN THE BLANK

Read each sentence and fill in the blank line with a word that complete the sentence. (Note: Hyphenated words get one line.)

1. A ___*client*___ is an individual cared for by a home health agency or provider.
2. A ___*resident*___ is an individual cared for in a long-term/extended care facility.
3. The more you learn about an individual's ___*cultural*___ ___*beliefs*___ and differences, the better you can provide sensitive care and services to your patients, residents, or clients.
4. A ___*need*___ is a requirement for survival.
5. Every person has basic ___*physical*___ and ___*psychological*___ needs.

MULTIPLE CHOICE

Choose the best answer for each question or statement.

1. Which of the following actions do not promote sleep and rest?
   A. Being aware of the noise around you
   (B.) Always turning off all the lights
   C. If possible, allowing the patient to use his own pillow
   D. Offering skin and mouth care as needed

Instructor Notes

2. Which of the following is not a good technique to try when dealing with a disruptive patient?
   (A.) Yell back at the patient.
   B. Be objective.
   C. Be alert.
   D. Remain calm, but firm.
3. Which of the following is considered a physiological need?
   A. Social groups
   B. Status, titles
   (C.) Shelter
   D. Family
4. Which of the following is not a guideline for appreciating cultural diversity?
   A. Treat everyone with respect.
   (B.) Take what the patient says literally.
   C. Be open, flexible, and adaptable.
   D. Thank others who help you to better understand about their culture.
5. Which of the following is true?
   (A.) Using flash cards and pictures with patients who do not speak English helps to reduce stress and anxiety.
   B. Use the universal "OK" sign to communicate with people of all cultures.
   C. Hold the patient's hand and look directly in her eyes when talking with people of all cultures.
   D. All of the above.

CRITICAL THINKING

CUSTOMER SERVICE

Encourage students to reflect and share their thoughts and experiences. Respect their privacy and confidentiality. Share your own viewpoints with the students.

CULTURAL CARE

Encourage students to reflect and share their thoughts and experiences. Respect their privacy and confidentiality. Share your own viewpoints with the students.

COOPERATION WITHIN THE TEAM

Encourage students to reflect and share their thoughts and experiences. Respect their privacy and confidentiality. Share your own viewpoints with the students.

Instructor Notes

NURSING ASSISTANT IN ACTION

You are caring for Mr. George, a seriously ill 32-year-old man. Following a head injury, he is being treated for an infection. When you come to assist him with lunch, he yells at you, "Get that slop out of here or I will throw the tray on the floor!"

What Is Your Response/Action?

Take the food out of the room. Check back in with Mr. George and ask him how he is feeling and if anything is bothering him. Ask if there is anything else you might be able to bring him. Then go talk with the nurse and express your concerns about Mr. George. Perhaps he is in pain, has had a worsening of his condition, or just needs to talk. Be aware of physical crisis management techniques because the patient is angry and has had a head injury.

4

Answers to Workbook Exercises

The following exercises will assist you to apply what you have read in Chapter 4, "Patients, Residents, and Clients." For each exercise, read the objective and use information you have read in Chapter 4 to answer the questions, complete the sentences, or label the diagrams.

EXERCISE 4-1

Objective: To recognize and correctly spell words related to the care of patients, residents, and clients.

Directions: Unscramble the words in the Word List at the left. Then circle the same words in the Word Search at the right.

Word List

1. TOMCSRUE ___*CUSTOMER*___
2. RSVEIEC ___*SERVICE*___
3. TNMUE SDNEE ___*UNMET NEEDS*___
4. TLUUCRE ___*CULTURE*___
5. NGLAAUGE ___*LANGUAGE*___
6. IBLEEFS ___*BELIEFS*___
7. HEBVIAOR ___*BEHAVIOR*___
8. TYREISIDV ___*DIVERSITY*___
9. PEELS ___*SLEEP*___

Word Search

R	G	T	P	I	K	P	S	F	D	L	C	M
K	S	I	K	N	E	Z	E	A	G	B	U	Y
Z	V	M	A	E	U	F	X	F	L	E	S	J
C	M	I	L	W	E	X	I	D	G	J	T	K
L	E	S	E	R	V	I	C	E	C	I	O	F
C	Q	D	O	G	L	P	J	A	H	B	M	A
U	N	M	E	T	N	E	E	D	S	Y	E	P
L	A	N	G	U	A	G	E	N	C	T	R	N
T	B	F	H	J	E	C	L	D	T	I	H	D
U	S	B	B	E	L	I	E	F	S	S	C	E
R	I	J	D	F	M	D	L	B	N	R	A	F
E	M	A	O	G	R	B	O	D	G	E	G	D
O	D	Q	H	D	J	A	F	I	J	V	I	B
I	B	E	H	A	V	I	O	R	K	I	H	K
F	K	C	O	H	L	B	R	A	G	D	L	O

EXERCISE 4-2

Objective: To apply what you have learned about patients, residents, and clients.

Directions: Read the following riddles carefully before writing the correct answer on the blank line.

1. What are the thoughts, beliefs, and values of a social group called? *Hint:* An alternative meaning is something that is very active in yogurt.
   culture
2. These are people who receive patient care. *Hint:* A salesperson values them.
   customers
3. If you are fearful, you may want this on at night when trying to sleep. *Hint:* The opposite of heavy.
   light

EXERCISE 4-3

Objective: To recognize the definitions of words related to the care of patients, residents, and clients.

Directions: Place the letter of the correct definition next to the matching word(s) from the word list below.

Word List

E 1. resident

C 2. ethnic diversity

G 3. service

B 4. need

H 5. physical crisis management

A 6. culture

F 7. client

I 8. patient

D 9. customer-focused care

Definitions

A. The thoughts, beliefs, and values of a social group

B. A requirement for survival

C. The variety of races, religions, and cultures in the world

D. Care designed to meet the needs of patients, residents, and clients (customers)

E. An individual cared for in a nursing home or other long-term/extended care facility

F. An individual cared for by a home health agency or provider

G. Factors, such as attentiveness, quality of food, and cleanliness of environment, that affect the care and comfort of the individual receiving health care

H. Methods for dealing with a dangerous situation involving a patient, resident, or client

I. An individual admitted to an inpatient or outpatient hospital, physician office, or clinic

EXERCISE 4-4

Objective: To recognize important components of care given to patients, residents, and clients.

Directions: Place the correct letters next to the matching phrase. More than one answer may apply.

CF = customer-focused care goal
FAS = factors affecting sleep
SS = sleep stages

CF, FAS **1.** Keep door closed at night to reduce noise.

CF **2.** Information is communicated to patients or to staff.

SS **3.** Body rests and restores.

CF, FAS **4.** Patient may not be comfortable with her roommate, so a change may be needed.

SS **5.** Muscles completely relax.

CF **6.** Care provided reflects respect for the individual.

FAS **7.** Avoid exertion less than 2 hours prior to sleeping time.

CF **8.** Family and friends are involved.

SS **9.** Vivid dreaming.

CF, FAS **10.** The patient is relieved of fear when possible.

SS **11.** Easily aroused.

FAS **12.** May be allowed to have own pillow from home.

SS **13.** Lower vital signs.

CF **14.** Caregivers work together in a planned way.

SS **15.** Sound sleep.

EXERCISE 4-5

Objective: To recognize the appropriate response to disruptive behavior.

Directions: Circle the correct response for the disruptive behavior.

1. Patient is angry:
   (A.) Remain calm.
   B. Frown and shout at them.

2. Patient is stressed:
   (A.) Be supportive.
   B. Ignore them.
3. Patient has emotional problems:
   A. Increase stimuli.
   (B.) Focus on safety.

EXERCISE 4-6

Objective: To apply what you have learned about patients, residents, and clients.

Directions: Circle the letter next to the word or statement that best completes the sentence or describes the sentence as true or false. If the sentence is false, draw a line through the incorrect part of the sentence and write the correction on the blank line.

1. Patients, families, and visitors will judge the care given to their loved ones based on all of the following *except*
   A. personal interactions and attentiveness.
   B. perceived helpfulness of the staff.
   C. employee behavior and quality of the food.
   (D.) location of the facility.
2. Dissatisfied customers may not complain, but they may ~~often~~ return to the same institution.
   A. True
   (B.) False
   Correct Answer: *not*
3. Dissatisfied customers will complain to an average of ________ other relatives, friends, or acquaintances.
   A. 4
   B. 7
   C. 200
   (D.) 20
4. There are ~~seventeen~~ goals of customer-focused care.
   A. True
   (B.) False
   Correct Answer: *seven*
5. Ethnic diversity is ~~decreasing~~ in the United States.
   A. True
   (B.) False
   Correct Answer: *increasing*

6. Currently, one in every four Americans is
- A. ethnically deprived.
- B. culturally defined.
- C. Hispanic, Chinese, or Asian.
- (D.) Hispanic, African American, or Asian.

7. Which level of need is the most basic according to Maslow?
- A. Esteem needs
- B. Belonging needs
- C. Security needs
- D. Physiological needs

8. "Different" ~~means~~ the wrong way of doing things.
- A. True
- (B.) False

Correct Answer: does not mean

9. To be respectful of your patient's cultural differences you should ________ rather than evaluate his behavior.
- A. listen
- B. observe
- C. describe
- (D.) all of the above

10. ________ are not easily translated into other languages, cultures, or value systems and are usually misunderstood.
- A. Directions
- B. Songs
- C. Poems
- (D.) Jokes

11. Part of the job of the nursing assistant is to try to show the patient that the health care institution is a friendly place and that the major concern is for their
- A. discharge.
- (B.) well-being.
- C. cure.
- D. cultural diversity.

12. It ~~is~~ a good idea to use culturally diverse gestures when communicating.
- A. True
- (B.) False

Correct Answer: is not

13. If your patient appears upset because of difficulty communicating, you should
- A. explain to him that the care team is friendly.
- (B.) report this to your immediate supervisor and reassure the patient.
- C. speak louder.
- D. write the directions on a flash card.

14. Because of cultural differences regarding modesty, it is a good idea to
- A. drape the patient's entire body at all times to be safe.
- (B.) ask your immediate supervisor for suggestions to protect the patient's modesty.
- C. ask the patient to stop being so different.
- D. keep the nursing assistant draped at all times.

15. All patient needs ~~must~~ be met every day by the nursing assistant.
- A. True
- (B.) False

Correct Answer: *do not have to*

16. In Maslow's hierarchy, ________ needs must be met before higher level needs.
- (A.) lower level
- B. middle level
- C. end level
- D. beginning level

17. An example of a lower level need is
- (A.) food.
- B. music.
- C. belonging.
- D. leaving.

18. Unmet needs can cause people to show physical reactions, such as
- A. anger.
- B. depression.
- C. weakness.
- (D.) all of the above.

19. Observe the patient's behavior carefully, so that you can report it
- A. subjectively.
- B. continually.
- (C.) objectively.
- D. quickly.

20. It is during sleep that
- A. work gets done.
- B. time stands still.
- (C.) tissues heal.
- D. life goes on.

21. Individuals have different ________ clocks.
- A. alarm
- B. body
- C. cultural
- (D.) biological

22. Whenever possible, plan care to accommodate the individual's sleep preferences.

(A.) True

B. False

Correct Answer: ______________________________

23. People need to spend enough time in ________ sleep each night to feel rested.

A. ABC

(B.) REM

C. RAP

D. EYE

24. The nursing assistant must make ____________ a priority when dealing with disruptive patients or families.

(A.) safety

B. humor

C. speed

D. sleep

25. Remember that many people want their "say," not their

A. "pay."

(B.) "way."

C. "day."

D. "play."

Infection Control

5

CHAPTER OVERVIEW

Instructor Notes

I. History of Infection Control
- A. Nosocomial or Health Care-Associated Infections

II. Nature of Microorganisms

III. Preventing the Spread of Infection
- A. Disinfection and Sterilization
- B. Asepsis

IV. Isolation Precautions
- A. Standard Precautions
- B. Transmission-based Precautions
  1. Contact Precautions
  2. Droplet Precautions
  3. Airborne Precautions
- C. A New Disease Called SARS
  1. Possible Cause of SARS
  2. Care of Patients with SARS
- D. Protective Equipment and Procedures
  1. Hand Hygiene
  2. Waterless Hand Hygiene
  3. Gloves
  4. The Mask
  5. Care and Cleaning of Noncritical Items
- E. Changes in Isolation Strategies

V. OSHA Standards for Occupational Exposure to Bloodborne Pathogens

VI. Asepsis and Sterile Technique

Instructor Notes

OBJECTIVES

When the students have completed this chapter, they will be able to:

- Differentiate between helpful and harmful microorganisms.
- List four conditions affecting the growth of bacteria.
- Summarize the history of infection control.
- List five ways microorganisms are spread.
- Explain how microorganisms are destroyed.
- Describe the three main purposes of asepsis.
- Identify what precautions are used for all patients.
- List the three elements necessary for transmission of infection.
- Demonstrate the procedures for handwashing and hand hygiene.
- Demonstrate the procedures for donning gloves, mask, and gown.
- Identify OSHA standards for occupational exposure to bloodborne pathogens.
- Identify recommendations for prevention and control of hepatitis C.
- Demonstrate sterile techniques.

KEY TERMS

Asepsis: The absence of microorganisms (germs)

Aseptic: Germ free, without disease-producing organisms

Autoclave: Device used to achieve sterility of an item through heat, pressure, and steam

Bacteria: Unicellular microorganism

Disinfection: The process of destroying as many harmful organisms as possible

Friction: The process of rubbing two surfaces together, such as skin

Hand Hygiene: A general term that applies to either handwashing, antiseptic handwash, antiseptic hand rub, or surgical hand antisepsis

Health Care-associated Infection (HAI): An infection acquired in a health care setting

Hepatitis B: Bloodborne disease that affects the liver and is easily transmitted within the health care setting following parenteral exposure

Hepatitis C: Prior to 1988 known as nonA-nonB hepatitis. Transmitted best through needle sticks and may result in chronic liver disease

Infection: Results from a pathogen producing a reaction that may cause soreness, tenderness, redness, and/or pus, fever, change in drainage, and so on

Infection Control: The effort to prevent the spread of pathogens

Isolation: To separate or set apart

Microorganism: A living thing that is so small it cannot be seen with the naked eye but only through a microscope

Instructor Notes

Normal Flora: Microorganisms that are necessary for health, and usually live and grow in specific locations; they are nonpathogenic when in or on a natural reservoir

Nosocomial Infection: Hospital-acquired infection

Pathogen: Disease-producing microorganism

Rickettsiae: An example of bacteria found in the tissues of fleas, lice, ticks, and other insects; Rickettsiae are transmitted to humans by insect bites

Severe Acute Respiratory Syndrome (SARS): A viral respiratory illness spread by close person-to-person contact

Spores: Bacteria that have formed hard shells around themselves as a defense

Sterile Field: An area created to work from when you are doing a sterile procedure

Sterilization: The process of killing all microorganisms, including spores

Transmission: The spread of microorganisms

Virus: A type of microorganism; much smaller than bacteria and can survive only in other living cells

CORE STUDENT ASSIGNMENTS

Students should:

- Read this chapter in their textbook, *Being a Nursing Assistant.*
- Underline any words or sentences they do not understand. Write down any questions they have.
- Complete the Chapter Review in their textbook.
- Read the Time Management Tip for this chapter and think about how they might use this tip in their work.
- Complete the Nursing Assistant in Action exercise.

OPTIONAL STUDENT ASSIGNMENTS

Students should:

- Complete all workbook assignments for this chapter in their copy of *Workbook for Being a Nursing Assistant.*
- Use the CD/CD-Rom disk enclosed with their textbook to hear the pronunciation of the key terms in the chapter.
- Watch the "Infection Control" video from the Care Provider Skills series.
- Use the Website address **(www.prenhall.com/wolgin)** to access the free, interactive Companion Website created for this textbook. Get hints, instant feedback, and textbook references to chapter-related multiple-choice questions. Read and react to the Nursing Assistant in Action exercise. Link to other interesting sites.

Instructor Notes

METHODOLOGY AND SUGGESTED ACTIVITIES

I. Lecture/Discussion

- Answer any questions the students may have.
- Discuss the key terms and related abbreviations. Repeat them out loud and practice using them in sentences.
- Discuss the Time Management Tip for this chapter.
- Discuss the Nursing Assistant in Action exercise.
- Discuss the Critical Thinking points for this chapter.
- Discuss personal safety and protection. Emphasize the importance of following Universal Precautions. Stress the need to wear protective equipment.
- Discuss conditions affecting growth of bacteria and offer many examples.
- Discuss OSHA-required training and its purposes.
- Discuss the function of the Centers for Disease Control and Prevention, the U.S. agency that traces the spread of infectious diseases.
- Explain the rationale for the Universal Precautions.
- Invite an infection-control nurse or epidemiologist to address the class.
- Go to a Central Supply Department to see how an autoclave is operated.
- Offer case studies involving reinfections, cross-infection, and self-inoculation.
- Acquire the standards for the disposal of biohazardous waste in your community. Discuss special federal, state, and local laws governing infectious waste materials.
- Discuss how hand hygiene plays a role in stopping the spread of infections.

II. Role Play/Lab

- Show the video for this chapter. Review principles of infection control. Have the students practice washing their hands. Have the students practice putting on and taking off a cover gown. Practice preparing a room for the different types of precautions.
- If possible, have microscopes in class or arrange a field trip to a lab so students can view microorganisms with a microscope.
- Practice putting on sterile gloves. Use a black light kit to show how germs spread.
- Have the students rub their hands together for a full minute to explain friction.
- Demonstrate personal care procedures. Provide ample opportunity for the students to practice these procedures.
- Demonstrate the correct use of various hand hygiene products.
- Display and explain all the isolation carts as appropriate, specifically those used in their individual facilities.
- Assign the students to teams of two. Have one student read one of the procedures out loud while the other student demonstrates. Have them trade places and repeat.
- Role play to reinforce the concept of clean versus dirty. Offer a variety of examples written on individual cards. Give one card to each student so that he or she can participate in the role play.

III. Evaluation

- Review the answers to the Chapter Review with students.
- Review the answers to the workbook exercises with students.
- Review the students' understanding of the Time Management Tip.
- To evaluate student comprehension, give a quiz.
- To evaluate student skills, administer the competency checklist.
- Have the students visit the interactive Companion Website and take the quiz.

Instructor Notes

ANSWERS TO CHAPTER REVIEW

FILL IN THE BLANK

Read each sentence and fill in the blank line with a word that completes the sentence. (Note: Hyphenated words get one line.)

1. If you wear contaminated gloves in public places, you risk spreading ___infection___.
2. A noncritical care item, such as a blood pressure cuff, can generally be ___cleaned___ versus disinfected.
3. ___Friction___ is the process of rubbing two surfaces together, such as skin.
4. Use ___Airborne___ Precautions when caring for a patient with TB.
5. When a patient is in Contact Precautions, you should always wear ___gloves___ when caring for the patient.

MULTIPLE CHOICE

Choose the best answer for each question or statement.

1. Normal flora means
   A. the normal plants seen around the hospital.
   (B.) the nonpathogenic microorganisms that live in our bodies.
   C. the pathogenic microorganisms that live in our bodies.
   D. All of the above.
2. Bacteria grow best in
   (A.) warm, moist, dark places.
   B. temperatures that are at or less than 76 degrees.
   C. dry, bright, surfaces.
   D. All of the above.
3. Sterilization means the
   (A.) process of killing all microorganisms.
   B. process of destroying as many microorganisms as possible.
   C. process of removing half of the microorganisms.
   D. All of the above.

Instructor Notes

4. In order for an infection to spread, all of the following factors need to be present *except*
   A. a source.
   B. a susceptible host.
   C. a means of transmission.
   (D.) a wet environment.
5. Which of the following types of precautions should be used for all patients?
   (A.) Standard Precautions
   B. Airborne Precautions
   C. Contact Precautions
   D. Droplet Precautions

CRITICAL THINKING

CUSTOMER SERVICE

Encourage students to reflect and share their thoughts and experiences. Respect their privacy and confidentiality. Share your own viewpoints with the students.

CULTURAL CARE

Encourage students to reflect and share their thoughts and experiences. Respect their privacy and confidentiality. Share your own viewpoints with the students.

COOPERATION WITHIN THE TEAM

Encourage students to reflect and share their thoughts and experiences. Respect their privacy and confidentiality. Share your own viewpoints with the students.

NURSING ASSISTANT IN ACTION

As part of your training you learned that handwashing is essential. You and a coworker happen to be in the restroom at the same time. Your coworker does not wash his hands after using the restroom. It is time for you both to assist feeding patients their lunches.

What Is Your Response/Action?

You should remind your coworker to wash his hands. This is a very important safety precaution for patients and other health care workers. Be direct or use a sense of humor, but do not just let the incident occur.

5

Answers to Workbook Exercises

The following exercises will assist you to apply what you have read in Chapter 5, "Infection Control." For each exercise, read the objective and use information you have read in Chapter 5 to answer the questions, complete the sentences, or label the diagrams.

EXERCISE 5-1

Objective: To recognize and correctly spell words related to infection control.

Directions: Unscramble the words in the Word List at the left. Then circle the same words in the Word Search at the right.

Word List

1. GNESHOPTA ___PATHOGENS___
2. THSO ___HOST___
3. SRECOU ___SOURCE___
4. RTSNAMSISION ___TRANSMISSION___
5. IONTLASIO ___ISOLATION___
6. DHWNASHAGNI ___HANDWASHING___
7. TCIFRNIO ___FRICTION___
8. TITPHEAIS ___HEPATITIS___
9. RELSIET ___STERILE___

Word Search

P	A	T	H	O	G	E	N	S	S	A	B	L	I	E	O
A	L	V	O	P	Y	Z	L	Q	C	K	M	K	Q	Z	A
E	N	V	S	O	U	R	C	E	F	G	H	Z	H	F	D
X	S	C	T	R	A	N	S	M	I	S	S	I	O	N	L
K	I	D	K	V	L	A	X	E	T	M	T	E	V	X	D
O	G	S	E	B	T	L	B	E	S	F	O	W	B	C	B
C	I	R	O	I	V	G	J	I	H	R	J	S	S	E	Y
A	K	M	E	L	H	G	L	S	B	I	A	J	I	G	Z
D	W	O	W	D	A	A	P	N	E	C	H	S	T	P	O
H	S	J	T	G	N	T	M	S	Z	T	N	I	I	C	H
D	T	X	B	S	D	K	I	B	E	I	E	K	T	M	B
M	E	K	M	Q	W	I	S	O	C	O	H	H	A	A	L
R	R	F	P	Z	A	N	P	G	N	N	D	F	P	L	E
A	I	L	C	R	S	L	D	H	V	T	T	Y	E	F	N
N	L	P	A	N	H	E	Y	V	L	D	N	A	H	I	K
H	E	W	H	S	I	S	G	M	X	S	F	R	P	E	G
J	C	F	T	S	N	H	C	A	K	J	C	M	B	D	E
F	O	D	K	J	G	N	T	D	P	S	G	H	Z	A	C
X	G	K	I	J	T	F	B	E	G	M	F	E	I	D	A

EXERCISE 5-2

Objective: To apply what you have learned about infection control.

Directions: Read the following riddles carefully before writing the correct answer on the blank line.

1. Put me on your skin or an object and I will kill many microorganisms as I disappear. *Hint:* Sometimes you will call me by a name that sounds like a woman's name but is spelled differently.

   ethyl alcohol

2. Without this process we would never be a host. *Hint:* An automobile has one of these.

   transmission

3. This word means "free of disease-producing organisms." *Hint:* The word would mean quite the opposite if you dropped the first letter.

   aseptic

EXERCISE 5-3

Objective: To recognize the definitions of words related to infection control.

Directions: Place the letter of the correct definition next to the matching word(s) from the Word List.

Word List

N	**1.** virus	F	**9.** hepatitis B
H	**2.** asepsis	D	**10.** disinfection
G	**3.** infection	L	**11.** spores
J	**4.** nosocomial infection	A	**12.** aseptic
C	**5.** bacteria	K	**13.** pathogen
E	**6.** friction	I	**14.** microorganism
B	**7.** autoclave	O	**15.** hand hygiene
M	**8.** sterilization	P	**16.** HAI

Definitions

A. Germ free, without disease-producing organisms
B. Device used to achieve sterility of an item through heat, pressure, and steam
C. Unicellular microorganism
D. The process of destroying as many harmful organisms as possible
E. The process of rubbing two surfaces together, such as skin

F. Bloodborne disease that affects the liver and is easily transmitted within the health care setting following parenteral exposure

G. Due to a pathogen producing a reaction that may cause soreness, tenderness, redness, and/or pus, fever, change in drainage, and so on

H. The absence of microorganisms

I. A living thing that is so small it cannot be seen with the naked eye but only through a microscope

J. Hospital acquired infection

K. Disease-producing microorganism

L. Bacteria that have formed hard shells around themselves as a defense

M. The process of killing all microorganisms, including spores

N. A type of microorganism that is much smaller than bacteria and can survive only in other living cells

O. Antiseptic hand rub, handwash, or surgical hand antisepsis

P. A health care-acquired infection

EXERCISE 5-4

Objective: To apply what you have learned about disinfection and sterilization.

Directions: Look at Figure 5-1; then circle the letter of the correct answer for each question.

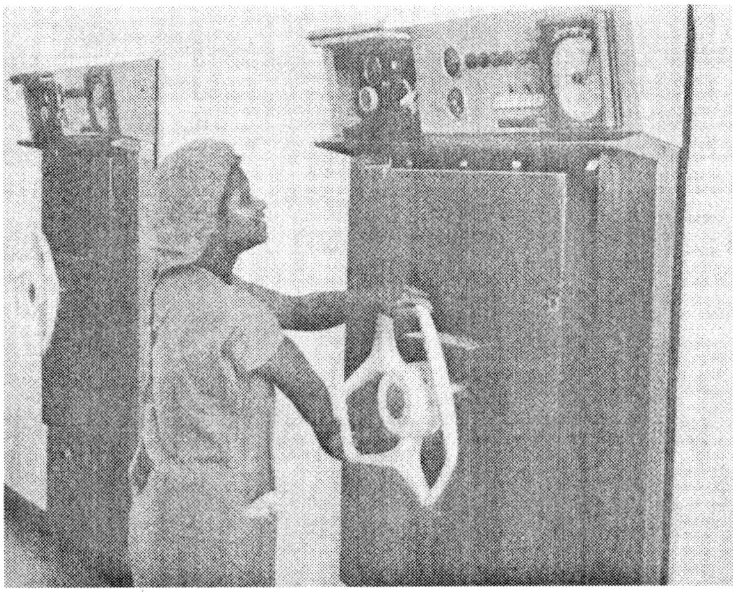

FIGURE 5-1

1. The machine in Figure 5-1 is called a(n)
   A. sterilizer.
   (B.) autoclave.
   C. pasteurizer.
   D. wheelchair.
   E. suction machine.

2. The autoclave sterilizes or completely destroys microorganisms by combining
   A. soap with hot water under pressure.
   B. acid with steam.
   C. ammonia with steam under pressure.
   D. heat with steam under pressure.
   E. water and bleach under pressure.

3. Autoclaves are used to kill
   A. bad germs only.
   B. all bacteria and viruses, including spores.
   C. parasites.
   D. time.

4. When an object is free of all ____________, it is sterile.
   A. grease
   B. worry
   C. wrinkles
   D. microorganisms

EXERCISE 5-5

Objective: To apply what you have learned about the use of patient care precautions and barrier devices, such as disposable gloves and a mask.

Directions: In Figure 5-2, label the steps in the order that you would perform them.

FIGURE 5-2

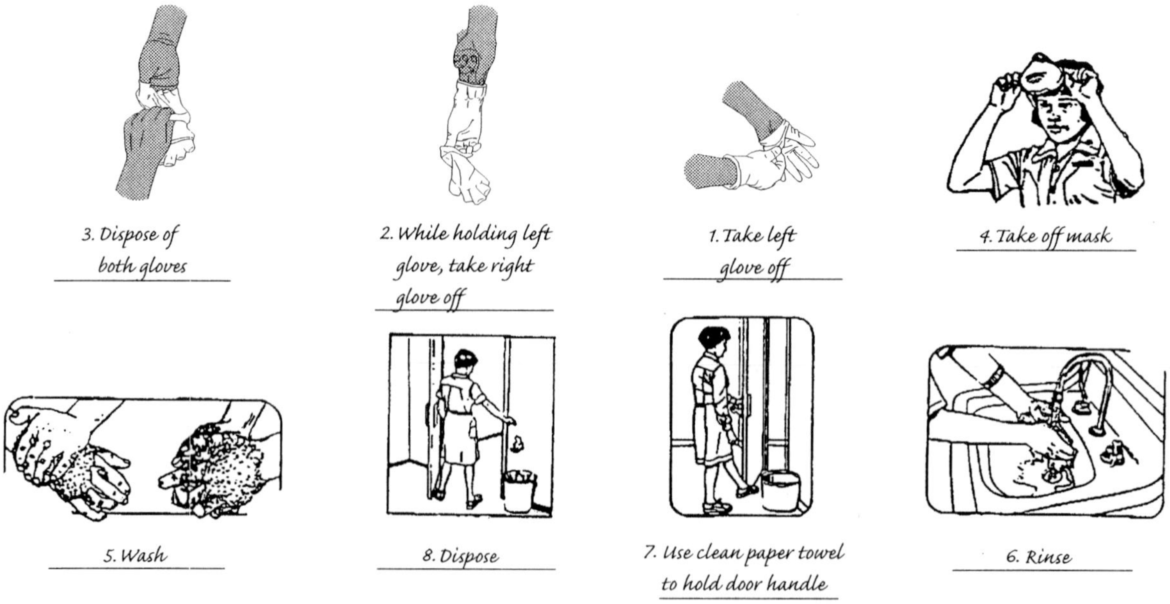

EXERCISE 5-6

Objective: To apply what you have learned about microorganisms and protective barriers.

Directions: Choose the correct method of mask use by putting a circle around either letter A or letter B in Figure 5-3.

FIGURE 5-3

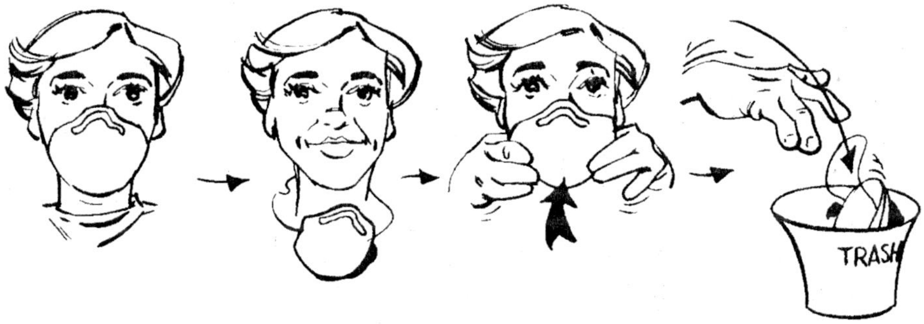

A:

To save money, wear the mask around your neck, and only put it on when you need it during the workday.

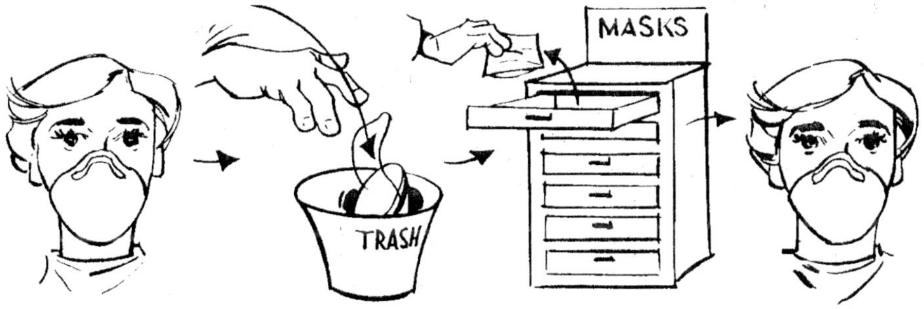

B:

Use each mask only once. Dispose of it when the procedure is complete, and get a clean mask the next time you need one.

EXERCISE 5-7

Objective: To apply what you have learned about infection control.

Directions: Circle the letter next to the word or sentence that best completes the sentence or describes the sentence as true or false. If the sentence is false, draw a line through the incorrect part of the sentence and write the correction on the blank line.

1. The source of microorganisms
   A. can only be the patient and the health care worker.
   B. is never really known.
   (C.) can be anyone, including objects in the environment.
   D. is a susceptible host only.

2. Standard Precautions are designed to provide safety to
   A. health care workers.
   B. patients.
   (C.) both A and B.
   D. nursing assistants who are in training.

3. To prevent or control the transmission of diseases, you
   A. must study very hard.
   B. must understand how a disease is spread.
   C. must protect yourself and your patient.
   (D.) both B and C.

4. Your ability to resist infections depends on your individual
   A. personality.
   B. income.
   C. age.
   (D.) health status and exposure to a pathogen.

5. To be reinfected means you or your patient have become infected a second time by the same microorganism.
   (A.) True
   B. False
   Correct Answer: ____________________

6. Cross-infection means becoming infected by a new microorganism from another patient or a health care worker.
   (A.) True
   B. False
   Correct Answer: ____________________

7. Standard Precautions apply to
   A. blood, all body fluids, nonintact skin, and mucous membranes.
   B. saliva, semen, and blood.
   C. care of the burned patient.
   (D.) all of the above.

8. Which of the following is not true about sterile fields?
A. Keep a 1-inch border around the field.
B. Do not cross your hand over a sterile field.
C. Do not turn your back on a sterile field.
(D.) Keep all used and unused pieces of equipment on the sterile field at all times.

9. Cleanliness is important, so be sure that your fingernails are
(A.) kept short and are cleaned frequently.
B. colorful and attractive at all times.
C. kept long to facilitate opening packages.
D. extended ½ inch beyond the ends of your fingers.

10. You have never had chicken pox and you discover your patient is infected with this disease. What do you do?
A. Hold your breath while caring for this patient.
B. Wear gloves and a mask to prevent infection in the patient.
C. You are over 21 and so cannot develop this disease.
(D.) Speak to your immediate supervisor about taking a different patient assignment.

11. The key to good handwashing is
(A.) washing long enough.
B. friction and hand cream to protect against chapping.
C. bar soap instead of dispensed soap.
D. adequate soap, lots of tepid water, and friction.

12. During handwashing, if your hands touched the inside of the sink you would
A. start over.
(B.) rinse 30 seconds longer, and use paper towels to wipe the sink.
C. use adequate paper towels and friction.
D. ignore it because you have soap on your hands to kill the germs.

13. Gloves ~~provide a complete barrier to~~ contamination.
A. True
(B.) False
Correct Answer: *may have small flaws so you should wash your hands after removing them to prevent*

14. ____________ is (are) a good technique to use during handwashing.
A. Transmission
(B.) Interlacing
C. Both A and B
D. Log-rolling

15. Hands must be washed after removing gloves.
(A.) True
B. False
Correct Answer: ______________________________

COMPETENCY CHECKLIST 5-1: INFECTION CONTROL

ACTIVITY	S	U	COMMENTS
1. Student correctly demonstrates proper handwashing procedure:			
A. Application of soap and water			
B. Use of friction			
C. Use of paper towel to shut off faucets			
2. Student correctly demonstrates proper procedure to open a sterile package:			
A. Verify supplies are sterile.			
B. Position and open the package.			
C. Add sterile items to sterile field.			
3. Student correctly demonstrates proper gloving procedure:			
A. Application of nonsterile disposable gloves			
B. Removal of nonsterile disposable gloves			
C. Application of sterile disposable gloves			
D. Removal of sterile disposable gloves			
4. Student correctly demonstrates proper gowning procedure:			
A. Application of gown			
B. Removal of gown			
5. Student correctly demonstrates proper procedure to clean noncritical items:			
A. Not visibly soiled			
B. Visibly soiled			

Safety

6

CHAPTER OVERVIEW

Instructor Notes

I. **General Safety Measures**

II. **Oxygen Safety**
   A. Oxygen Therapy

III. **Fire Safety and Prevention**
   A. Major Causes of Fire
      1. Smoking
      2. Misuses of Electricity
   B. In Case of a Fire

IV. **Patient Safety**
   A. Disasters
   B. Protective Devices

V. **Patient Restraint Policy Example**
   A. Alternatives to Restraints
   B. When Restraints Are Clearly Indicated
   C. Key Points for Restraint Orders
   D. Types of Restraints Used
   E. Restraint and Seclusion Standards Do Not Apply in the Following Situations
   F. Emergency Application for Restraint and/or Seclusion
   G. Events Preceding and Leading up to Restraint and/or Seclusion
   H. Psychiatry Departments/Behavioral Health
   I. Application of Restraints
   J. Patient Care
   K. Physical Management
      1. Team Roles and Responsibilities
      2. Management of Behavior Problems Related to Delirium and Dementia
   L. Falls and Restraints
      1. Modifying Risk Factors for a Fall
      2. Bed Rails and Restraints

Instructor Notes

M. Physician Responsibilities: Patient Assessment and Orders
   1. Patient Assessment
   2. Orders
N. OBRA Regulations
O. Restraint Alternatives
P. Restraining the Pediatric Patient
   1. Applying Elbow Restraints
Q. Ambulation Safety with a Cane, Walker, or Crutches

OBJECTIVES

When the students have completed this chapter, they will be able to:

- List the general rules of safety in a health care setting.
- List safety precautions in caring for older adults and children.
- Describe the special safety precautions necessary when oxygen is being used.
- Explain what can be done to prevent fires and what to do in case of fire.
- Practice restraint application.
- Discuss restraint alternatives.
- Discuss and document care of patients in restraints.
- Identify OBRA regulations regarding the use of restraints.
- List the safety rules for patient ambulation.

KEY TERMS

Ambulate: To walk or move about

Ambulation: To walk or move about in an upright position

Bed Alarm: A control unit that activates an audible alarm and the nurse call system when the patient's weight leaves a pressure-sensitive mat for a preselected amount of time

Cannula: A flexible tube that can be inserted into a body cavity and used to draw fluids out or give oxygen or fluids

Chair Alarm: A battery-operated control unit that activates an audible alarm immediately if the patient tries to get up out of the chair

Clove Hitch: A type of knot that can be easily released in case of emergency

Cognition: Awareness; the mental processes by which knowledge is acquired

Confusion: Bewilderment; the state of being disoriented to person, place, or time

Delirium: A disordered mental state that develops over a short period of time

Dementia: A progressive medical condition characterized by personality change; decline in intellectual capacity, judgment, and memory; and impairment of impulse control

Flowmeter: A device used to control and regulate the flow of oxygen

Gait Training: Rehabilitative exercise to help patients improve their walking ability

Instructor Notes

Nasal: Pertaining to the nose and nasal cavity

OBRA Regulations: Federal rules and requirements established by the Omnibus Budget Reconciliation Act of 1987

Oxygen: A colorless, odorless, tasteless gaseous element that is essential for respiration; air is 21 percent oxygen

Pressure-sensitive Mat: A disposable mat that is connected to a bed or chair alarm

Protective Devices: Measures taken to keep a patient safe or to prevent injury

Restraint Alternative: Protective measures, such as a saddle or wedge cushion, self-releasing belt, or lap tray, that are used to help prevent falls but do not physically restrain an individual

Restraints: A protective measure ordered by a physician to prevent patients from harming themselves or others

CORE STUDENT ASSIGNMENTS

Students should:

- Read this chapter in their textbook, *Being a Nursing Assistant.*
- Underline any words or sentences they do not understand. Write down any questions they have.
- Complete the Chapter Review in their textbook.
- Read the Time Management Tip for this chapter and think about how they might use this tip in their work.
- Complete the Nursing Assistant in Action exercise.

OPTIONAL STUDENT ASSIGNMENTS

Students should:

- Complete all workbook assignments for this chapter in their copy of *Workbook for Being a Nursing Assistant.*
- Use the CD/CD-Rom disk enclosed with their textbook to hear the pronunciation of the key terms in the chapter.
- Watch the "Complying with Legal Standards" and the "Being Reliable" sections of the "Focus on Professionalism" video and the "Patient's Right to Refuse Care" section of the "Patient's Rights" video from the Care Provider Skills series.
- Use the Website address **(www.prenhall.com/wolgin)** to access the free, interactive Companion Website created for this textbook. Get hints, instant feedback, and textbook references to chapter-related multiple-choice questions. Read and react to the Nursing Assistant in Action exercise. Link to other interesting sites.

Instructor Notes

METHODOLOGY AND SUGGESTED ACTIVITIES

I. Lecture/Discussion

- Answer any questions the students may have.
- Discuss the key terms and related abbreviations. Repeat them out loud and practice using them in sentences.
- Discuss the Time Management Tip for this chapter.
- Discuss the Nursing Assistant in Action exercise.
- Discuss the Critical Thinking points for this chapter.
- Discuss personal safety and protection. Emphasize the importance of following Universal Precautions. Stress the need to wear protective equipment.
- Familiarize the students with the Medicare law dealing with "Specified Rights," from the House Congressional Record, H12989, December 22, 1987, Omnibus Budget Reconciliation Act of 1987.
- Identify the exit routes in the facilities and the home setting.
- Discuss evacuation procedures both in a facility and in the home setting.
- Stress the RACE system.
- Discuss the pros and cons of patient restraint: safety versus personal freedom.

II. Role Play/Lab

- Show the videos for this chapter. Discuss why hospitals and health care institutions need safety regulations. Role play what you would do in a fire, tornado, or hazardous spill in your institution.
- Display oxygen equipment. Explain the rationale for its use and safety measures.
- Display and describe a regulation flowmeter.
- Invite a respiratory therapist to speak and demonstrate equipment.
- Practice scenarios with upset patients and families. Try out the physical management techniques.
- Distribute handouts on electrical safety obtained from your local electric company.
- Invite a local firefighter to discuss fire safety and prevention.
- Invite a physical therapist to demonstrate equipment and stress ambulatory safety using a walker, cane, and crutches.
- Assign role play scenarios requiring the students to use appropriate equipment.
- Practice applying the restraints among students. Practice restraint alternatives as well as what to say to families about restraints and safety precautions.

III. Evaluation

- Review the answers to the Chapter Review with students.
- Review the answers to the workbook exercises with students.
- Review the students' understanding of the Time Management Tip.
- To evaluate student comprehension, give a quiz.
- To evaluate student skills, administer the competency checklist.
- Have the students visit the interactive Companion Website and take the quiz.

ANSWERS TO CHAPTER REVIEW

Instructor Notes

FILL IN THE BLANK

Read each sentence and fill in the blank line with a word that completes the sentence. (Note: Hyphenated words get one line.)

1. Be sure to lock the ___brakes___ on wheelchairs, stretchers, and commode chairs.

2. The special device used with oxygen that controls and regulates the amount of oxygen is called the ___flowmeter___ .

3. An ___ABC___ extinguisher can be used on all types of fires.

4. ___Smoking___ is the number one cause of fires in health care institutions.

5. Never tie or secure a restraint device to a ___movable___ part of a bed or chair.

MULTIPLE CHOICE

Choose the best answer for each question or statement.

1. All of the following are true about oxygen *except*
   A. it is a colorless, odorless, tasteless gas.
   (B.) the more oxygen a patient has the better.
   C. oxygen is one of the key elements needed for fire.
   D. room air is 21 percent oxygen.

2. The *P* in the acronym **PASS** means
   A. pass me the fire extinguisher.
   B. panic.
   C. push people out of the way.
   (D.) pull the safety pin or seal at the top of the extinguisher.

3. All of the following are misuses of electricity *except* which one?
   A. Electrical equipment in contact with water
   B. Use of numerous extension cords
   C. Use of frayed cords and plugs
   (D.) Use of three-pronged plugs

4. Which of the following is not a restraint alternative?
   A. Chair alarm
   B. A positioning device like a cushion or pad
   (C.) Lap belt
   D. Constant staff or family supervision

Instructor Notes

5. When ambulating a patient,
   A. apply good body mechanics.
   B. be sure of the patient's ability to ambulate before you attempt to move him.
   C. always communicate to the patient what you expect of him.
   (D.) All of the above.

CRITICAL THINKING

CUSTOMER SERVICE

Encourage students to reflect and share their thoughts and experiences. Respect their privacy and confidentiality. Share your own viewpoints with the students.

CULTURAL CARE

Encourage students to reflect and share their thoughts and experiences. Respect their privacy and confidentiality. Share your own viewpoints with the students.

COOPERATION WITHIN THE TEAM

Encourage students to reflect and share their thoughts and experiences. Respect their privacy and confidentiality. Share your own viewpoints with the students.

NURSING ASSISTANT IN ACTION

Mrs. Smith is an elderly woman with Alzheimer's disease living in an assistive care unit. She frequently wanders into other patients' rooms and then uses their bathrooms or looks in their drawers for belongings she has lost. The other residents are becoming impatient and angry with her. One resident asks you to lock Mrs. Smith in her own room because she is tired of finding her belongings and bathroom messed up by Mrs. Smith. Would locking Mrs. Smith in her room be considered a restraint?

What Is Your Response/Action?

Yes, locking Mrs. Smith in her room would be considered a restraint and false imprisonment. One idea would be to try more restraint alternatives with Mrs. Smith. One alternative to try first is distraction. Perhaps some sorting activities like folding towels or wash cloths. If that is not successful, a chair alarm might work for portions of the day.

Answers to Workbook Exercises

6

The following exercises will assist you to apply what you read in Chapter 6, "Safety." For each exercise, read the objective and use information you have read in Chapter 6 to answer the questions, complete the sentences, or label the diagrams.

EXERCISE 6-1

Objective: To recognize and correctly spell words related to safety.

Directions: Unscramble the words in the Word List on the left. Then circle the same words in the Word Search at the right.

Word List

1. YTEFAS ______ *SAFETY*
2. STANISTRER ______ *RESTRAINTS*
3. ROAB ______ *OBRA*
4. RFEI ______ *FIRE*
5. YXENOG ______ *OXYGEN*
6. TNEPVER ______ *PREVENT*
7. SKEABR ______ *BRAKES*
8. ZOARSR ______ *RAZORS*
9. NIFCONUOS ______ *CONFUSION*

Word Search

A	N	O	R	C	A	D	P	E	J	M	K	K	F	A	H	C
K	S	Q	U	A	Z	L	J	L	G	Q	F	A	L	E	C	D
R	M	V	E	Q	R	F	B	X	H	O	L	J	S	M	F	Z
J	V	S	A	F	E	T	Y	D	F	I	T	D	A	H	I	E
Z	A	F	G	H	S	F	M	I	N	B	J	C	R	O	B	D
P	B	F	C	D	T	J	B	K	A	H	Z	T	V	A	H	G
D	C	I	J	N	R	C	E	N	D	P	E	N	U	X	J	H
X	I	O	B	R	A	H	D	B	R	A	K	E	S	I	G	H
J	K	X	L	F	I	R	E	I	A	D	A	V	M	H	D	B
K	P	Y	R	H	N	F	A	C	Z	F	V	E	J	A	H	K
L	S	G	L	I	T	S	P	J	O	H	S	R	A	Z	L	I
O	M	E	V	C	S	A	I	T	R	L	N	P	P	R	S	D
H	T	N	H	J	G	J	K	S	S	H	L	D	J	V	D	G
M	V	G	Z	A	M	V	O	G	X	I	M	G	F	A	N	A
B	O	D	I	Q	R	A	K	C	O	N	F	U	S	I	O	N

EXERCISE 6-2

Objective: To recognize safety issues and immediate actions to be taken.

Directions: Place the correct letters that would apply to the situation next to the matching phrase, *then* circle the correct response you should take immediately. More than one set of letters can be selected for each situation.

OS = oxygen safety	RS = restraint safety	CS = child safety
FS = fire safety	AS = ambulation safety	PS = patient safety

1. Your patient has nasal oxygen on at 3 liters and there is a NO SMOKING—OXYGEN IN USE sign on the wall above his bed. His wife is preparing to light a candle at the bedside and say a prayer for his recovery.

Letters: ___OS, FS, PS___ **What would you do?**

A. You grab the fire extinguisher and Pull the pin, Aim low, Squeeze the handle, and Sweep from side to side, aiming at the base of the candle.

(B.) You put out the candle and explain to her that open flames are dangerous when oxygen is running. You offer to show her where the chapel is located.

C. You turn off the oxygen for 20 minutes until she is done praying.

D. You ignore the situation because such a small flame is harmless.

2. You are ready to leave for the day and stop in to say goodbye to your patient. She tells you that the floor in the bathroom is wet. You realize that the housekeeping staff has gone home for the day.

Letters: ___PS, AS___ **What would you do?**

(A.) You clean up the floor immediately or get someone else to do it.

B. You leave immediately, because you must take your sick child to the doctor.

C. You provide the patient with a call light and instruct her to ask someone on the new shift to do it because you are leaving.

D. You tell the patient to stay out of the bathroom until someone else comes to clean it up.

3. You are coming on your new shift and notice that one of your patients is wearing a chest restraint that is on backwards. The patient is sleeping at this time.

Letters: ___RS, PS___ **What would you do?**

A. Let him sleep for now.

B. Make a note to change the restraint later on when you have more time.

C. Leave a call light within reach.

(D.) Check with your immediate supervisor to determine if help is needed when changing the restraint, based on the patient's condition and reason for wearing the restraint. You change the restraint immediately.

4. You notice that your patient, a 7-year-old, is picking at the IV site on his arm.

Letters: ____CS____ **What would you do?**

A. You restrain him immediately.

B. You report this to your immediate supervisor.

C. You sit with the child, give him some toys to play with, and report this to your immediate supervisor later that day.

(D.) You report this to your supervisor immediately. You stop by often to distract him as you sit with him, give him some toys, and explain how important it is to not disturb the IV.

5. When getting a patient up to sit at the bedside in a reclining chair, you notice the chair's wheel brakes do not work well. This causes the chair to slide backward about 6 inches across the floor as the patient sits down. The patient is not injured.

Letters: ____PS____ **What would you do?**

A. Make out a work repair form and send it to the proper person.

B. Notify your immediate supervisor, and tell your coworkers to be careful.

(C.) Get another chair for your patient. Get help transferring him to the new chair, and remove the broken chair from the patient care area after labeling it "broken." Report this to your immediate supervisor.

D. Make sure the chair is always up against the wall in the future when you transfer the patient to it, so that he will not be injured when it moves.

6. As you prepare to take Mr. O'Shea for a walk, you notice that the walker he brought from home to use in the hospital has two rubber tips missing from the feet.

Letters: ____AS, PS____ **What would you do?**

A. Make a note to have the medical equipment staff take a look at it next time they are in.

(B.) Obtain another walker that is the same size and that has all four rubber tips in place before you ambulate him.

C. Tell his wife to buy some new tips for the walker.

D. Let him use it this time because he is too impatient to wait for his walk, and you don't want him to complain to the immediate supervisor about you.

EXERCISE 6-3

Objective: To apply what you have learned about safety.

Directions: Circle the letter next to the word or statement that best completes the sentence or describes the sentence as true or false. If the sentence is false, draw a line through the incorrect part of the sentence and write the correction on the blank line.

1. **RACE** stands for
   A. **R**un **A**way and **C**all **E**MS.
   B. **R**emove yourself **A**nd **C**all "**E**xit!"
   C. **R**un **A**nd **C**orrect the **E**mergency.
   (D.) **R**emove the patient; **A**ctivate the alarm; **C**ontain the fire; **E**xtinguish the fire, if safe to do so.
2. It takes three things to have a fire: heat, fuel, and ~~wind~~.
   A. True
   (B.) False
   Correct Answer: *oxygen*
3. It is important to ~~change~~ the evacuation plan of your facility.
   A. True
   (B.) False
   Correct Answer: *follow*
4. The Omnibus Budget Reconciliation Act (OBRA) calls any device a restraint that keeps a patient from moving freely or keeps the patient from reaching parts of her body.
   (A.) True
   B. False
   Correct Answer: ____________________
5. It should be noted that there is sometimes an increase in injury to patients in restraints.
   (A.) True
   B. False
   Correct Answer: ____________________
6. When the patient is utilizing nasal oxygen, the areas where skin irritation may occur are
   (A.) any area where the plastic cannula may touch.
   B. only behind the ears.
   C. the nostrils and the eyelids.
   D. behind the neck and the forehead.
7. ___________ is the number one cause of fires in health care institutions.
   A. A sleepy patient
   B. A broken electrical cord
   C. Too much oxygen
   (D.) Smoking

8. A fire extinguisher may be labeled
A. A for all, B for wood, C for combustion.
B. only A for paper fires and B for electrical fires.
C. ABC for "all burning clothing."
(D.) ABC for use on any type of fire.

9. Always place used disposable razors
A. in a red waste basket.
(B.) in approved containers.
C. in recycling bins.
D. where they can be quickly found for reuse later.

10. Room cleaning supplies should
A. be left at the bedside at all times.
B. be labeled and dated before leaving at the bedside.
(C.) be stored away from the patient care area.
D. be kept in the patient's bathroom.

11. Electrical equipment must never come in contact with
A. heat, fuel, or oxygen.
B. patients.
C. the nursing assistant.
(D.) water.

COMPETENCY CHECKLIST 6-1: SAFETY

ACTIVITY	S	U	COMMENTS
1. Student will demonstrate the correct method for applying a waist restraint.			
2. Student will demonstrate the correct method for applying a vest restraint.			

IMPORTANT CRITERIA

1. The nurse or therapist will decide what type of restraint is to be used.			
2. Never tie or secure a restraint to any movable part of a bed or chair.			
3. The patient must be checked at least every 30 minutes while restrained, or more often according to the institution's policy.			
4. Carefully check pressure points for redness or irritation of the skin.			
5. The patient must be released to offer food and liquids, toilet, and exercise, and to reposition him.			

7

Body Mechanics: Positioning, Moving, and Transporting Patients

CHAPTER OVERVIEW

Instructor Notes

I. **Proper/Protective Body Mechanics**

II. **Positioning and Draping the Patient**
   A. Knee-Chest Position
   B. Dorsal Lithotomy Position

III. **Moving and Lifting Patients**

IV. **Transporting a Patient by Wheelchair**

V. **Using a Stretcher**

VI. **Assisting the Patient to Ambulate**
   A. Using a Gait Belt
   B. Using a Cane, Walker, or Crutches

VII. **Assisting a Falling Patient**

Instructor Notes

OBJECTIVES

When the students have completed this chapter, they will be able to:

- Describe techniques for proper/protective body mechanics.
- Lift, hold, or move an object or patient using techniques for proper/protective body mechanics.
- List the different positions for patients, assist patients into those positions, and drape for privacy.
- List the guidelines for moving and lifting patients.
- Move a helpless patient up in bed.
- Move a patient up in bed with the patient's help.
- Move the mattress to the head of the bed with the patient's help.
- Move a helpless patient to one side of the bed on the patient's back.
- Log roll the patient.
- Turn a patient on either side.
- Transport and reposition a patient in a wheelchair; move the patient from the bed to a wheelchair and back into bed.
- Move the helpless patient using a portable mechanical patient lift.
- Transport a patient by stretcher, and move the patient from the bed to a stretcher and back into bed.
- Assist a patient to ambulate.
- Assist a falling patient.

KEY TERMS

Ambulation: The act or process of walking

Bedridden: Unable to get out of bed

Body Alignment: The correct, or anatomical, positioning of a patient's body; also the arrangement of the body in a straight line

Dorsal Lithotomy Position: The position in which a patient lies on the back, with legs spread apart and knees bent

Dorsal Recumbent Position: Lying down or reclining; refers to the back or the back part of an organ

Drape: A covering used to provide privacy during an examination or operation

Draping: Covering a patient or parts of a patient's body with a sheet, blanket, bath blanket, or other material during a physical examination or prior to surgery

Fowler's Position: The position in which the head of the patient's bed is at a 45°–90° angle

Incontinent: Unable to control the bowels or bladder

Knee-Chest Position: A bent posture with the knees and chest touching the examining table, sometimes used for examining the rectum or for women who have recently given birth, to allow the uterus to fall forward into its natural position

Instructor Notes

Nonambulatory: Unable to walk

Prone Position: Lying on one's stomach

Proper/Protective Body Mechanics: Special ways of standing and moving one's body to make the best use of strength and to avoid fatigue

Semi-Fowler's Position: The position in which the head of the patient's bed is at a 30°–45° angle

Side-lying (Lateral) Positions: Lying on one's left or right side

Sims's Position: Position in which the patient lies on the left side with the right knee and thigh drawn up, often used for a rectal examination

Stretcher: A wheeled cart on which patients are moved from one place to another

Supine Position: Lying on one's back

Transporting: Moving something or someone from one place to another

Trendelenburg's Position: Position in which the bed or operating table on which a patient is lying is tilted so that the patient's head is about one foot below the level of his knees to allow more blood flow to the head and prevent shock; also called *shock position*

CORE STUDENT ASSIGNMENTS

Students should:

- Read this chapter in their textbook, *Being a Nursing Assistant.*
- Underline any words or sentences they do not understand. Write down any questions they have.
- Complete the Chapter Review in their textbook.
- Read the Time Management Tip for this chapter and think about how they might use this tip in their work.
- Complete the Nursing Assistant in Action exercise.

OPTIONAL STUDENT ASSIGNMENTS

Students should:

- Complete all workbook assignments for this chapter in their copy of *Workbook for Being a Nursing Assistant.*
- Use the CD/CD-Rom disk enclosed with their textbook to hear the pronunciation of the key terms in the chapter.
- Watch the "Body Mechanics" and the "Transfer and Ambulation" video from the Care Provider Skills series.
- Use the Website address **(www.prenhall.com/wolgin)** to access the free, interactive Companion Website created for this textbook. Get hints, instant feedback, and textbook references to chapter-related multiple-choice questions. Read and react to the Nursing Assistant in Action exercise. Link to other interesting sites.

Instructor Notes

METHODOLOGY AND SUGGESTED ACTIVITIES

I. Lecture/Discussion

- Answer any questions the students may have.
- Discuss the key terms and related abbreviations. Repeat them out loud and practice using them in sentences.
- Discuss the Time Management Tip for this chapter.
- Discuss the Nursing Assistant in Action exercise.
- Discuss the Critical Thinking points for this chapter.
- Discuss personal safety and protection. Emphasize the importance of following Universal Precautions. Stress the need to wear protective clothing.
- Discuss principles related to body mechanics in positioning, moving, and transporting patients.
- Discuss ways to protect nursing assistants' bodies: time versus safety.
- Discuss ways to have the patient participate safely in transfers.

II. Role Play/Lab

- Show the videos for this chapter. Have the students practice lifting techniques and transfer and ambulation techniques with each other. To promote back safety, emphasize caregiver planning and communication to the patient about what to do prior to any lifting, transferring, or ambulating technique.
- Demonstrate all proper/protective body mechanics.
- Have the students practice correct body mechanics and return demonstrations.
- Have the students draw a picture of a stick figure on a bed to clarify their concept of body alignment.
- Demonstrate positioning a patient with and without lift equipment.
- Write the names of the positions on slips of paper. Give one to each student. Give each student a turn to model his or her position while the rest of the class tries to name the position and arrange the drape.
- Ask one student to play the part of the patient. Stress rules as you demonstrate the use of a pull sheet.
- Demonstrate using a stretcher, gait belt, cane, walker, and crutches. Have students return the demonstration.
- Demonstrate the proper method for assisting a falling patient. Have students return the demonstration.

III. Evaluation

- Review the answers to the Chapter Review with students.
- Review the answers to the workbook exercises with students.
- Review the students' understanding of the Time Management Tip.
- To evaluate student comprehension, give a quiz.
- To evaluate student skills, administer the competency checklist.
- Have the students visit the interactive Companion Website and take the quiz.

ANSWERS TO CHAPTER REVIEW

Instructor Notes

FILL IN THE BLANK

Read each sentence and fill in the blank line with a word that completes the sentence. (Note: Hyphenated words get one line.)

1. ___Proper___ ___body___ ___mechanics___ are special ways of standing and moving to make the best use of strength and to avoid fatigue.
2. A ___drape___ is a covering used to provide privacy during an examination or operation.
3. Right or left ___side-lying___ positions are used to promote comfort and to relieve pressure points.
4. Whenever you are pushing a stretcher, you should be at the end where the patient's ___head___ is.
5. Use of a ___gait___ ___belt___ positioned snugly around the patient's waist will help you to control the patient while walking.

MULTIPLE CHOICE

Choose the best answer for each question or statement.

1. Which one of the following is not a guideline for proper body mechanics?
   A. Position your body close to the load.
   (B.) Lift and carry rather than push an object.
   C. Use good posture.
   D. Keep your feet slightly apart for better balance.
2. The supine position refers to which patient position?
   (A.) Lying on back
   B. Head of the bed up 45–90 degrees
   C. Lying down or reclining with the knees bent, soles of the feet flat on the bed
   D. None of the above
3. Trendelenburg's position is used to treat patients who are experiencing
   A. cardiac arrest.
   B. diabetes.
   (C.) shock.
   D. seizures.

Instructor Notes

4. The dorsal lithotomy position is used for
   A. shock.
   (B.) physical exams of the bladder or vagina.
   C. physical exam of the patient's back.
   D. physical exam of the rectum.
5. Which of these activities is not a follow-up activity to report to the nurse?
   A. Reporting that the patient's position has been changed.
   (B.) How many people were required to move the patient.
   C. How the patient tolerated the move.
   D. The time of the position change.

CRITICAL THINKING

CUSTOMER SERVICE

Encourage students to reflect and share their thoughts and experiences. Respect their privacy and confidentiality. Share your own viewpoints with the students.

CULTURAL CARE

Encourage students to reflect and share their thoughts and experiences. Respect their privacy and confidentiality. Share your own viewpoints with the students.

COOPERATION WITHIN THE TEAM

Encourage students to reflect and share their thoughts and experiences. Respect their privacy and confidentiality. Share your own viewpoints with the students.

NURSING ASSISTANT IN ACTION

You are assigned to assist Mr. Bigg, a helpless 320-pound patient up from a wheelchair to his bed. You bring the mechanical lift to his room and have requested a coworker to help you. When you start explaining what you plan to do, Mr. Bigg resists. He says: "You are not going to use that contraption on me! The last time I was in that thing, the staff person did not know how to work it and frightened me. I am staying right where I am!"

What Is Your Response/Action?

Reassure Mr. Bigg that you know how to use the lift equipment. Point out that your coworker is also well trained and will be there to further assist Mr. Biggs. Tell Mr. Biggs that using the lift is the safest way to move him with for his own safety and for the safety of the nursing assistants.

7

Answers to Workbook Exercises

The following exercises will assist you to apply what you have read in Chapter 7, "Body Mechanics: Positioning, Moving, and Transporting Patients." For each exercise, read the objective and use information you have read in Chapter 7 to answer the questions, complete the sentences, or label the diagrams.

EXERCISE 7-1

Objective: To recognize and correctly spell words related to body mechanics utilized while positioning, moving, and transporting a patient.

Directions: Unscramble the words in the Word List at the left. Then circle the same words in the Word Search at the right.

Word List

1. ICMHENACS ___MECHANICS___
2. YOBD ___BODY___
3. GEIUAFT ___FATIGUE___
4. JYNUIR ___INJURY___
5. TNIGFLI ___LIFTING___
6. PLHEESSL ___HELPLESS___
7. RNATSPTOR ___TRANSPORT___
8. LALF ___FALL___
9. NUSIPE ___SUPINE___

Word Search

M	E	A	B	C	D	O	X	F	J	A	K	L	M
D	E	F	I	J	O	K	B	K	Q	Y	D	I	H
W	D	C	S	I	W	A	J	R	Z	B	E	F	V
S	N	K	H	E	L	P	L	E	S	S	G	T	I
U	A	N	F	A	T	I	G	U	E	R	A	I	L
P	L	P	K	M	N	X	Q	A	J	Z	C	N	U
I	V	A	C	L	E	I	N	J	U	R	Y	G	Y
N	P	M	L	E	X	V	C	F	D	W	D	B	L
E	F	S	C	Z	F	W	U	S	L	A	V	L	H
X	Q	R	T	P	B	O	D	Y	X	E	A	G	Y
T	R	A	N	S	P	O	R	T	B	F	C	E	Z

EXERCISE 7-2

Objective: To apply what you have learned about using good body mechanics to position, move, and transport patients.

Directions: Read the following riddles carefully before writing the correct answer on the blank line.

1. These two words refer to use of the proper techniques for standing and moving one's body. What are they? *Hint:* If your car was damaged in a collision, you would ask these skilled workers to fix it.
body mechanics ______________________

2. This term can refer to the way a patient walks, or it can describe a device used to support the patient while walking. What is it? *Hint:* It sounds like part of a fence.
gait ______________________

EXERCISE 7-3

Objective: To recognize the definitions of words used in applying good body mechanics to the positioning, moving, and transporting of patients.

Directions: Complete the sentences with the words from the Word List below.

Word List

Trendelenburg's	body mechanics	Fowler's
body alignment	side-lying	Sims's
knee-chest	supine	bedridden
dorsal recumbent	lithotomy	draping
nonambulatory	drape	prone

1. ___*Nonambulatory*___ means not able to walk.

2. ___*Body*___ ___*alignment*___ refers to the arrangement of the body in a straight line and the placing of portions of the body in correct anatomical position.

3. Bedbound or ___*bedridden*___ means the patient is unable to get out of bed.

4. ___*Body*___ ___*mechanics*___ are special ways of standing and moving one's body to make the best use of strength and avoid fatigue.

5. The patient is in ___*Fowler's*___ position when the head of the bed is at a 45°–90° angle.

6. Covering the patient or parts of the patient's body with a sheet, blanket, or other material is called ___*draping*___ the patient.

7. The patient is in ___*lithotomy*___ position when he lies on his back with his legs spread apart and knees bent.

8. When the patient is lying down on his back he is in the dorsal recumbent position.

9. In the supine position the patient is lying on his back.

10. In the side-lying position the patient is lying on his side.

11. The patient is in Trendelenburg's position when the bed or operating table is tilted so that the patient's head is about a foot below the level of his knees.

12. When the patient is lying on his left side with his right knee and thigh drawn up, he is in Sim's position.

13. A(n) drape is a covering used to provide privacy during an examination or operation.

14. In the knee-chest position the patient assumes a bent posture with the knees and chest touching the examination table or bed.

15. In the prone position the patient is lying on his stomach.

EXERCISE 7-4

Objective: To demonstrate an understanding of correct body mechanics to use when lifting and/or changing position.

Directions: Circle the letters of the pictures in Figure 7-1 that illustrate correct body mechanics.

1.

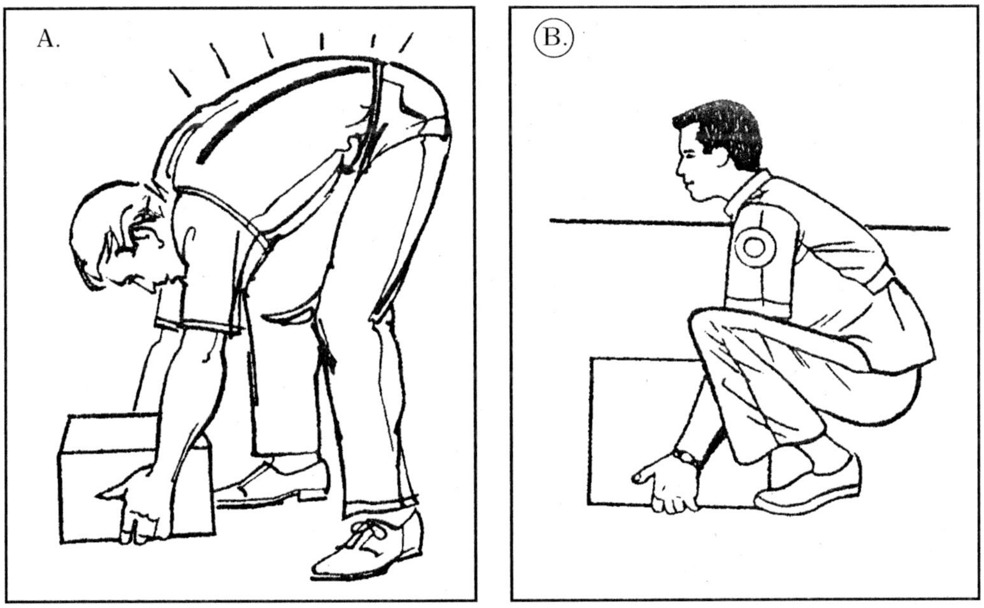

FIGURE 7-1

FIGURE 7-1 (cont.)

2.
3.

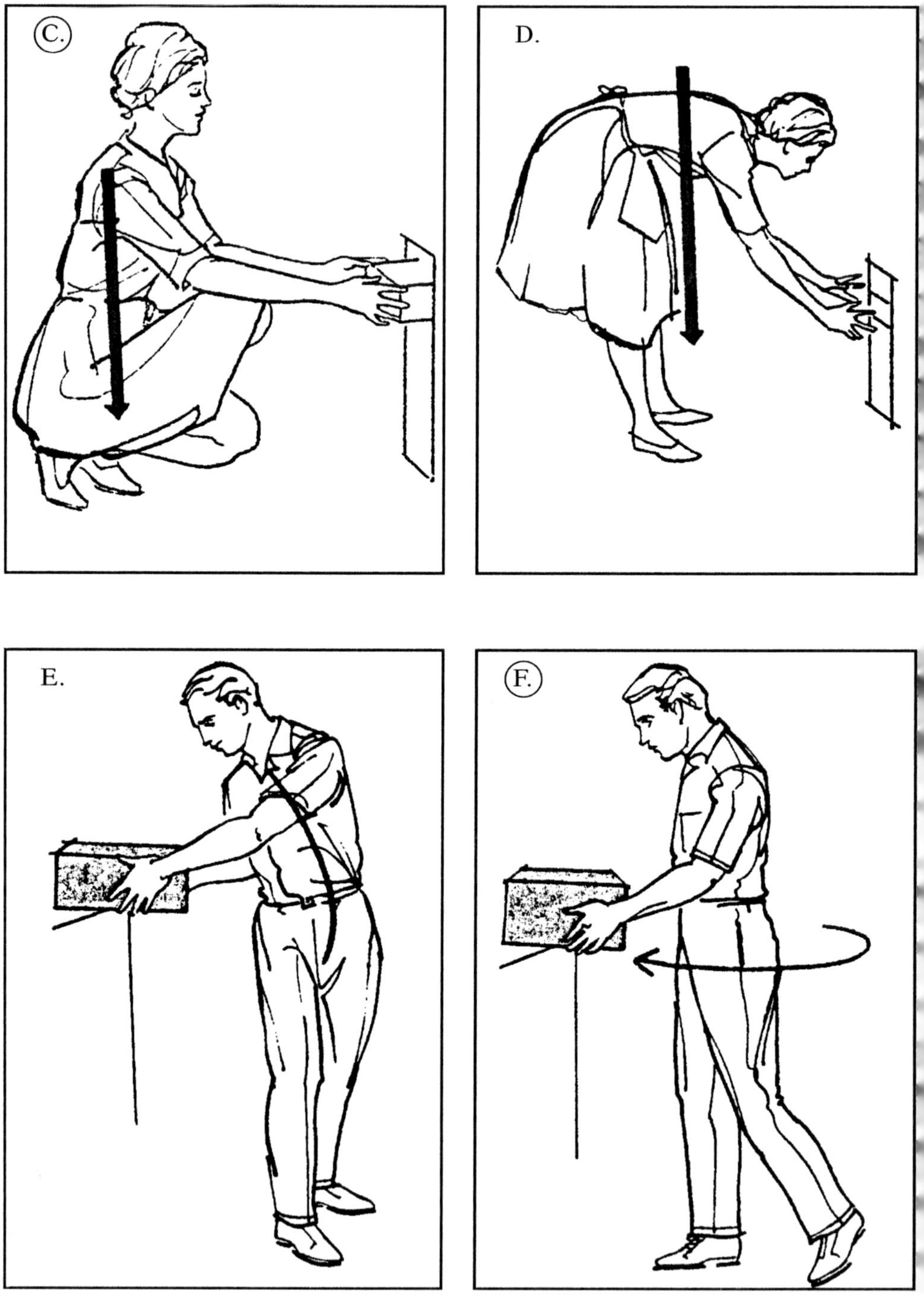

EXERCISE 7-5

Objective: To recognize methods of moving a patient using proper body mechanics.

Directions: Label the pictures in Figure 7-2 with the correct letter from the list that describes the type of moving procedure shown.

List

A. Turning a patient on his side away from you
B. Moving the mattress to the head of the bed with the patient's help
C. Moving a helpless patient to one side of the bed on his back
D. Moving the nonambulatory patient up in bed
E. Turning a patient on his side toward you
F. Moving a patient up in bed with his help

FIGURE 7-2

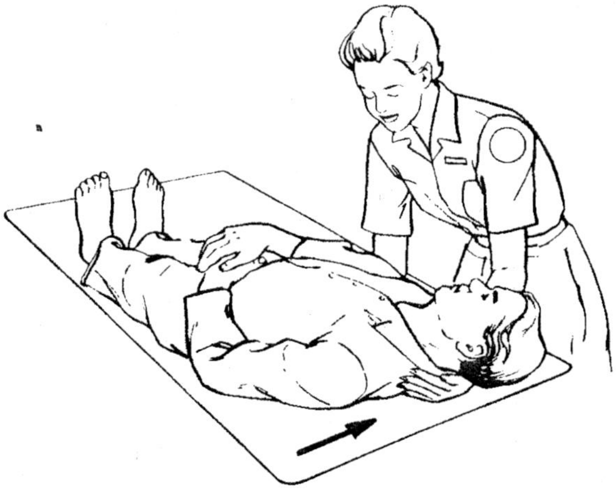

1. C

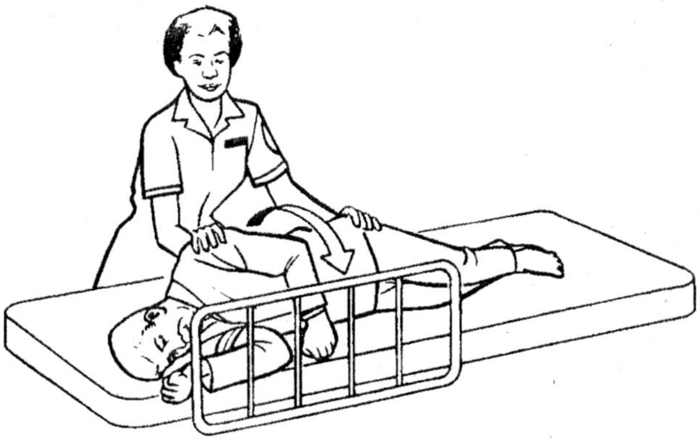

2. A

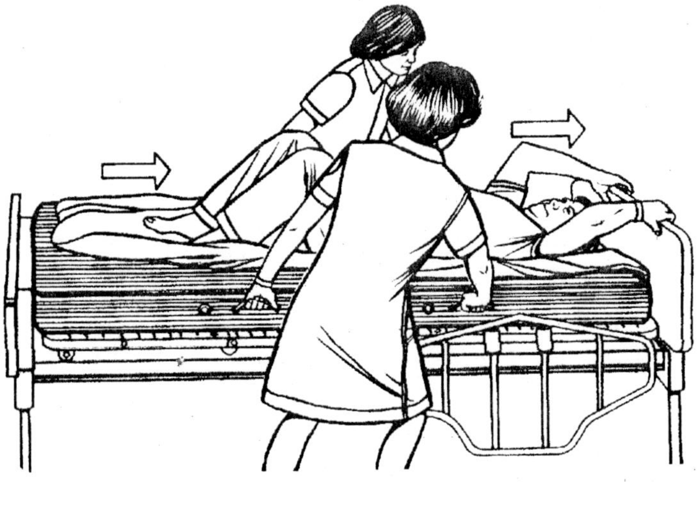

3. B

FIGURE 7-2 (cont.)

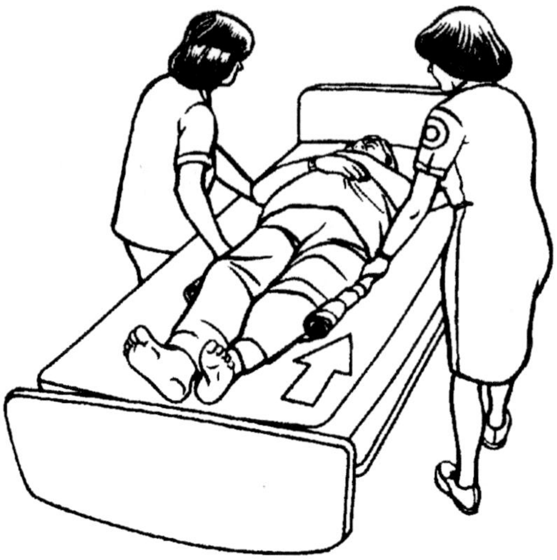

4. ___D___

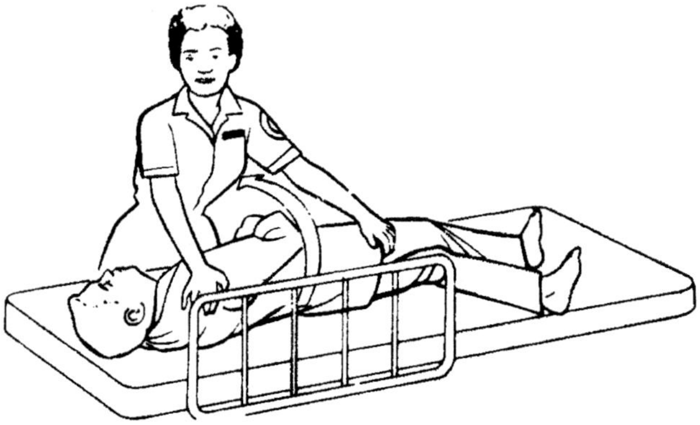

5. ___E___

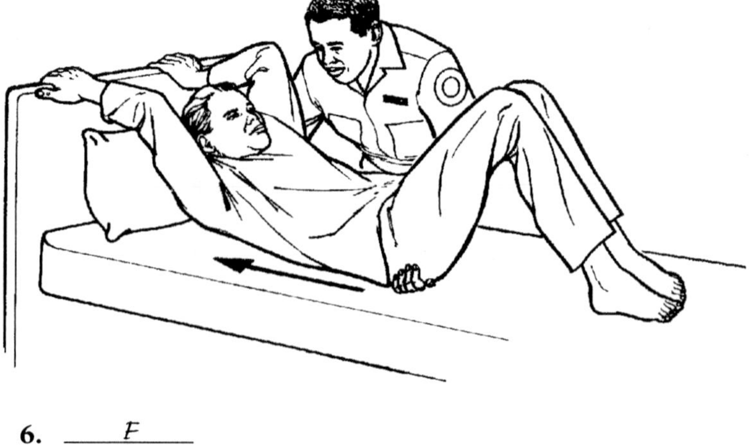

6. ___F___

EXERCISE 7-6

Objective: To recognize the proper methods of draping and positioning the patient.

Directions: Label the pictures in Figure 7-3 with the letter from the list that describes the correct method of draping and positioning the patient.

List

A. Horizontal recumbent position
B. Side-lying (lateral) position
C. Dorsal recumbent position
D. Trendelenburg's position
E. Prone position
F. Reverse Trendelenburg's position
G. Dorsal lithotomy position
H. Fowler's position at 45°
I. Left Sims's position
J. Knee-chest position
K. Left lateral position

FIGURE 7-3

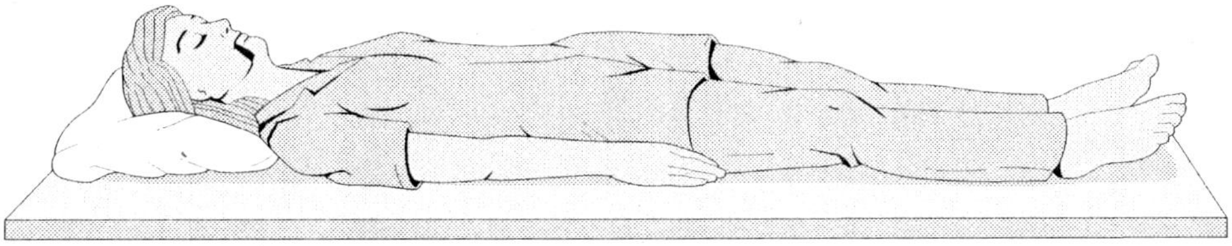

1. ___A___

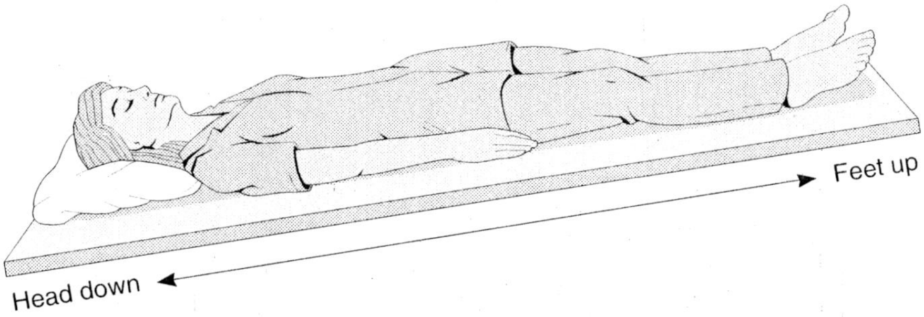

2. ___D___

FIGURE 7-3 (cont.)

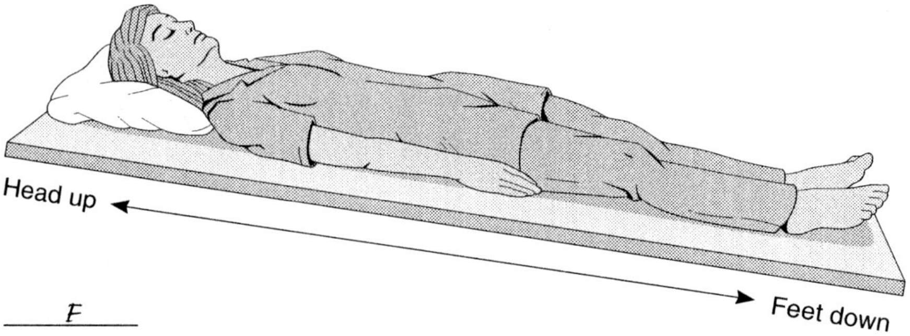

3. ___F___

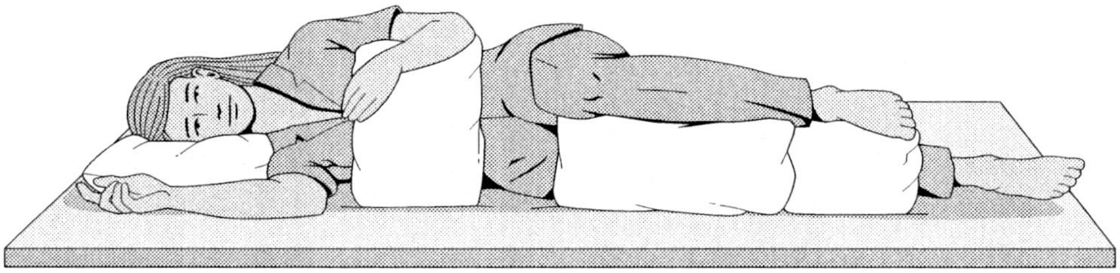

4. ___B___

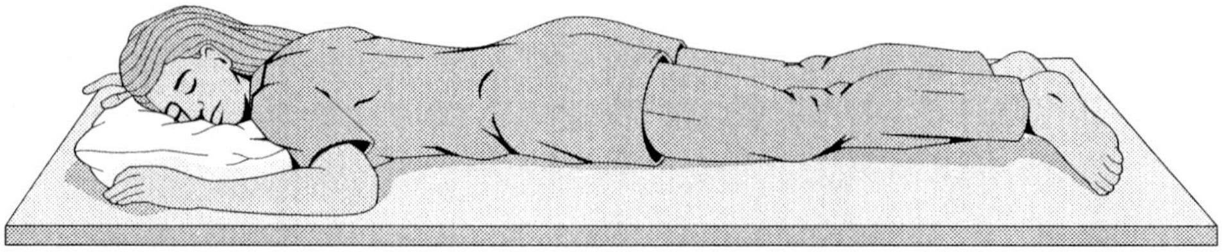

5. ___E___

FIGURE 7-3 (cont.)

6. G

7. C

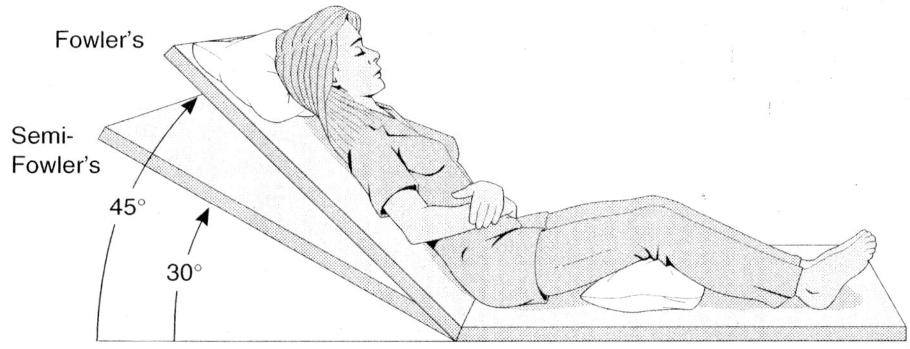

8. H

FIGURE 7-3 (cont.)

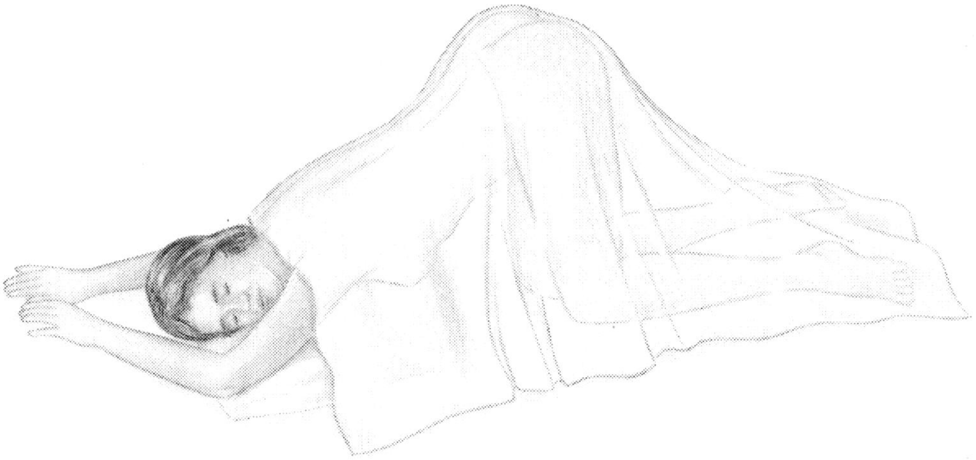

9. J

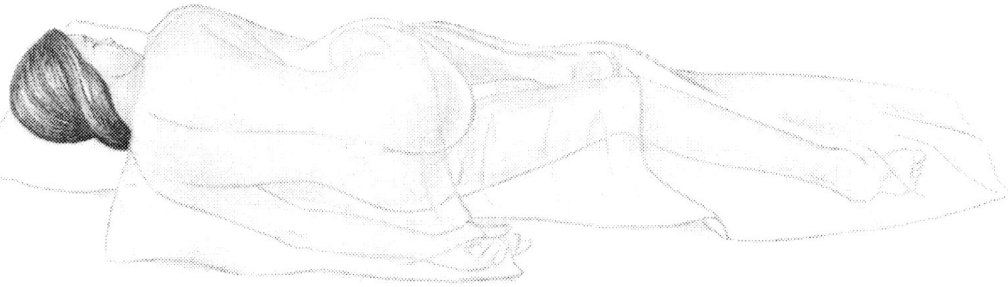

10. I

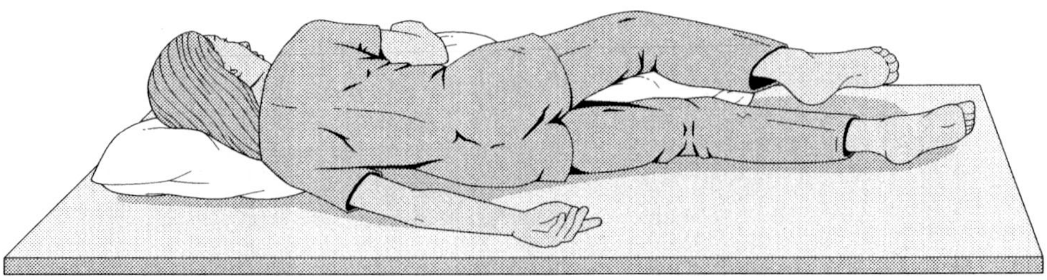

11. K

EXERCISE 7-7

Objective: To apply what you have learned about using good body mechanics to position, move, and transport patients.

Directions: Circle the letter next to the statement that best completes the sentence.

1. The term *body mechanics* refers to
- A. the correct positioning of the patient's body.
- B. the bones and joints.
- (C.) special ways of standing and moving one's body.
- D. artificial arms or legs.
- E. rolling the patient like a log.

2. The purpose of good body mechanics is
- A. to rest comfortably in a hospital bed.
- (B.) to make the best use of your own strength and avoid injury.
- C. to feel good while losing weight.
- D. to avoid friction and irritation to the patient's skin.
- E. to become stronger and more agile.

3. When an action requires physical effort, you should
- A. get close to the load that is being lifted.
- B. use good posture.
- C. try to use as many muscles or groups of muscles as possible.
- D. ask a friend to do it.
- (E.) A, B, and C.

4. When lifting an object, you should
- A. keep your feet slightly more than hip width apart.
- B. avoid twisting your arms.
- C. squat close to the load.
- D. maintain the natural curves in your back.
- (E.) all of the above.

5. When you have to move a heavy object,
- A. it is better to push it than to lift it.
- B. it is better to pull it than to lift it.
- C. it is better to roll it than to carry it.
- D. it is best to get help from another nursing assistant.
- (E.) all of the above.

6. The correct positioning of a patient's body is referred to as
- A. body mechanics.
- (B.) body alignment.
- C. body position.
- D. special patient care treatments.
- E. body arrangement.

EXERCISE 7-8

Objective: To apply what you have learned about lifting and moving patients.

Directions: Fill in the blank spaces with the words from the Word List below.

Word List

friction	position	slide	folded	grip
draw sheet	irritation	roll	bed	under

A pull sheet can help you move the patient in ____bed____ more easily. A regular sheet ____folded____ over many times and placed ____under____ the patient can be used as a pull sheet. The cotton ____draw sheet____ can also be used as a pull sheet. When moving the patient, ____roll____ the pull sheet up tightly on each side next to the patient's body. ____Grip____ the rolled portion to ____slide____ the patient into the desired ____position____. Use of the pull sheet avoids ____friction____ and ____irritation____ to the patient's skin that touches the bedding.

EXERCISE 7-9

Objective: To apply what you have learned about using good body mechanics to position, move, and transport patients.

Directions: Circle the letter next to the statement that best completes the sentence or describes the sentence as true or false. If the sentence is false, draw a line through the incorrect part of the sentence and write the correction on the blank line.

1. When using a gait belt you should position yourself
   A. about 12 inches from the patient.
   B. in front of the patient's stronger side.
   C. in the dorsal recumbent position.
   (D.) slightly behind the weaker side of the patient.
2. A stretcher should be pushed with the patient's ~~head~~ moving first.
   A. True
   (B.) False
   Correct Answer: ____feet____
3. If a patient begins to fall when you are ambulating him,
   A. bend your back and lower yourself to the floor.
   B. quickly drop to the floor to cushion the patient's fall with your body.
   C. bend your knees and flex your arms.
   (D.) bend your knees and lower your body to the floor with the patient.

4. When moving a patient in a wheelchair down a steep ramp, you should ~~push~~ the chair down ~~frontwards~~.
   A. True
   (B.) False
   Correct Answer: take, backwards

5. Which of the following is not a patient position?
   A. Supine
   B. Lateral
   (C.) Foley's
   D. Sims's

6. Many conditions and injuries make it dangerous for a patient to be in certain positions.
   (A.) True
   B. False
   Correct Answer: ______

7. All members of the nursing team are required to know the prescribed position the patient should be in
   (A.) as ordered by the doctor.
   B. as requested by the family.
   C. as preferred by the patient.
   D. within 2 hours of starting their shift.

8. Before moving the patient, all ______ must be placed where it won't be pulled.
   A. visitors
   B. sheets
   (C.) tubing (such as catheters and IVs)
   D. pillows

9. A general rule when moving patients is to
   A. drop the arms and legs over the edge of the stretcher.
   B. pull with a quick, jerky movement.
   C. remove all catheters and other tubing.
   (D.) give the most support to the heaviest parts of the body.

10. Before moving any patient you must
   (A.) always check the identification bracelet.
   B. rest by taking a break.
   C. notify your immediate supervisor.
   D. be fitted for a gait belt.

COMPETENCY CHECKLIST 7-1: BODY MECHANICS

ACTIVITY	S	U	COMMENTS
1. Student will correctly demonstrate the proper method to move and lift patients:			
A. Moving the helpless patient			
B. Moving a patient up in bed with his help			
C. Moving the mattress to the head of the bed with the patient's help			
D. Moving the helpless patient to one side of the bed on his back			
E. Log rolling the patient			
F. Turning a patient onto his side toward you			
G. Turning a patient onto his side away from you			
H. Repositioning a patient in a chair or wheelchair			
I. Moving the nonambulatory patient into a wheelchair or arm chair from the bed			
J. Helping a nonambulatory patient back into bed from a wheelchair or arm chair			
K. Helping a patient who can stand and is ambulatory back into bed from a chair or a wheelchair			
L. Using a portable mechanical patient lift to move the helpless patient			
M. Moving a patient from the bed to a stretcher			
2. Student will demonstrate the correct method of ambulating a patient:			
A. Using a gait belt			
B. Using a cane, walker, or crutches			
C. Walking a patient			
3. Student will demonstrate the correct method of assisting a falling patient.			

8

Admitting, Transferring, and Discharging a Patient

CHAPTER OVERVIEW

Instructor Notes

I. **Admitting the Patient**
   A. Patient Plan of Care
   B. Weighing and Measuring

II. **Transferring the Patient**

III. **Discharging the Patient**
   A. Discharge and Health Teaching
   B. Discharge Planning

Instructor Notes

OBJECTIVES

When the students have completed this chapter, they will be able to:

- Explain their role in following the patient plan of care.
- Admit a patient to the nursing unit by following the correct procedure.
- Weigh and measure a patient.
- Follow the correct procedure to transfer a patient to another room or unit within the institution.
- Describe the components of a discharge and patient health education plan and explain the importance of the plan.
- List the discharge planning activities.
- Discharge a patient from the institution following the correct procedure.
- Help make the patient feel comfortable and secure during all activities.

KEY TERMS

Admission: The administrative process that covers the period from the time the patient enters the institution door to the time the patient is settled

Assessing: Gathering facts to identify needs and problems

Convalescence: The period of recovery after illness or surgery

Discharge: The official procedure for helping patients to leave the health care institution, including teaching them how to care for themselves at home

Evaluating: Determining whether a plan (such as the patient care plan) has been effective

Holistic: An approach that reflects the four dimensions of a "whole" person: physiological, psychological, sociocultural, and spiritual

Implementing: Carrying out or accomplishing a given plan

Patient Plan of Care: A written plan stating the nursing diagnosis, the patient goals or expected outcomes, and the nursing orders, interventions, or actions to be taken

Physiological: Referring to a person's biological response to alterations in the body's structures and functions

Planning: Deciding what to do and how to do it

Psychological: Referring to a person's cognitive and emotional responses to the self and the surrounding environment

Sociocultural: Referring to a person's interpersonal responses to socialization practices in the family and community

Spiritual: Referring to an individual's personal responses to inspirational forces

Transfer: Moving a hospital patient from one room, unit, or facility to another

CORE STUDENT ASSIGNMENTS

Instructor Notes

Students should:

- Read this chapter in their textbook, *Being a Nursing Assistant.*
- Underline any words or sentences they do not understand. Write down any questions they have.
- Complete the Chapter Review in their textbook.
- Read the Time Management Tip for this chapter and think about how they might use this tip in their work.
- Complete the Nursing Assistant in Action exercise.

OPTIONAL STUDENT ASSIGNMENTS

Students should:

- Complete all workbook assignments for this chapter in their copy of *Workbook for Being a Nursing Assistant.*
- Use the CD/CD-Rom disk enclosed with their textbook to hear the pronunciation of the key terms in the chapter.
- Watch the "Body Mechanics" and the "Transfer and Ambulation" videos from the Care Provider Skills series.
- Use the Website address **(www.prenhall.com/wolgin)** to access the free, interactive Companion Website created for this textbook. Get hints, instant feedback, and textbook references to chapter-related multiple-choice questions. Read and react to the Nursing Assistant in Action exercise. Link to other interesting sites.

METHODOLOGY AND SUGGESTED ACTIVITIES

I. Lecture/Discussion

- Answer any questions the students may have.
- Discuss the key terms and related abbreviations. Repeat them out loud and practice using them in sentences.
- Discuss the Time Management Tip for this chapter.
- Discuss the Nursing Assistant in Action exercise.
- Discuss the Critical Thinking points for this chapter.
- Discuss personal safety and protection. Emphasize the importance of following Universal Precautions.
- Discuss the importance of the care plan for the patient because it acts as a communication tool for staff and the patient.
- Invite a home care nurse to speak to the students.
- Discuss the information the nurse will teach the patient before discharge, for example, diabetes education or cardiac care.
- Discuss the feelings the patient may have upon being admitted or discharged. Discuss how this attitude varies with age and techniques the nursing assistant can use to put the patient at ease.

Instructor Notes

II. Role Play/Lab

- Show the videos for this chapter. Have the students practice the lifting techniques and the transfer and ambulation techniques with each other. To promote back safety, emphasize caregiver planning and communication to the patient about what to do prior to any lifting, transferring or ambulating technique.
- Have the students paired into teams to practice admitting, transferring, and discharging a patient. Discuss whose "space" it is—the patient's or the staff's.
- Have the students practice telling the nurse the admission and discharge information.
- Have the students practice moving each other around on stretchers or in wheelchairs.
- Discuss the importance of securing and retrieving patient valuables.

III. Evaluation

- Review the answers to the Chapter Review with students.
- Review the answers to the workbook exercises with students.
- Review the students' understanding of the Time Management Tip.
- To evaluate student comprehension, give a quiz.
- To evaluate student skills, administer the competency checklist.
- Have the students visit the interactive Companion Website and take the quiz.

ANSWERS TO CHAPTER REVIEW

FILL IN THE BLANK

Read each sentence and fill in the blank line with a word that completes the sentence. (Note: Hyphenated words get one line.)

1. The process that covers the time when patients enter the institution until she is settled in is called ___admission___.
2. Do not use an adult's first name without first being given ___permission___.
3. Using a ___mechanical___ lift is often a good idea for patients who cannot stand by themselves.
4. ___Written___ permission is needed from a physician prior to a patient being discharged.
5. The ___holistic___ approach to care includes the physiological, psychological, sociocultural, and spiritual aspects of the patient.

MULTIPLE CHOICE

Instructor Notes

Choose the best answer for each question or statement.

1. Which of the following does not create a favorable first impression for a patient being admitted to a facility
   A. Being greeted warmly
   B. A clean environment
   (C.) Staff wearing dirty shoes
   D. A quiet relaxed environment

2. The patient plan of care serves as a guide for the care a patient will receive and is written by the
   (A.) RN.
   B. MD.
   C. CNA.
   D. RD.

3. The weight of the patient is very important because
   A. it will determine the final cost of care.
   B. it will determine who is treated first.
   (C.) it will be used to determine the dose of some medications.
   D. All of the above.

4. When discharging a patient, do all of the following *except*
   A. wash your hands.
   B. help the patient collect and pack their belongings.
   (C.) have the patient take their dirty bed linen home.
   D. make sure the patient takes home all their written instructions.

5. Which of the following is not a part of discharge instructions?
   A. Explanation of medications the patient will take at home
   B. Follow-up appointments
   C. Activity or diet restrictions
   (D.) How to ignore signs and symptoms of pain

CRITICAL THINKING

CUSTOMER SERVICE

Encourage students to reflect and share their thoughts and experiences. Respect their privacy and confidentiality. Share your own viewpoints with the students.

CULTURAL CARE

Encourage students to reflect and share their thoughts and experiences. Respect their privacy and confidentiality. Share your own viewpoints with the students.

Instructor Notes

COOPERATION WITHIN THE TEAM

Encourage students to reflect and share their thoughts and experiences. Respect their privacy and confidentiality. Share your own viewpoints with the students.

NURSING ASSISTANT IN ACTION

Mr. Jolly has been your patient for the past 4 days. He is now being transferred to a nursing home. He is not looking forward to the move because he feels comfortable with the staff on your unit and is concerned that staff at the new facility will ignore him or be unable to take care of him. He says, "You know I am right!"

What Is Your Response/Action?

Reassure Mr. Jolly that the staff members on the new unit are excellent care givers and that he will get good care there. You may reinforce why he is being transferred—to get the next level of care that he needs. Tell him you have enjoyed caring for him and you know the next staff will too.

8

Answers to Workbook Exercises

The following exercises will assist you to apply what you have read in Chapter 8, "Admitting, Transferring, and Discharging a Patient." For each example, read the objective and use information you have read in Chapter 8 to answer the questions, complete the sentences, or label the diagrams.

EXERCISE 8-1

Objective: To recognize the definitions of words related to admitting, transferring, and discharging a patient.

Directions: Place the letter of the correct definition next to the matching word(s) from the Word List.

Word List

H	**1.** implementing	N	**8.** psychological
I	**2.** transfer	B	**9.** assessing
L	**3.** sociocultural	M	**10.** holistic
J	**4.** physiological	F	**11.** patient plan of care
C	**5.** discharge	E	**12.** planning
G	**6.** admission	A	**13.** evaluating
D	**7.** spiritual	K	**14.** convalescence

Definitions

A. Determining whether a plan (such as the patient care plan) has been effective

B. Gathering facts to identify needs and problems

C. The official procedure for helping patients to leave the health care institution, including teaching them how to care for themselves at home

D. Referring to an individual's personal response to inspirational forces

E. Deciding what to do and how to do it

F. A written plan stating the nursing diagnosis, the patient goals or expected outcomes, and the nursing orders, interventions, or actions to be taken

G. The administrative process that covers the period from the time the patient enters the institution door to the time the patient is settled

H. Carrying out or accomplishing a given plan

I. Moving a hospital patient from one room, unit, or facility to another

J. Referring to a person's biological response to alterations in the body's structures and functions

K. The period of recovery after illness or surgery

L. Referring to a person's interpersonal responses to socialization practices in the family and community

M. An approach that reflects the four dimensions of a "whole" person: physiological, psychological, sociocultural, and spiritual

N. Referring to a person's cognitive and emotional responses to the self and the surrounding environment

EXERCISE 8-2

Objective: To apply what you have learned about admitting, transferring, and discharging a patient.

Directions: Read the following riddles carefully before writing the correct answer on the blank line.

1. All nursing care plans have these to achieve. What are they? *Hint:* In hockey, you keep score by counting these. ____goals____
2. This word describes the nursing care plan. What is it? *Hint:* A carpenter has more than one of these in his box. ____tool____
3. These are used to weigh a patient. What are they? *Hint:* Most fish have these. ____scales____

EXERCISE 8-3

Objective: To apply what you have learned about admitting, transferring, and discharging a patient.

Directions: Circle the letter next to the word or statement that best completes the sentence or describes the sentence as true or false. If the sentence is false, draw a line through the incorrect part of the sentence and write the correction on the blank line.

1. At the time of admission, the nursing assistant is very important to the patient because
   A. the patient may be frightened and uncomfortable.
   B. the patient may be in pain.
   C. the patient may be seriously ill.
   (D.) all of the above.

2. The nursing assistant, by being ________ and ________, will make the patient's admission process easier.
   A. irate, hasty
   B. slow, disorganized
   C. confused, sleepy
   (D.) pleasant, courteous

3. It ~~is not~~ a good idea to introduce yourself to a patient being admitted even if he is in a lot of pain.
   A. True
   (B.) False
   Correct Answer: is

4. The nursing assistant should address the adult patient
   A. with his first name to be informal and friendly.
   B. with his initials only.
   C. as grandma or grandpa to make them feel part of the health care family.
   (D.) As Mr., Miss, or Ms. and the patient's last name.

5. If it is possible, allow the parents to stay with a child during admission to a health care facility.
   (A.) True
   B. False
   Correct Answer: ________________

6. When admitting a patient, you should keep in mind
   A. the reason for her admission.
   B. the remaining work to be done with other patients.
   C. the tasks the nurse has asked you to do for this patient.
   (D.) A and C.

7. The nursing assistant is a representative of the institution.
   (A.) True
   B. False
   Correct Answer: ________________

8. An important tool for 24-hour communication for the health care team is the
   A. care strategy log.
   B. physician's log.
   (C.) nursing care plan.
   D. Internet.

9. The nursing care plan helps the team deliver
   A. the mail.
   (B.) continuous and consistent care.
   C. floral bouquets.
   D. uncoordinated care.

10. The registered nurse ________ the care plan on admission.
   A. finishes
   (B.) begins
   C. rejects
   D. approves

11. The registered nurse will identify patient problems and nursing diagnoses.
   (A.) True
   B. False
   Correct Answer: ________________________________

12. The registered nurse reevaluates the plan of care each day to reflect
   A. the sun.
   B. the changing needs of the team.
   C. the staffing limits.
   (D.) the changing needs of the patient.

13. It is important that the nursing assistant review the plan of care each day to
   A. see what information on the plan has changed.
   B. make suggestions, as a way to contribute to the plan.
   C. identify goals the patient is achieving.
   (D.) all of the above.

14. The plan of care will influence how the nursing assistant
   A. organizes his work.
   B. plans his work.
   C. observes and reports the patient's activities.
   (D.) all of the above.

15. The nursing assistant is responsible for
   A. gathering data objectively.
   B. reporting data in a timely manner.
   C. documenting the care given to the patient.
   (D.) all of the above.

16. The patient must be identified by ________ before preparing to transfer him.
   A. asking the family or visitors who he is
   B. asking him if he is the one to be transferred
   (C.) checking the identification bracelet
   D. calling the doctor

17. The nursing assistant should be aware that some patients will be ________ that they must be transferred to another facility or even to another unit.

A. alarmed
B. angry
C. anxious
(D.) all of the above

18. The nursing assistant can give the patient emotional support after transferring him by

A. reassuring him that his family will find him eventually.
B. telling him he shouldn't worry so much because he could be moved again tomorrow.
C. telling him about other patients you have transferred today.
(D.) reassuring him that his family and visitors will be given the new room number.

19. A common way to transfer the patient is

A. on a wheelchair scale.
B. on a draw sheet.
(C.) on a stretcher or in a wheelchair.
D. all of the above.

20. After the transfer, the immediate supervisor will want to know all of the following *except*

A. the time of the transfer.
B. the patient's reaction to the transfer.
(C.) the number of patients discharged that day.
D. observations of anything unusual.

21. If the patient is discharged to another health care facility,

(A.) the patient may require a caregiver or nurse to accompany her.
B. the nursing assistant will not be involved in this kind of transfer.
C. an ambulance is never used.
D. there will be no special instructions from the nurse.

22. Today, patients tend to have ~~shorter~~ convalescent periods at home than in the past.

A. True
(B.) False

Correct Answer: longer

23. Teaching patients how to care for themselves at home is the responsibility of

A. the nursing assistant only.
B. the nurse only.
(C.) the entire nursing team.
D. the person who chooses to take on that responsibility.

24. The patient's family must be included in the discharge education process because

A. it's nice to be included.
(B.) the family may be the primary caregivers at home.
C. they want to be included.
D. they are paying the bill.

25. The best approach to discharge teaching is the

A. partial approach.
B. complete approach.
(C.) holistic approach.
D. discharge approach.

26. The discharge instructions will include

A. detailed housekeeping instructions.
B. detailed travel arrangements.
(C.) details on diet, activity, and medications.
D. information on how to discharge a patient.

27. Explanation of care in the home environment will include information on

A. available transportation and elimination of hazards in the home.
B. available housekeeping services.
C. economic support agencies.
(D.) all of the above.

28. The nursing assistant should ask the patient if he has the written discharge information before wheeling him off the floor.

(A.) True
B. False
Correct Answer: ______________________________

29. It is the nursing assistant's responsibility to read and understand the institution's policies and procedures for __________ of the patient.

A. admission
B. discharge
C. transfer
(D.) all of the above

30. By following the plan of care, the nursing assistant will contribute to the nursing team's goal for quality patient care.

(A.) True
B. False
Correct Answer: ______________________________

COMPETENCY CHECKLIST 8-1: ADMITTING, TRANSFERRING, AND DISCHARGING A PATIENT

ACTIVITY	S	U	COMMENTS
1. The student will demonstrate the correct method for:			
A. Admitting a patient			
B. Weighing and measuring the height of a patient			
C. Transferring a patient			
D. Discharging a patient			

The Patient's Room

9

CHAPTER OVERVIEW

Instructor Notes

I. The Patient's Unit
- A. Equipment
  - 1. Disposable Equipment

II. Creating a Safe and Comfortable Patient Room

III. Caring for a Patient in a Home Setting
- A. Safety
- B. Fire Safety and Burn Prevention
- C. Reporting an Accident or Emergency by Telephone

Instructor Notes

OBJECTIVES

When the students have completed this chapter, they will be able to:

- Describe the typical patient's unit and list the equipment it contains.
- Check the unit for convenience to the patient, organization, and safety.
- Describe the purpose of each piece of equipment.
- Create an appropriate environment in the home in which to provide care for the patient.
- Provide a safe environment for the patient by eliminating safety hazards and anticipating safety needs.
- Describe how to contact emergency assistance.

KEY TERMS

Alternating-Pressure Mattress: A pad similar to an air mattress that can be placed beneath the patient to reduce pressure on the head, shoulders, back, heels, elbows, and bony prominences

Bed Cradle: A frame shaped like a barrel cut in half lengthwise used to keep bed linens off a part of the patient's body

Bedpan: A pan used by patients who must defecate or urinate while in bed

Disposable Equipment: Equipment that is used one time only or for one patient only and then thrown away

Emesis Basin: A pan used for catching material that a patient spits out, vomits, or expectorates

Equipment: Materials, tools, devices, supplies, furnishings, and necessary things used to perform a task

Flammable: Capable of burning quickly and easily

Intravenous Pole: A tall pole, also called IV pole, that attaches to a bed or is on rollers or casters; this pole is used to hold the containers or tubes needed, for example, during a blood transfusion

Lamb's Wool: A wide strip of lamb's hide with the fleece attached or an imitation material used to increase patient comfort

Patient Lift: A mechanical device with a sling seat used for lifting a patient into and out of such equipment as the hospital bed, bathtub, or wheelchair

Patient Unit: The space for one patient, including the hospital bed, bedside table, chair, and other equipment

Specialty Bed: A bed that constantly changes pressure under the patient. Used to minimize pressure points in the treatment or prevention of pressure ulcers

Stretcher: A narrow rolling table with or without a mattress or simply a canvas stretched over a frame used to transport patients; the latter may also be called a litter, gurney, or cart

Urinal: A portable container given to male patients in bed so they can urinate without getting out of bed

Instructor Notes

Walker: A stable frame made of metal tubing used to support the unsteady patient while walking; the patient holds the walker while taking a step, moves it forward, and takes another step

Wheelchair: A chair on wheels used to transport patients

CORE STUDENT ASSIGNMENTS

Students should:

- Read this chapter in their textbook, *Being a Nursing Assistant.*
- Underline any words or sentences they do not understand. Write down any questions they have.
- Complete the Chapter Review in their textbook.
- Read the Time Management Tip for this chapter and think about how they might use this tip in their work.
- Complete the Nursing Assistant in Action exercise.

OPTIONAL STUDENT ASSIGNMENTS

Students should:

- Complete all workbook assignments for this chapter in their copy of *Workbook for Being a Nursing Assistant.*
- Use the CD/CD-Rom disk enclosed with their textbook to hear the pronunciation of the key terms in the chapter.
- Watch the "Patient's Rights" video from the Care Provider Skills series.
- Use the Website address **(www.prenhall.com/wolgin)** to access the free, interactive Companion Website created for this textbook. Get hints, instant feedback, and textbook references to chapter-related multiple-choice questions. Read and react to the Nursing Assistant in Action exercise. Link to other interesting sites.

METHODOLOGY AND SUGGESTED ACTIVITIES

I. Lecture/Discussion

- Answer any questions the students may have.
- Discuss the key terms and related abbreviations. Repeat them out loud and practice using them in sentences.
- Discuss the Time Management Tip for this chapter.
- Discuss the Nursing Assistant in Action exercise.
- Discuss the Critical Thinking points for this chapter.
- Discuss personal safety and protection. Emphasize the importance of following Universal Precautions. Stress the need to wear protective equipment.
- Students can make a checklist of everything that belongs in the unit.
- Visit a pediatric unit or arrange to talk with a home care nurse.
- Discuss similarities and differences between caring for a patient in a health care facility versus at the patient's home.

Instructor Notes

- Discuss what makes each of the students feel comfortable when ill.
- Discuss cultural differences in perceptions of illness and pain.
- Discuss how to make an emergency call in the student's institution.

II. Role Play/Lab

- Show the video for this chapter. Have the students try and name all of the patient rights. Discuss how it would feel to be in a place that did not honor these rights. Have the students role play interactions that incorporate honoring patient rights, such as admitting a patient.
- Display many pieces of equipment. (Include both disposable equipment and nondisposable equipment.) Put labels in a box. Have each student pick a label and attach it to the proper piece of equipment. Also, ask the student to demonstrate and/or explain the proper use of the equipment.
- Have the students match the names and descriptions of various pieces of equipment.
- Play a word game. The leader says, "I'm thinking of a . . . " and reads the description from the text. The other students guess the name.
- Play a game where the student names a piece of equipment and states how it could help a patient and then how it could hurt a patient if used incorrectly.

III. Evaluation

- Review the answers to the Chapter Review with students.
- Review the answers to the workbook exercises with students.
- Review the students' understanding of the Time Management Tip.
- To evaluate student comprehension, give a quiz.
- To evaluate student skills, administer the competency checklist.
- Have the students visit the interactive Companion Website and take the quiz.

ANSWERS TO CHAPTER REVIEW

FILL IN THE BLANK

Read each sentence and fill in the blank line with a word that completes the sentence. (Note: Hyphenated words get one line.)

1. An ___*alternating*___ ___*pressure*___ mattress is a device placed beneath a bedridden patient to decrease the risk for pressure ulcers.

2. Equipment that is used for one patient only is called ___*disposable*___ equipment.

3. A(n) ___*bed*___ ___*cradle*___ is a frame-shaped device used to keep linens off the bed.

4. Lamb's wool is a piece of material used to increase the patient's ___*comfort*___.

Instructor Notes

5. When working in the home, you must respect the patient's beliefs and attitudes even if they are ___different___ from yours.

MULTIPLE CHOICE

Choose the best answer for each question or statement.

1. The unit should be arranged for the convenience of the
(A.) patient.
B. staff.
C. family.
D. physician.

2. All of the following are pieces of patient equipment *except*
A. binders.
B. foot board.
C. walkers.
(D.) covers.

3. All of the following are examples of a piece of disposable equipment *except*
A. cups.
(B.) foot board.
C. bedpan.
D. tissues.

4. To create a comfortable room setting for the patient, do all of the following *except*
A. put the TV on a channel the patient likes.
B. keep the lights and heat at a level comfortable for the patient.
(C.) keep the side rails up at all times.
D. provide privacy for the patient.

5. Provide a safe environment for your patient by
A. removing loose rugs that slip.
B. keeping hallways uncluttered.
C. cleaning up spills.
(D.) All of the above.

CRITICAL THINKING

CUSTOMER SERVICE

Encourage students to reflect and share their thoughts and experiences. Respect their privacy and confidentiality. Share your own viewpoints with the students.

Instructor Notes

CULTURAL CARE

Encourage students to reflect and share their thoughts and experiences. Respect their privacy and confidentiality. Share your own viewpoints with the students.

COOPERATION WITHIN THE TEAM

Encourage students to reflect and share their thoughts and experiences. Respect their privacy and confidentiality. Share your own viewpoints with the students.

NURSING ASSISTANT IN ACTION

Mrs. Estes has been admitted for asthma and she has many allergies. She tells you the pillow on her bed needs to go because it is bothering her. You are not sure if there is any other type of pillow available for her to use. She tells you to take the pillow out of her room, but you are ordered to have her head elevated.

What Is Your Response/Action?

Tell Mrs. Estes that you wish to make her as comfortable as possible and keep her head elevated so that she can heal safely. You could consider offering a blanket or towel for a pillow or raising the head of the bed without a pillow. Check with the nurse to be sure the bed elevation requirement is being met. Also, inform the nurse of the dilemma. She may be able to check Mrs. Estes's pain level and/or offer her some other pain relief measure.

Answers to Workbook Exercises

9

The following exercises will assist you to apply what you have read in Chapter 9, "The Patient's Room." For each example, read the objective and use information you have read in Chapter 9 to answer the questions, complete the sentences, or label the diagrams.

EXERCISE 9-1

Objective: To recognize the definitions of words related to the patient's environment.

Directions: Place the letter of the correct definition next to the matching word(s) from the word list.

Word List

D **1.** alternating-pressure mattress

N **2.** lamb's wool

G **3.** equipment

H **4.** bedpan

L **5.** stretcher

K **6.** walker

M **7.** patient lift

A **8.** flammable

E **9.** patient unit

O **10.** specialty bed

C **11.** wheelchair

B **12.** bed cradle

I **13.** urinal

P **14.** emesis basin

J **15.** disposable equipment

F **16.** intravenous pole

R **17.** foot board

S **18.** bed board

Q **19.** binders

Definitions

A. Capable of burning quickly and easily

B. A frame shaped like a barrel cut in half lengthwise and used to keep bed linens off a part of the patient's body

C. A chair on wheels used to transport patients

D. A pad similar to an air mattress that can be placed beneath the patient to reduce pressure on the head, shoulders, back, heels, elbows, and bony prominences

E. The space for one patient, including the hospital bed, bedside table, chair, and other equipment

F. A tall pole, also called an IV pole, that attaches to a bed or is on rollers or casters; this pole is used to hold the containers or tubes needed, for example, during a blood transfusion

G. Materials, tools, devices, supplies, furnishings, and necessary things used to perform a task

H. A pan used by patients who must defecate or urinate while in bed

I. A portable container given to male patients in bed so they can urinate without getting out of bed

J. Equipment that is used one time only or for one patient only and then thrown away

K. A stable frame made of metal tubing used to support the unsteady patient while walking; the patient holds it while taking a step, moves it forward, and takes another step

L. A narrow rolling table with or without a mattress, or simply a canvas stretched over a frame, used to transport patients; the latter may also be called a litter or a gurney

M. A mechanical device with a sling seat used for lifting a patient into and out of such equipment as the hospital bed, bathtub, or wheelchair

N. A wide strip of lamb's hide with the fleece attached, or an imitation material, used to increase patient comfort

O. A bed that constantly changes pressure under the patient; used to minimize pressure points in the treatment or prevention of pressure ulcers

P. A pan used for catching material that a patient spits out, vomits, or expectorates

Q. Strips of heavy cotton cloth with Velcro fasteners; these are wrapped securely around the patient's body over the abdomen to give support and comfort following abdominal surgery

R. A small board placed upright at the foot of the bed and used to keep the patient's feet aligned properly to prevent foot drop

S. A large board placed beneath the mattress to provide additional support for patients with back, muscle, or bone problems

EXERCISE 9-2

Objective: To recognize important actions to take in accident prevention and reporting.

Directions: The five categories listed below (HFS, HSH, CFH, RET, BP) are about accident prevention and reporting. For each of the specific safety items listed below, select an appropriate category. You may select more than one category for each item.

HFS = home fire safety
HSH = home safety hazards
CFH = calling for help
RET = reporting an emergency by telephone
BP = burn prevention

Possible answers include:

HFS, BP, CFH, RET **1.** If a fire occurs, get the patient out of the area.

RET, HFS, CFH **2.** The fire department emergency number is kept near the telephone.

HSH, HFS **3.** Cluttered hallways and walkways

HSH **4.** Loose rugs that slip or do not have a nonskid backing

HFS, BP, HSH **5.** Avoid using flammable liquids.

BP, HSH **6.** Check the temperature of water before using it on the patient.

HSH, CFH, RET **7.** Wet floor

RET **8.** Have handy the telephone number of the poison control center.

CFH, RET **9.** Give the name of the patient and identify your location, room number, or address.

HSH **10.** Dimly lit hallways and walkways

CFH, RET **11.** Give your name first when you call.

HFS, BP, HSH **12.** Keep matches away from children and confused adults.

HSH **13.** Sharp objects such as knives, razors, and hypodermic needles

HSH **14.** Poisons (such as cleaning solutions)

CFH, RET **15.** Clearly state the problem: Objectively state exactly what has happened or what help you need.

HSH, HFS **16.** Faulty or uneven stairs or loose debris on stairs

RET, CFH **17.** Have the number of your home care supervisor near the telephone.

EXERCISE 9-3

Objective: To apply what you have learned about the patient's environment.

Directions: Circle the letter next to the word or statement that best completes the sentence or describes the sentence as true or false. If the sentence is false, draw a line through the incorrect part of the sentence and write the correction on the blank line.

1. ~~Disposable~~ equipment requires washing and disinfecting.
   A. True
   (B.) False
   Correct Answer: *Reusable*
2. When the nursing assistant is unfamiliar with the equipment used, he must ask for assistance from the nurse or
   A. must ask the patient how others have used it.
   B. make a wild guess and try to figure it out by himself.
   C. quickly try to get the equipment to work.
   (D.) review instructions prior to working with the item.
3. Disposable equipment ~~may~~ be reused by other patients it is washed in hot soapy water.
   A. True
   (B.) False
   Correct Answer: *must not, even if*
4. When working in a patient's home do all of the following *except*
   A. do not disturb the patient's personal things.
   B. be respectful of differences in food, cleanliness, or lifestyle.
   (C.) perform heavy labor like window washing.
   D. suggest moving items that are a safety risk.
5. A primary goal is to make the patient feel
   A. comfortable in the hallway.
   (B.) comfortable in her environment.
   C. more important than other patients.
   D. busy and occupied after surgery.
6. An emergency phone list should include the police and fire departments, the patient's physician and the responsible family member.
   (A.) True
   B. False
   Correct Answer: ____________________
7. If the patient has belongings from home, the nursing assistant
   (A.) should demonstrate respect for the articles.
   B. should borrow the articles if needed.
   C. should rearrange them to suit his own preferences.
   D. should instruct the family to take them back home.

8. The nursing assistant should create a
(A.) safe environment for his patients.
B. complex and busy environment for the patient.
C. list of environmental rules for the patient and family to follow.
D. risky environment to keep the patient alert to danger.

9. The unit should be arranged
A. for the comfort of the nursing assistant.
(B.) for the convenience of the patient.
C. by the immediate supervisor only.
D. in a complex and mazelike pattern.

10. A key word to remember when rearranging furniture is
(A.) anticipation.
B. drudgery.
C. speed.
D. obstacle course.

11. If the patient is right handed, place the call light near
A. the doorway.
B. the left ear.
C. the telephone.
(D.) the right hand.

12. A unit designed for a child is ~~the same~~ as for an adult.
A. True
(B.) False
Correct Answer: *not the same*

13. The two most important factors that will determine how a pediatric unit is arranged and the equipment that will be needed are
A. the age of the child and the parents.
B. the diagnosis only.
C. the age of the nursing assistant.
(D.) the age of the child and the reason for hospitalization.

14. If there is more than one unit in a room, draw curtains can be used for privacy.
(A.) True
B. False
Correct Answer: ____________________

Bedmaking

10

CHAPTER OVERVIEW

Instructor Notes

I. Bedmaking

II. Four Basic Beds

A. Closed Bed
B. Open, Fan-folded, or Empty Bed
C. Postoperative or Surgical Bed
D. Occupied Bed

Instructor Notes

OBJECTIVES

When the students have completed this chapter, they will be able to:

- Explain the reason for making the patient's bed with great care.
- Identify and describe the four basic methods of making a bed.
- List the guidelines to follow for bedmaking.
- Make the closed bed.
- Make the open, fan-folded bed.
- Make the postoperative bed (surgical, OR [operating room], stretcher, and recovery room bed).
- Make the occupied bed.

KEY TERMS

Closed Bed: Bed made with bedspread in place

Decubitus Ulcers: Tissue breakdown resulting from pressure or reduced blood flow (often called pressure sores or bed sores)

Draw Sheet: Small sheet made of plastic, rubber, or cotton placed across the middle of the bed to cover and protect the bottom sheet and assist in moving the patient

Fan-fold: Method of arranging bed linens so that the covers and bedspread are folded at the foot of the bed out of the way

Occupied Bed: One with a patient in it

Open Bed: Bed made with top sheet folded so as to give patient easy entrance

Postoperative Bed: Bed made with top sheet folded lengthwise and positioned to one side, allowing transfer of the patient from the surgical stretcher to the bed without unnecessary movement

CORE STUDENT ASSIGNMENTS

Students should:

- Read this chapter in their textbook, *Being a Nursing Assistant.*
- Underline any words or sentences they do not understand. Write down any questions they have.
- Complete the Chapter Review in their textbook.
- Read the Time Management Tip for this chapter and think about how they might use this tip in their work.
- Complete the Nursing Assistant in Action exercise.

OPTIONAL STUDENT ASSIGNMENTS

Students should:

- Complete all workbook assignments for this chapter in their copy of *Workbook for Being a Nursing Assistant.*
- Use the CD/CD-Rom disk enclosed with their textbook to hear the pronunciation of the key terms in the chapter.

- Watch the "Infection Control" video from the Care Provider Skills series.
- Use the Website address **(www.prenhall.com/wolgin)** to access the free, interactive Companion Website created for this textbook. Get hints, instant feedback, and textbook references to chapter-related multiple-choice questions. Read and react to the Nursing Assistant in Action exercise. Link to other interesting sites.

Instructor Notes

METHODOLOGY AND SUGGESTED ACTIVITIES

I. Lecture/Discussion

- Answer any questions the students may have.
- Discuss the key terms and related abbreviations. Repeat them out loud and practice using them in sentences.
- Discuss the Time Management Tip for this chapter.
- Discuss the Nursing Assistant in Action exercise.
- Discuss the Critical Thinking points for this chapter.
- Discuss personal safety and protection. Emphasize the importance of following Universal Precautions. Stress the need to wear protective equipment.
- Stress any institution-specific guidelines to follow.
- Review body mechanics and ergonomic tips for use with bedmaking.

II. Role Play/Lab

- Show the video for this chapter. Discuss ways that making and changing beds can spread or contain germs. Demonstrate how to keep the linen off of the caregiver's uniform while changing beds.
- Demonstrate and provide ample opportunity for the students to practice these procedures.
- If you use a volunteer student as a patient, remember that they cannot see what you are doing and may need additional instruction later.
- Assign the students to teams to practice the bedmaking procedures. One will read and/or observe while the other performs the skills. Then they trade places.
- As they practice, the student (patient) should become aware of the need for side rails. Discuss when the use of side rails is appropriate.
- Some students enjoy competition. If your students do, allow them to have bedmaking contests. Consider their time and performance.
- Reinforce body mechanics, infection control, and customer service perspectives with bedmaking.

III. Evaluation

- Review the answers to the Chapter Review with students.
- Review the answers to the workbook exercises with students.
- Review the students' understanding of the Time Management Tip.
- To evaluate student comprehension, give a quiz.
- To evaluate student skills, administer the competency checklist.
- Have the students visit the interactive Companion Website and take the quiz.

Instructor Notes

ANSWERS TO CHAPTER REVIEW

FILL IN THE BLANK

Read each sentence and fill in the blank line(s) with the word or words that complete the sentence. (Note: Hyphenated words get one line.)

1. Tissue breakdown resulting from pressure or reduced blood flow is called a *decubitus* *ulcer*.
2. A *closed* bed is one that is made with the bedspread in place.
3. An *occupied* bed is one made with the patient in it.
4. *plastic* should never touch a patient's skin.
5. By *fan-folding* a bed, you make it easy for the patient to get in and out.

MULTIPLE CHOICE

Choose the best answer for each question or statement.

1. Bedmaking is important because
   A. it increases the patient's comfort.
   B. getting the wrinkles out is good for the skin.
   C. many patients spend a great deal of time in their beds.
   (D.) All of the above.
2. Never shake the linen when changing the bed in order to
   (A.) prevent the spread of germs.
   B. avoid knocking things over.
   C. save time.
   D. prevent distracting the patient.
3. When making a patient's bed, you should do all of the following *except*
   A. do not let dirty linen touch your uniform.
   B. avoid taking extra linen in the room.
   (C.) use pins to fix ripped linen.
   D. fold linen in on itself when removing it.
4. The use of a draw sheet is helpful
   A. to cover and protect the patient's bed.
   B. to move a patient in bed.
   C. to increase patient's comfort during moves.
   (D.) All of the above.
5. Use the open, empty, or fan-folded type of bed when
   (A.) the patient can get out of bed.
   B. the patient is confined to bed.
   C. the patient is going to surgery.
   D. None of the above.

CRITICAL THINKING

Instructor Notes

CUSTOMER SERVICE

Encourage students to reflect and share their thoughts and experiences. Respect their privacy and confidentiality. Share your own viewpoints with the students.

CULTURAL CARE

Encourage students to reflect and share their thoughts and experiences. Respect their privacy and confidentiality. Share your own viewpoints with the students.

COOPERATION WITHIN THE TEAM

Encourage students to reflect and share their thoughts and experiences. Respect their privacy and confidentiality. Share your own viewpoints with the students.

NURSING ASSISTANT IN ACTION

Mr. Jacobs is an elderly man whose bed sheets require frequent changes. You have already changed his bed once on your shift when you notice he has soiled his sheets again. You are already late to leave for your scheduled lunch break. It crosses your mind that you could pretend you did not notice and leave his room.

What Is Your Response/Action?

You have several options to consider. It is not ethically a good idea to leave Mr. Jacobs without assistance. You could change the bed for Mr. Jacobs yourself, but be sure not to display any signs of frustration or inconvenience to him. You could also ask for assistance with the bed change from a coworker or ask the coworker to assist Mr. Jacobs. Be sure to return the favor later. Finally, it would be a good idea to report the frequent soiling of the bed to the nurse who could check into any underlying medical problems or solutions.

Instructor Notes

Answers to Workbook Exercises

10

The following exercises will assist you to apply what you have read in Chapter 10, "Bedmaking." For each exercise, read the objective and use information you have read in Chapter 10 to answer the questions, complete the sentences, or label the diagrams.

EXERCISE 10-1

Objective: To apply what you have learned about the different methods of bedmaking.

Directions: Choose terms from the Word List to label the four methods of bedmaking in Figure 10-1. Then, next to each Practice Description, write the number of the correct method of bedmaking you would use.

Word List

occupied postoperative open closed

FIGURE 10-1

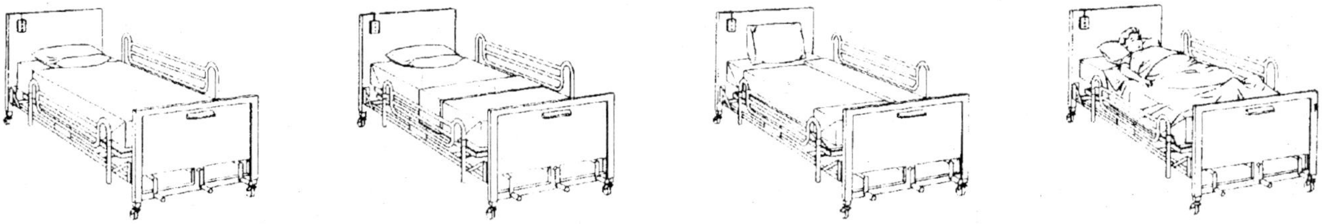

1. *Closed*
2. *open*
3. *postperative*
4. *occupied*

Practice Description

3 **1.** Mrs. O'Shea will be returning from surgery in the next 2 hours.

4 **2.** You have finished giving Mr. Garcia a complete bath. He has had a stroke and is too weak to get out of bed.

2 **3.** Mrs. Chang is being ambulated in the hallway, so you decide to make her bed now.

1 **4.** Your patient has been discharged, the room and bed have been cleaned, and your immediate supervisor asks you to make the bed.

EXERCISE 10-2

Objective: To be able to correctly recall bedmaking guidelines.

Directions: Circle the letter next to the statement that best completes the sentence.

1. By fan-folding the top of the bed, you make it easier for the patient to
   A. roll out of bed in the morning.
   B. bathe himself.
   C. make his own bed.
   (D.) get back into the bed.

2. Shaking the bed linen
   A. can be done safely in the hallway.
   B. should not be done because it disturbs the doctors.
   C. should be done daily.
   (D.) spreads germs and should not be done.

3. When a cotton draw sheet is not available,
   A. you do not need to use one.
   B. reuse the one that was taken off earlier.
   C. use a large sheet that has been folded in half lengthwise. Avoid wrinkles.
   (D.) use a large sheet that has been folded in half widthwise. Avoid wrinkles.

4. Torn or damaged linen should
   A. be disposed of in red bags.
   B. be used to make the bed.
   C. be torn into strips and used for cleaning.
   (D.) be sent for repair according to the policy of your institution.

5. Wrinkles in the sheet indent the skin and
   A. promote good circulation by stimulating the skin.
   (B.) may be avoided by pulling the sheet tightly to smoothe it.
   C. can be removed by the patient lying on it for 2 hours.
   D. will not occur if it is made of cotton fabric.

6. You can save time and energy when making a bed if you
A. get someone else to do it.
B. stand either at the head or at the foot of the bed.
C. make one side of the bed and then quickly crawl across to the other side.
(D.) use good body mechanics to make as much of the bed as possible on one side before going to the other side.

7. The ________ side of a bed protector should never touch a patient's skin.
A. cotton
B. wet
(C.) plastic
D. white

8. A rubber or plastic bed protector can be used if it
A. is clean.
B. is covered by a cotton sheet.
C. is dry.
(D.) all of the above.

9. Wrinkles in the sheets can
A. make the patients sleep soundly.
(B.) cause skin breakdown, leading to decubitus ulcers.
C. be ignored.
D. be removed by shaking them vigorously.

10. Taking extra linen into a patient's unit
A. is a good idea because if it is not used it can be put back on the linen cart and used later for someone else.
(B.) is a wasteful practice.
C. makes the patient feel cared for.
D. is convenient because you will have extra linen if you need it.

COMPETENCY CHECKLIST 10-1: BEDMAKING SKILLS

ACTIVITY	S	U	COMMENTS
1. Student correctly demonstrates the open method of bedmaking.			
2. Student correctly demonstrates the closed method of bedmaking.			
3. Student correctly demonstrates the postoperative method of bedmaking.			
4. Student correctly demonstrates the occupied method of bedmaking.			

Home Health Care

11

CHAPTER OVERVIEW

Instructor Notes

I. **Working in the Home Health Care Field**
   - A. Home Health Care Agencies and Other Employees
   - B. The Home Health Aide

II. **Helpful Personal Qualities of the Home Health Aide**
   - A. The Importance of Efficiency and Punctuality
   - B. Transcultural Nursing in the Home

III. **The Family Unit**

IV. **Duties of the Home Health Aide**
   - A. Basic Nursing Assistant Tasks and Procedures
   - B. Using the Discharge Plan
   - C. Procedures the Home Health Aide May Not Do in the Home

V. **Safety in the Home**
   - A. Safety Hazards
   - B. Fire Safety and Burn Prevention

VI. **Reporting an Accident or Emergency by Telephone**
   - A. Phone Numbers to Keep Handy
   - B. Calling for Help

VII. **Care of the Infant in the Home**
   - A. Preparing Formula
   - B. Different Types of Formula
     1. Ready-to-feed (Prepared) Formula
     2. Powdered Formula
     3. Concentrated Liquid Formula

VIII. **Housekeeping Responsibilities in the Home**
   - A. Cleaning Responsibilities May Include
   - B. Infection Control in the Home
   - C. Nutrition and Food Service

IX. **Reporting and Recording**

Instructor Notes

OBJECTIVES

When the students have completed this chapter, they will be able to:

- Differentiate between working in the home and in the health care institution.
- Describe the four categories of home health care providers.
- Define the role of the home health aide.
- Show respect for the beliefs, opinions, culture, and customs of patients and their families.
- List 26 basic tasks and procedures they may be assigned to perform in the home.
- Assist in the implementation of the discharge plan by communicating with the home care team.
- List nine procedures the home health aide may *not* do in the home.
- Describe 11 potential safety hazards in the home.
- Write a list of the phone numbers that should always be kept next to the phone for use in reporting an accident or emergency.
- List rules to follow for storing infant formula.
- List three types of infant formula.
- Sterilize water, bottles, nipples, and caps.
- Identify eight housekeeping responsibilities the home health aide may be assigned to perform in the home.
- Discuss how to apply at least five principles of infection control to the home setting.
- Discuss nutrition and food service as it applies to the home setting.
- Record their activities and those of the patient during their scheduled home visit.
- Describe the types of patient information that should be reported to the supervisor immediately.

KEY TERMS

Bed-bound: Unable to get out of bed

Caregiver: The family member or significant other who is taking the major responsibility for the care of the patient

Efficiency: Getting all of one's duties completed in an organized fashion within a designated work period

Family Unit: A group brought together by shared needs, interests, and mutual concern for the well-being of all its members

Flammable: Capable of burning quickly and easily

Formula: A liquid food prescribed for an infant containing most required nutrients

Hospice Care: The care of patients with terminal conditions who choose to remain at home until their death

Infection Control: Restraining or curbing the spread of microorganisms

Instructor Notes

Long-term Supportive Care: The care of chronically ill patients who are unable to care for themselves and live alone or have limited family support

Microorganism: A living thing so small it cannot be seen with the naked eye but only through a microscope

Punctuality: Arriving at one's planned destination on time

Responsibility: A duty or obligation; that for which one is accountable

Short-term Intermittent Skilled Nursing Care: The care provided to acutely ill patients or those with an exacerbated illness with the purpose of educating the patients to become independent in self-care and functional ability

Sterilize: Destroy all microorganisms

Time/Travel Record: Record or log describing how time is spent in a patient's home and/or account of travel time it took to and from the patient's home or running errands

CORE STUDENT ASSIGNMENTS

Students should:

- Read this chapter in their textbook, *Being a Nursing Assistant.*
- Underline any words or sentences they do not understand. Write down any questions they have.
- Complete the Chapter Review in their textbook.
- Read the Time Management Tip for this chapter and think about how they might use this tip in their work.
- Complete the Nursing Assistant in Action exercise.

OPTIONAL STUDENT ASSIGNMENTS

Students should:

- Complete all workbook assignments for this chapter in their copy of *Workbook for Being a Nursing Assistant.*
- Use the CD/CD-Rom disk enclosed with their textbook to hear the pronunciation of the key terms in the chapter.
- Watch the "Dealing with Dementia" and the "Patient's Rights" videos from the Care Provider Skills series.
- Use the Website address **(www.prenhall.com/wolgin)** to access the free, interactive Companion Website created for this textbook. Get hints, instant feedback, and textbook references to chapter-related multiple-choice questions. Read and react to the Nursing Assistant in Action exercise. Link to other interesting sites.

Instructor Notes

METHODOLOGY AND SUGGESTED ACTIVITIES

I. Lecture/Discussion

- Answer any questions the students may have.
- Discuss the key terms and related abbreviations. Repeat them out loud and practice using them in sentences.
- Discuss the Time Management Tip for this chapter.
- Discuss the Nursing Assistant in Action exercise.
- Discuss the Critical Thinking points for this chapter.
- Discuss personal safety and protection. Emphasize the importance of following Universal Precautions. Stress the need to wear protective equipment.
- Emphasize that all procedures, rules, skills, and Universal Precautions are applied when working in the home setting.
- Discuss appropriate safeguards to prevent accidents in the home.
- Invite a social worker to speak to the class to elaborate on family structure.
- Contact your local fire department to invite a firefighter to speak on home fire safety.
- Invite a dietitian or nutritionist to discuss therapeutic diets and food management in the home.
- Invite a local home health agency nursing supervisor to speak on time management.
- Discuss the importance of infection control in the home setting.
- Review and discuss procedures allowed and not allowed in the home.
- Discuss the importance of reviewing the discharge plan.
- Emphasize professional traits needed in the workplace when working alone.

II. Role Play/Lab

- Show the videos for this chapter. Discuss ways of dealing with dementia in the home environment. Have the students practice role playing scenarios with difficult or dementia patients in the home setting. Review how the nursing assistant will honor the patient's rights in the home setting.
- Display different types of formula and demonstrate preparation and storage.
- Demonstrate the procedure for sterilizing tap water and discuss commercially bottled water.
- Demonstrate the procedure for sterilizing bottles and display various types of feeding bottles.
- Arrange a field trip to a local postpartum infant care class.
- Request sample flow sheets from local agencies to display and discuss documentation modes with the class.
- Have the students develop emergency contact lists for their local areas.
- Write each of the chapter tasks on individual cards. Distribute one card to each student. Have each student discuss or role play how they would accomplish this task in the home setting.

Instructor Notes

- Have the students role play clinical situations of potential conflict between patient/family and the home health aide.
- Have the students role play reporting clinical situations to the supervisor.
- Have the students practice mixing formula and sterilizing feeding bottles and water.
- Role play the act of calling for help in the home setting.

III. Evaluation

- Review the answers to the Chapter Review with students.
- Review the answers to the workbook exercises with students.
- Review the students' understanding of the Time Management Tip.
- To evaluate student comprehension, give a quiz.
- To evaluate student skills, administer the competency checklist.
- Have the students visit the interactive Companion Website and take the quiz.

ANSWERS TO CHAPTER REVIEW

FILL IN THE BLANK

Read each sentence and fill in the blank line with a word that completes the sentence. (Note: Hyphenated words get one line.)

1. A group of people brought together by shared needs, interests, and mutual concerns for the well-being of all its members is a ___family___.
2. ___Infection___ ___control___ involves restraining or curbing the spread of microorganisms.
3. A patient who is unable to get our of bed is ___bed-bound___.
4. If an accident or medical emergency occurs in the home, call ___Emergency___ ___Medical___ ___Service___.
5. One of the principal concerns of the home health aide is patient ___safety___.

MULTIPLE CHOICE

Choose the best answer for each question or statement.

1. When caring for a person in his or her home, home health aides generally refer to that person as a
   (A.) client.
   B. patient.
   C. sir or madam.
   D. diagnosis.

Instructor Notes

2. Which of the following is not a helpful characteristic of a home health aide?
   A. Polite
   B. Trustworthy
   (C.) Inconsiderate
   D. Careful

3. Which of the following is not a reason why a person may need home health assistance?
   A. Family works outside the home.
   (B.) Patient does not want help.
   C. The client cannot shop and prepare meals.
   D. The client cannot provide transportation.

4. Which of the following is not a duty of the home health aide?
   A. Preparing bottles
   B. Shopping for food for the client
   (C.) Changing sterile dressings
   D. Collect specimen samples

5. Which of the following phone numbers does not need to be kept handy?
   A. Fire station
   B. Police station
   (C.) Pizza delivery
   D. Pharmacy delivery

CRITICAL THINKING

CUSTOMER SERVICE

Encourage students to reflect and share their thoughts and experiences. Respect their privacy and confidentiality. Share your own viewpoints with the students.

CULTURAL CARE

Encourage students to reflect and share their thoughts and experiences. Respect their privacy and confidentiality. Share your own viewpoints with the students.

COOPERATION WITHIN THE TEAM

Encourage students to reflect and share their thoughts and experiences. Respect their privacy and confidentiality. Share your own viewpoints with the students.

NURSING ASSISTANT IN ACTION

Instructor Notes

You are assigned to care for Mr. McCollum in his home. He is an elderly man dying from lung cancer. Your supervisor informed you that he is not supposed to smoke because he is receiving oxygen. Mr. McCollum asks you to please bring him cigarettes and let him smoke anyway because he is already dying so why not give him the one thing he really needs to make him feel better?

What is Your Response/Action?

You could agree with Mr. McCollum that the desire for a cigarette is very strong. Explain or reinforce to him that the oxygen is helping him to breathe easier and feel better. Cigarettes would get in the way of that relief.

Instructor Notes

Answers to Workbook Exercises

11

The following exercises will assist you to apply what you have read in Chapter 11, "Home Health Care." For each exercise, read the objective and use information you have read in Chapter 11 to answer the questions, complete the sentences, or label the diagrams.

EXERCISE 11-1

Objective: To recognize and correctly spell words related to home health care.

Directions: Unscramble the words in the Word List at the left. Then circle the same words in the Word Search at the right.

Word List

1. EBD-BNDUO ______ BED-BOUND
2. FYAILM NTIU ______ FAMILY UNIT
3. NOGL RMTE ______ LONG TERM
4. EARCVEGIR ______ CAREGIVER
5. MREENGCYE ______ EMERGENCY
6. MOEH LEHTHA ______ HOME HEALTH
7. EIAD ______ AIDE
8. EGRAHCSID ______ DISCHARGE

Word Search

B	E	D	B	O	U	N	D	C	E	P	B	E	D	X
A	L	E	S	G	Z	W	G	L	M	T	R	A	C	D
P	F	T	R	Z	A	C	A	B	E	S	V	X	D	L
G	A	B	X	T	L	Q	G	J	R	B	H	W	S	N
X	M	W	N	U	S	I	C	P	G	I	T	B	I	G
K	I	X	V	D	A	O	A	J	E	A	L	E	N	T
S	L	O	N	G	T	E	R	M	N	V	A	I	D	E
Q	Y	E	S	F	Y	Z	E	L	C	B	E	Y	C	X
L	U	I	R	T	Z	Y	G	E	Y	C	H	L	D	V
B	N	T	C	O	A	H	I	B	B	R	E	M	J	U
C	I	L	A	D	R	M	V	D	I	O	M	E	C	L
S	T	F	M	X	S	D	E	G	T	X	O	A	G	D
O	D	S	W	F	L	Z	R	D	B	C	H	F	S	O
D	I	S	C	H	A	R	G	E	O	A	S	T	W	P

EXERCISE 11-2

Objective: To be able to recognize the variety of important duties you will perform as a home health nursing assistant.

Directions: Place the correct letters next to the matching phrase. More than one set of letters may be selected for some of the phrases.

ADL	= activities of daily living	PMT	= positioning, moving, transporting the patient
C	= communication	SKC	= skin care
CE	= care of the environment	SP	= special procedures
IC	= infection control	SPC	= specimen care
N	= nutrition	VS	= vital signs
PC	= personal care		

Answers may vary; possible answers include:

C **1.** Informing the patient of procedures you perform

IC, CE **2.** Washing the bathtub before and after use

SPC **3.** Recording intake and output

CE, IC **4.** Washing the dishes used to prepare the meals

SKC, IC, PC **5.** Keeping the patient's skin clean and dry

CE, IC, PC **6.** Making the patient's bed and changing the linen as needed

IC, SKC, SP **7.** Changing simple dressings and applying nonmedicated ointment

ADL, PMT **8.** Transporting the patient to the doctor's office

PMT, ADL **9.** Assisting the patient to use a bedside commode

SP **10.** Applying an elastic bandage to the patient's leg

ADL, N **11.** Shopping for the patient's groceries

ADL, PC **12.** Helping the patient brush his teeth and get dressed

VS **13.** Taking the patient's temperature, pulse, respirations, and blood pressure

PMT **14.** Positioning the patient in the bed

IC **15.** Using good handwashing skills and wearing disposable gloves

SP **16.** Performing range-of-motion exercises

C **17.** Making an accurate record of duties performed for the patient

CE, IC, PC **18.** Washing the patient's clothing and linens

N, ADL **19.** Cooking and preparing nutritious meals for the patient

SP **20.** Applying a binder to the patient

PC **21.** Offering in-between and meal nourishment

CE, IE **22.** Cleaning patient equipment

EXERCISE 11-3

Objective: To demonstrate appropriate responses to family situations.

Directions: Read the situation description and then choose the appropriate response.

1. You are assigned to provide home care 3 hours a day for a patient who is terminally ill with advanced lung cancer. She and her husband smoke heavily each time you are there. You are a nonsmoker and do not like being exposed to the smoke. Although the doctor has encouraged the family to not smoke, they choose to continue. **What would you do?**
   A. You continue to inform them about the dangers of smoking.
   B. You repeatedly inform them of your dislike of smoking.
   C. You tell them, "It's me or the cigarettes! Make your choice!"
   (D.) You arrange to have the husband leave the room when he smokes, and you leave the room when the patient smokes.

2. You are uneasy around your home care patient's pet, a large dog. Each time you visit the home, he follows you around, growling occasionally, and watches you closely as you care for the patient. **What would you do?**
   A. Bring the dog a bone to occupy him each time you visit.
   B. Take him by the collar and put him outside.
   (C.) Explain how you feel to the patient, and ask that the dog be put in another room or outside when you visit.
   D. Ignore the dog and pretend it doesn't bother you.

3. The family members begin to argue with each other about whose turn it is to do the laundry for your patient. **What would you do?**
   A. Because you know who should be doing the laundry, you point him out to the group.
   B. Offer to do the laundry for the family.
   (C.) Continue to care for the patient and do not get involved in the argument.
   D. Ask the family to stop arguing.

4. When working at a patient's home, you observe that it is very dusty, dirty, and cluttered. **What would you do?**
   A. You decide to be nice and stay late one day to clean the entire house so that it meets your standards.
   B. You offer to clean up the mess for pay.
   (C.) You ignore the condition of the house and focus on the patient.
   D. You call up some of the patient's relatives and ask them to clean the house before your next visit.

5. You notice that the locked security grates over all the windows would not allow escape in case of a fire. **What would you do?**
   A. Talk to the family about a plan of escape in case of fire.
   B. Bring this situation to the attention of your supervisor immediately.
   C. Talk to the family about the danger posed by the grates on the windows.
   (D.) All of the above.

EXERCISE 11-4

Objective: To recognize the definitions of words related to the nursing assistant and home health care.

Directions: Place the letter of the correct definition next to the matching word(s) from the Word List.

Word List

O **1.** time/travel record

M **2.** short-term intermittent skilled nursing care

N **3.** sterilize

E **4.** flammable

C **5.** efficiency

A **6.** bed-bound

H **7.** infection control

J **8.** punctuality

D **9.** family unit

K **10.** microorganism

B **11.** caregiver

G **12.** hospice care

L **13.** responsibility

F **14.** formula

I **15.** long-term supportive care

Definitions

A. Unable to get out of bed

B. The family member or significant other who is taking the major responsibility for care of the patient

C. Getting all of one's duties completed in an organized fashion within a designated work period

D. A group brought together by shared needs, interests, and mutual concern for the well-being of all its members

E. Capable of burning quickly and easily

F. A liquid food prescribed for an infant containing most required nutrients

G. The care of patients with terminal conditions who choose to remain at home until their death

H. Restraining or curbing the spread of microorganisms

I. The care of chronically ill patients who are unable to care for themselves and live alone or have limited family support

J. Arriving at one's planned destination on time

K. A living thing so small it cannot be seen with the naked eye but only through a microscope

L. A duty or obligation; that for which one is accountable

M. The care provided to acutely ill patients or those with an exacerbated illness, with the purpose of educating the patients to become independent in self-care and functional ability

N. Destroying all microorganisms

O. A record or log describing how time is spent in a patient's home and/or an account of the time it took to and from the patient's home or running errands

EXERCISE 11-5

Objective: To apply what you have learned about home health care.

Directions: Circle the letter next to the word or statement that best completes the sentence or describes the sentence as true or false. If the sentence is false, draw a line through the incorrect part of the sentence and write the correction on the blank line.

1. Helpful personal qualities of the home health aide are all of the following *except*
   A. the ability to be a self-starter.
   B. dependability and punctuality.
   C. an ethical approach to patient care.
   (D.) musical ability.

2. By not discussing the patient's condition with your own family you show
   A. respect for the privacy of your patient.
   B. respect for the confidentiality of the patient.
   (C.) both A and B.
   D. a lack of interest in your patient.

3. In your role as a home health care aide, it is important to maximize your time by
   A. balancing time and money.
   (B.) balancing patient preferences with travel distances.
   C. driving at high speeds, when necessary, to be on time.
   D. leaving your patient assignment early, so that you can be on time for the next patient.

4. If you are delayed ________, you must call the patient to set a new arrival time.
   A. more than 30 minutes
   B. more than 45 minutes
   C. more than 2 days
   (D.) for any amount of time

5. The number one complaint of ~~home health care aides~~ is lack of punctuality by the ~~patient~~.
   A. True
   (B.) False
   Correct Answer: *patients, home health care aides*

6. As a member of the health care team, you are expected to maintain _________ in the home.
   A. the status quo
   B. a sense of humor
   C. complete silence
   (D.) a professional attitude

7. While working in the home, you are part of the health care team, but an important difference is that you will usually not have another member of the team
   A. to whom you can refer problems.
   B. to whom you can speak if you have questions.
   (C.) physically present in the home with you while you care for the patient.
   D. to act as a supervisor.

8. An example of demonstrating honesty and accuracy when handling the patient's money is to
   (A.) attach all receipts to the shopping list.
   B. mix it with your own money.
   C. simply tell the patient what you have spent, because you know she has a good memory.
   D. keep the loose change for yourself.

9. In most cases, the goal of patient care in the home is to promote ~~increasing~~ dependence of the patient on the home health aide.
   A. True
   (B.) False
   Correct Answer: *decreasing*

10. The ~~home health aide~~ is responsible for making the first home evaluation and developing the plan of care to be followed by caregivers.
   A. True
   (B.) False
   Correct Answer: *nurse*

11. The discharge planning process requires communication with the home health care team by all members *except*
   A. the patient.
   (B.) the banker.
   C. the home health aide.
   D. the nurse.

12. It is important that all team members understand what the _________ are for each patient's plan of care.
   A. outcome prices
   (B.) outcome goals
   C. outcome costs
   D. insurance benefits

13. The home health aide must be alert to prevent accidents in the patient's home by ________ unsafe conditions.

A. creating, berating, and aggregating
B. improvising, supervising, and relating
C. maintaining, prolonging, and inventing
(D.) eliminating, preventing, and correcting

14. When all the outcome goals have been met, the patient will

A. receive the bill.
B. be cured.
C. be hospitalized.
(D.) be discharged from home care services.

15. If you are not sure how long a baby's formula has been in the refrigerator,

A. taste it yourself.
B. boil it for 10 minutes.
C. leave it in there for another time.
(D.) discard it and make fresh formula.

16. The use of boiled and then cooled water to make formula is important because boiling will kill the microorganisms in the water. These microorganisms may make the baby sick.

(A.) True
B. False
Correct Answer: ______________________________

17. There are several different kinds of formulas, but in all cases it is important to

A. wash your hands, as well as the containers before opening them.
B. read the instructions for preparation.
C. shake all containers of liquid and concentrated formulas before opening.
(D.) do all of the above.

18. Once formula is prepared it must be

A. fed to the infant immediately.
B. fed to the infant after boiling for 10 minutes.
(C.) kept refrigerated until ready to use.
D. kept at room temperature.

19. The home health aide may have housekeeping responsibilities in addition to care of the patient.

(A.) True
B. False
Correct Answer: ______________________________

20. ________ is an inexpensive disinfectant found in most homes that can be used to clean sinks, bathtubs, and toilets.
   A. Isopropyl alcohol
   B. A mixture of vinegar and oil
   C. Baking soda and vinegar
   (D.) Laundry bleach

21. When preparing food for the patient, remember to consider
   A. your likes and dislikes.
   B. the cultural and religious preferences of the patient.
   C. special dietary restrictions the patient may have.
   (D.) both B and C.

22. It is very important to arrange your visit during the mealtime hours if part of your duties are to
   A. eat three meals a day.
   B. bathe the patient only.
   C. do the laundry.
   (D.) prepare a meal and record the amount eaten.

23. To be a self-starter means to be able to
   A. carry out duties with much assistance.
   B. accomplish only tasks you started yourself.
   (C.) work independently and effectively.
   D. start working only when by yourself.

24. If a patient has no toothpaste or denture cleaner, you may use ________ in its place.
   A. salt
   B. handsoap
   (C.) baking soda
   D. vinegar

25. When you show respect for the cultural beliefs and customs of the patient and his family, you
   (A.) make them feel valued as individuals.
   B. will make them like you.
   C. will change their daily habits.
   D. will make them happy.

COMPETENCY CHECKLIST 11-1: INFANT CARE

ACTIVITY	S	U	COMMENTS
1. The student will demonstrate the proper procedure for sterilizing tap water.			
2. The student will demonstrate the proper procedure for sterilizing bottles, nipples, and caps.			
3. The student will demonstrate the proper procedure for preparing:			
A. Ready-to-feed formula			
B. Powdered formula			
C. Concentrated liquid formula			

12

Personal Care of the Patient

CHAPTER OVERVIEW

Instructor Notes

I. **Daily Care of the Patient**
   A. Early Morning Care: Before Breakfast (Sometimes called Early A.M. Care)
   B. Morning Care: After Breakfast (Sometimes called A.M. Care)
   C. Afternoon Care: After Lunch
   D. Evening Care: After Supper, Before Bedtime (Sometimes called P.M. Care)
   E. Activities of Daily Living: The Flow Sheet

II. **Oral Hygiene**

III. **Helping the Patient to Bathe**

IV. **Perineal Care**

V. **Care of Nails and Feet**

VI. **The Back Rub**

VII. **Changing the Patient's Gown**

VIII. **Hair Care**

IX. **Shaving the Patient's Beard**

X. **Elimination Needs**

XI. **The Incontinent Patient**

Instructor Notes

OBJECTIVES

When the students have completed this chapter, they will be able to:

- Establish a schedule of personal care.
- Record what they have done for the patient on the activities of daily living (ADL) flow sheet (or other appropriate form).
- Care for the patient's mouth using good oral hygiene techniques.
- Bathe the patient.
- Give perineal care.
- Care for the patient's nails and feet as instructed.
- Give a back rub.
- Change the patient's gown.
- Care for the patient's hair.
- Shave the patient's beard; remove facial hair.
- Help the patient use a bedpan, a urinal, or a bedside commode.
- Care for the incontinent patient.

KEY TERMS

Activities of Daily Living (ADL): The activities or tasks usually performed every day, such as toileting, washing, eating, and dressing

Bedpan: A pan used by patients who must defecate or urinate while in bed

Commode: A movable chair enclosing a bedpan or with an opening that can fit over a toilet

Dentures: Artificial teeth. Dentures may replace some or all of a person's teeth; they are described as being partial or complete and upper or lower

Eliminate (Defecate): To rid the body of waste products; to excrete, expel, remove, put out; to have a bowel movement; to excrete waste matter from the bowels

Flow Sheet: A checklist or chart for recording the activities of daily living

Fracture Pan: A bedpan with a flat end that goes under the patient

Incontinence: The inability to control the bowels or bladder

Oral Hygiene: Cleanliness of the mouth

Perineum (Perineal Area): The body area between the thighs (external genitalia and rectal area)

Self-care: Activities or care tasks performed by the patient

Urinal: A portable container given to male patients so they can urinate without getting out of bed

Urinate: To discharge urine from the body; other words for this function are void, micturate, and pass water

CORE STUDENT ASSIGNMENTS

Instructor Notes

Students should:

- Read this chapter in their textbook, *Being a Nursing Assistant.*
- Underline any words or sentences they do not understand. Write down any questions they have.
- Complete the Chapter Review in their textbook.
- Read the Time Management Tip for this chapter and think about how they might use this tip in their work.
- Complete the Nursing Assistant in Action exercise.

OPTIONAL STUDENT ASSIGNMENTS

Students should:

- Complete all workbook assignments for this chapter in their copy of *Workbook for Being a Nursing Assistant.*
- Use the CD/CD-Rom disk enclosed with their textbook to hear the pronunciation of the key terms in the chapter.
- Watch the "Personal Care" video and the "Bed Bath" video from the Care Provider Skills series.
- Use the Website address **(www.prenhall.com/wolgin)** to access the free, interactive Companion Website created for this textbook. Get hints, instant feedback, and textbook references to chapter-related multiple-choice questions. Read and react to the Nursing Assistant in Action exercise. Link to other interesting sites.

METHODOLOGY AND SUGGESTED ACTIVITIES

I. Lecture/Discussion

- Answer any questions the students may have.
- Discuss the key terms and related abbreviations. Repeat them out loud and practice using them in sentences.
- Discuss the Time Management Tip for this chapter.
- Discuss the Nursing Assistant in Action exercise.
- Discuss the Critical Thinking points for this chapter.
- Discuss personal safety and protection. Emphasize the importance of following Universal Precautions. Stress the need to wear protective equipment.
- Discuss the importance of good documentation and reference to the nursing care plan for individual patient preferences.
- Discuss how personal care can improve the comfort, dignity, and well-being of the patient.
- Have the students discuss what helps make them feel better.
- Discuss the effect different cultures have on patient care, personal grooming, and modesty.

Instructor Notes

II. Role Play/Lab

- Show the videos for this chapter. Have the students practice providing personal care to mannequins. Discuss the various types of partial baths in addition to a full bed bath.
- Emphasize the points listed in the text as you demonstrate the procedures.
- Demonstrate each procedure. Then have the students demonstrate each procedure.
- Assign the students to teams to practice the procedures. The first student will read and/or observe while the second student performs the skills. Then they should change roles. The third student will be the patient.
- Have the student teams role play the experience of being bathed, receiving a back rub, and receiving the bedpan.
- Obtain unsalable dentures from a dental lab for practice use.
- Role play ways to maintain patient dignity, privacy, and comfort during personal care activities.
- Long-term facilities usually have a beautician in-house. If your clinical facility has an in-house beautician, ask the beautician to demonstrate the procedures for shampooing the patient's hair and for combing the patient's hair.
- Have the students record care on the ADL flow sheet as they practice the procedures.
- Arrange demonstrations of the procedures during clinical training within a facility.

III. Evaluation

- Review the answers to the Chapter Review with students.
- Review the answers to the workbook exercises with students.
- Review the students' understanding of the Time Management Tip.
- To evaluate student comprehension, give a quiz.
- To evaluate student skills, administer the competency checklist.
- Have the students visit the interactive Companion Website and take the quiz.

ANSWERS TO CHAPTER REVIEW

FILL IN THE BLANK

Read each sentence and fill in the blank line with a word that completes the sentence. (Note: Hyphenated words get one line.)

1. Care of a person's mouth and teeth is called ___*oral*___ ___*hygiene*___.
2. Activities that can be performed by the patient are called ___*self-care*___ activities.
3. ___*Incontinence*___ is the inability to control the bowels or bladder.

Instructor Notes

4. You would give your patients a ___urinal___ or a ___bedpan___ if they needed to urinate in bed.

5. Providing ___hair___ ___care___ helps a patient feel better and look better.

MULTIPLE CHOICE

Choose the best answer for each question or statement.

1. Helping the patient with oral hygiene, bathing, and making the bed are all part of
   A. early A.M. care.
   (B.) A.M. care.
   C. afternoon care.
   D. evening care.
2. Helping a patient with oral hygiene, offering a bedpan, and giving a back rub are all part of
   A. early A.M. care.
   B. A.M. care.
   C. afternoon care.
   (D.) evening care.
3. Which of the following will not allow you to accurately measure urine output?
   A. Urinal
   B. Bedside commode
   (C.) Toilet
   D. Bedpan
4. When cleaning dentures, do all of the following *except*
   A. wear gloves.
   B. provide privacy.
   (C.) take the dentures to the sink in your hands.
   D. moisten the dentures to put them back in place.
5. Which of the following is not a type of bath?
   A. Complete bed bath
   B. Partial bed bath
   C. Shower
   (D.) All of the above are types of baths.

CRITICAL THINKING

CUSTOMER SERVICE

Encourage students to reflect and share their thoughts and experiences. Respect their privacy and confidentiality. Share your own viewpoints with the students.

Instructor Notes

CULTURAL CARE

Encourage students to reflect and share their thoughts and experiences. Respect their privacy and confidentiality. Share your own viewpoints with the students.

COOPERATION WITHIN THE TEAM

Encourage students to reflect and share their thoughts and experiences. Respect their privacy and confidentiality. Share your own viewpoints with the students.

NURSING ASSISTANT IN ACTION

You are assigned to wash and style the hair of Mrs. Williams, an African American woman. You have never seen or used the hair products she has on hand for you to use. You want Mrs. Williams to think you know what you are doing, and are unsure what she will think if you tell her the truth. You attended a class at the beginning of your orientation, but today you do not remember anything now that you need the information! She says, "Well what are you waiting for? I thought you came in here to help me do my hair?"

What Is Your Response/Action?

You must be truthful with Mrs. Williams and tell her that you have not used the products before and that you will call your supervisor for instructions because you want her hair to look very nice when you are finished helping her.

12

Answers to Workbook Exercises

The following exercises will assist you to apply what you have read in Chapter 12, "Personal Care of the Patient." For each exercise, read the objective and use information you have read in Chapter 12 to answer the questions, complete the sentences, or label the diagrams.

EXERCISE 12-1

Objective: To recognize and correctly spell words related to helping the patient take a shower.

Directions: Unscramble the words in the Word List at the left. Then circle these same words in the Word Search at the right.

Word List

1. HICAR ____ *CHAIR*
2. THAB LOSTEW ____ *BATH TOWELS*
3. PASO ____ *SOAP*
4. WASHPEROC ____ *SHOWERCAP*
5. HASTLOWCH ____ *WASHCLOTH*
6. HBTA TMA ____ *BATH MAT*
7. NECLA NOWG ____ *CLEAN GOWN*
8. FEDINISTANTC NOISTULO ____ *DISINFECTANT SOLUTION*
9. NAYLDUR AGB ____ *LAUNDRY BAG*
10. ABLEDSIPOS SOGLEV ____ *DISPOSABLE GLOVES*
11. OAAMPSO ____ *SHAMPOO*

Word Search

R	U	N	O	D	P	G	S	I	T	W	R	Y	J	U	P
O	K	Y	D	I	P	R	U	S	H	A	M	P	O	O	A
N	N	O	T	S	U	W	Q	P	B	A	C	T	S	U	S
J	C	H	A	I	R	Q	J	E	F	Z	R	T	Z	T	K
F	A	U	P	N	L	L	I	A	M	J	B	B	U	W	E
L	T	K	J	F	O	G	J	U	O	D	B	U	D	C	Z
W	H	T	H	E	V	C	K	U	M	A	A	D	R	A	N
W	A	S	H	C	L	O	T	H	H	D	T	B	A	T	U
A	J	O	I	T	I	C	O	U	T	C	H	R	T	D	P
L	K	I	K	A	A	T	W	O	K	L	T	A	I	C	J
A	O	A	S	N	M	H	E	L	P	E	O	K	T	G	B
U	T	Z	O	T	O	B	R	E	A	A	W	E	A	J	C
N	O	B	A	S	I	B	I	W	R	N	E	S	N	T	D
D	I	S	P	O	S	A	B	L	E	G	L	O	V	E	S
R	U	N	N	L	J	T	H	E	K	O	S	X	Y	Z	Z
Y	Q	W	H	U	O	H	S	H	O	W	E	R	C	A	P
B	I	D	E	T	O	M	P	T	I	N	K	U	W	T	J
A	U	U	N	I	O	A	A	A	D	T	J	W	A	T	T
G	Y	M	U	O	U	T	S	M	E	O	Q	T	Y	O	S
O	T	P	U	N	T	T	T	E	L	W	P	T	Q	T	V

EXERCISE 12-2

Objective: To be able to apply the correct meaning of words used to describe the personal care of patients.

Directions: Place the letter of the correct definition next to the matching word(s) from the Word List.

Word List

K	**1.** dentures	D	**7.** urinate
H	**2.** bedpan	E	**8.** flow sheet
G	**3.** self-care	C	**9.** oral hygiene
B	**4.** urinal	A	**10.** defecate
I	**5.** ADL	F	**11.** incontinence
J	**6.** commode	L	**12.** fracture pan

Definitions

A. To rid the body of waste matter from the bowels
B. A portable container given to male patients so they can urinate without getting out of bed
C. Cleanliness of the mouth
D. To discharge urine from the body
E. A checklist or chart for recording the activities of daily living
F. The inability to control the bowels or bladder
G. Activities or care tasks performed by the patient
H. A pan used by patients who must defecate or urinate while in bed
I. The activities or tasks usually performed every day, such as toileting, washing, eating, or dressing
J. A movable chair enclosing a bedpan or having an opening that can fit over a toilet
K. Artificial teeth
L. A shallow bedpan used by patients with mobility limitations

EXERCISE 12-3

Objective: To recognize when to discuss a change in patient condition or activity with your immediate supervisor. Example: Patient requires a change in the bathing procedure.

Directions: For each of the situations described below, identify the *change* in bathing procedure you think should be considered and discussed with your immediate supervisor. Place the correct letters next to the situation described.

CBB = Complete bed bath PBB = Partial bed bath
TB = Tub bath S = Shower

___S___ **1.** Mr. Thompson has had a partial bed bath ordered for the last 2 days. He will be discharged soon, and he walks to the bathroom and in the hallway with assistance. He tells you he usually takes showers at home.

___S___ **2.** Mrs. James will be going home tomorrow with her new baby. Yesterday, she received a partial bed bath. She is able to use the bathroom and dress herself with no difficulty today.

___TB___ **3.** Mrs. Sun, a new nursing home resident, tells you that at home she liked to take tub baths. You check your list and see that you have been assigned to have her take a shower.

___CBB___ **4.** You are assigned to give Mr. Sims a partial bath. You notice that he does not wash himself thoroughly and complains of being very tired today.

___TB___ **5.** Mrs. James likes to walk in her bare feet and has to be frequently reminded to put on her slippers. Her feet and toenails are quite dirty, and she has many callouses. She says that at home she likes to put a chair in the tub to sit on while she soaks her feet and washes. She has been taking partial bed baths.

EXERCISE 12-4

Objective: To apply what you have learned about giving personal care to a patient.

Directions: Circle the letter next to the statement that best completes the sentence or describes the sentence as true or false. If the sentence is false, draw a line through the incorrect part of the sentence and write the correction on the blank line.

1. Patient care must be unhurried and ________ to meet each patient's special needs.
- A. uninterrupted
- B. fast
- (C.) personalized
- D. worthwhile

2. A patient scheduled for surgery should
- A. brush his teeth after eating.
- (B.) perform mouth care to reduce bacteria in the mouth.
- C. never have mouth care done within 1 hour of the operation.
- D. cancel his mouth care.

3. Always wear ________ when giving a patient mouth care.
- A. a mask
- B. a raincoat and boots
- (C.) disposable gloves
- D. a gown

4. Perineal care is done for which of the following reasons?
   A. Cleanse perineal area
   B. Prevent skin breakdown
   C. Promote healing of perineal stitches
   (D.) All of the above

5. Bath water ~~should never be changed once you have started the bath~~.
   A. True
   (B.) False
   Correct Answer: *should be changed if too soapy or cool*

6. Perineal care is specific care given to the
   A. arms and legs.
   B. periorbital arches.
   C. ears and mouth.
   (D.) external genitalia and rectal area.

7. If the patient's fingernails or toenails need trimming,
   (A.) follow the policy of your institution regarding care of patient's nails.
   B. tell them to cut their nails.
   C. soak them in warm water.
   D. do nothing because this is not part of personal care.

8. Giving the patient hair care will make him
   A. hungry and tired.
   B. slim and trim.
   (C.) look better and feel better.
   D. want to go home.

9. Before shaving a patient's face,
   A. get advice from his wife.
   (B.) get permission from the patient and your immediate supervisor.
   C. make sure he is sleeping.
   D. wait until he is eating breakfast.

10. Incontinent patients should be checked to see if they are clean and dry ~~only at the beginning and at the end of each shift~~.
   A. True
   (B.) False
   Correct Answer: *frequently during the shift.*

11. Decubitus ulcers can result if the patient's skin is not kept clean and dry.
   (A.) True
   B. False
   Correct Answer: ______________________

12. Mouth care is needed only when the patient is expecting visitors.

A. True

(B.) False

Correct Answer: is

13. Each patient is to be treated

A. as if he were family.

B. according to the flow sheet.

C. to a reward if he follows orders.

(D.) as an individual.

14. Your observations while helping patients are important to other members of the health care team.

(A.) True

B. False

Correct Answer: ______

15. Providing personal care of the patient in a skillful and respectful manner will

A. take too much time.

B. prevent avoidance of ADLs.

(C.) increase her comfort and well-being.

D. decrease her appetite.

16. When performing personal care for the small child, include the parent or have them remain close by.

(A.) True

A. False

Correct Answer: ______

17. Babies lose body heat more quickly than adults, so be sure to

A. turn all fans on high when bathing them.

(B.) dry their skin quickly.

C. keep them undressed until the skin is dry to the touch.

D. bathe them only during the summer months.

18. Adults and geriatric patients like to

A. have all personal care performed for them.

(B.) maintain control over their own care.

C. have the nursing assistant make all decisions for them.

D. give up as much freedom to choose their care as possible.

COMPETENCY CHECKLIST 12-1: PERSONAL CARE

ACTIVITY	S	U	COMMENTS
1. Student correctly states the steps involved in:			
A. Early morning care			
B. Morning care			
C. Afternoon care			
D. Evening care			
2. Student correctly demonstrates oral hygiene:			
A. Mouth care			
B. Denture care			
3. Student correctly demonstrates how to bathe a patient:			
A. Complete bed bath			
B. Partial bed bath			
C. Tub bath			
D. Shower			
4. Student correctly demonstrates how to give perineal care:			
A. Male perineal care			
B. Female perineal care			
5. Student correctly demonstrates how to care for nails and feet:			
A. Foot care for the elderly and diabetic patient			
B. Routine foot care			
6. Student correctly demonstrates how to give a back rub:			
A. Routine care			
B. Special care			
7. Student correctly demonstrates how to change a patient's gown:			
A. Routine change			
B. Change when arm injured or patient has IV			

COMPETENCY CHECKLIST 12-1: PERSONAL CARE (CONTINUED)

ACTIVITY	S	U	COMMENTS
8. Student correctly demonstrates how to give hair care:			
A. Washing the hair			
B. Combing the hair			
9. Student correctly demonstrates how to shave a patient's beard:			
A. Using a safety razor			
B. Using an electric razor			
10. Student correctly demonstrates how to meet patient's elimination needs:			
A. Offering bedpan			
B. Offering urinal			
C. Offering commode			
D. Incontinent patient care			

CORE ELEMENTS OF PERSONAL CARE

1. Wash hands and wear gloves.
2. Provide privacy and dignity.
3. Meet patient's individual needs.
4. Care is unhurried.
5. Provide safety.
6. Follow all steps of the procedure.

Emergency Care

13

CHAPTER OVERVIEW

Instructor Notes

I. **What to Do in an Emergency**
   A. Legal Issues
   B. Emergency Medical Services

II. **Shock**
   A. Types of Shock

III. **Heart Attack, Chest Pain, and Cardiac Arrest**

IV. **Cardiopulmonary Resuscitation (CPR)**
   A. Airway
   B. Breathing
   C. Circulation

V. **Choking**

VI. **Stroke or Cerebrovascular Accident**

VII. **Seizures**

VIII. **Hemorrhage**

IX. **Burns**

X. **Poisoning**

Instructor Notes

OBJECTIVES

When the students have completed this chapter, they will be able to:

- List the guidelines to follow in an emergency.
- Describe the signs of shock and guidelines for care of a patient in shock.
- Explain the purpose of CPR and list its three basic elements.
- List the signs of heart attack, cardiac arrest, and stroke, and explain what should be done to help the person in crisis.
- Explain the purpose of the Heimlich maneuver.
- Demonstrate how to assist someone who is having a seizure.
- Demonstrate the most effective way to control bleeding.
- Demonstrate first aid for a burn victim.
- Explain what to do for someone who has been poisoned.

KEY TERMS

Bioterrorism: Terrorist attacks using chemical or biological materials

Cardiac Arrest: The unexpected stopping of the heartbeat and circulation

Cardiopulmonary Resuscitation (CPR): An emergency procedure used to reestablish effective circulation and respiration in order to prevent irreversible brain damage

Cardiovascular System: Circulatory system which includes heart, arteries, veins, and capillaries

Emergency: Events that call for immediate action

First Aid: The first action taken to help a person who is in crisis

Heart Attack: Interruption or damage to the blood supply to the heart muscle; myocardial infarction

Hemorrhage: The extreme or unexpected loss of blood; heavy bleeding

Poison: Any substance ingested, inhaled, injected, or absorbed into the body that will interfere with normal physiological functions

Seizure: An episode either partial or generalized, which may include altered consciousness, motor activity, or sensory phenomena and convulsions

Shock: The failure of the cardiovascular system to provide sufficient blood circulation to every part of the body

Stroke: Interruption or damage to the blood supply to the brain; a cerebrovascular accident

CORE STUDENT ASSIGNMENTS

Students should:

- Read this chapter in their textbook, *Being a Nursing Assistant*.
- Underline any words or sentences they do not understand. Write down any questions they have.

- Complete the Chapter Review in their textbook.
- Read the Time Management Tip for this chapter and think about how they might use this tip in their work.
- Complete the Nursing Assistant in Action exercise.

Instructor Notes

OPTIONAL STUDENT ASSIGNMENTS

Students should:

- Complete all workbook assignments for this chapter in their copy of *Workbook for Being a Nursing Assistant.*
- Use the CD/CD-Rom disk enclosed with their textbook to hear the pronunciation of the key terms in the chapter.
- Watch the "Handling Infectious Waste" section of the "Infection Control" video from the Care Provider Skills series.
- Use the Website address **(www.prenhall.com/wolgin)** to access the free, interactive Companion Website created for this textbook. Get hints, instant feedback, and textbook references to chapter-related multiple-choice questions. Read and react to the Nursing Assistant in Action exercise. Link to other interesting sites.

METHODOLOGY AND SUGGESTED ACTIVITIES

I. Lecture/Discussion

- Answer any questions the students may have.
- Discuss the key terms and related abbreviations. Repeat them out loud and practice using them in sentences.
- Discuss the Time Management Tip for this chapter.
- Discuss the Nursing Assistant in Action exercise.
- Discuss the Critical Thinking points for this chapter.
- Discuss personal safety and protection. Emphasize the importance of following Universal Precautions. Stress the need to wear protective equipment.
- Review and discuss the role of the nursing assistant in each of the emergency situations and the corresponding guidelines for care.
- Emphasize the importance of a calm manner during emergencies.
- Explain how signs and symptoms lead to the correct actions.
- Invite an emergency medical technician to speak to the class.
- Review the disaster responsibilities of your agency as they relate to bioterrorism. Review the nursing assistant's role.

II. Role Play/Lab

- Show the video for this chapter. Have the students practice responding to emergencies with the appropriate personal protective equipment. Review with the students who to contact in their institution if they do become exposed to a patient's body fluids.
- Role play emergency scenarios and have the students practice their responses.

Instructor Notes

- Have the students practice being the patient and the nursing assistant.
- Have a CPR instructor lead a class for the students.
- Have the students survey their homes for poisonous substances.
- Have the students practice calling "911" in mock bioterrorism situations as well as for poison control situations.

III. Evaluation

- Review the answers to the Chapter Review with students.
- Review the answer to the workbook exercises with students.
- Review the students' understanding of the Time Management Tip.
- To evaluate student comprehension, give a quiz.
- To evaluate student skills, administer the competency checklist.
- Have the students visit the interactive Companion Website and take the quiz.

ANSWERS TO CHAPTER REVIEW

FILL IN THE BLANK

Read each sentence and fill in the blank line with a word that completes the sentence. (Note: Hyphenated words get one line.)

1. An ___emergency___ is a situation or event that requires immediate action.
2. Failure of the cardiovascular system to provide sufficient blood circulation to every part of the body results in ___shock___.
3. ___Cardiac___ ___arrest___ is the unexpected stopping of the heartbeat and circulation.
4. The "A" in "ABC" stands for ___airway___.
5. Apply ___direct___ pressure with the palm of the hand over an area that is bleeding.

MULTIPLE CHOICE

Choose the best answer for each question or statement.

1. All of the following may be signs of shock *except*
   A. eyes appear dull and lackluster.
   B. pupils may be dilated.
   (C.) the patient is not breathing.
   D. face appears pale and cyanotic.

Instructor Notes

2. Signs of a cardiac arrest may include all of the following *except*
A. loss of consciousness.
B. absence of pulse.
(C.) bleeding.
D. absence of breathing.

3. When initiating CPR, you first determine unresponsiveness and then
(A.) call for assistance.
B. open the airway.
C. check for breathing.
D. check for pulse.

4. If a choking person can still speak a little
A. go ahead and perform the Heimlich maneuver.
B. wait before performing CPR.
(C.) wait before performing the Heimlich maneuver.
D. leave and come back and check on the person in 10 minutes.

5. If your patient is having a seizure, you should
A. try to force a tongue blade between his teeth.
B. ask "Can you speak?"
(C.) not attempt to restrain the patient's movements.
D. leave the patient and go get help.

CRITICAL THINKING

CUSTOMER SERVICE

Encourage students to reflect and share their thoughts and experiences. Respect their privacy and confidentiality. Share your own viewpoints with the students.

CULTURAL CARE

Encourage students to reflect and share their thoughts and experiences. Respect their privacy and confidentiality. Share your own viewpoints with the students.

COOPERATION WITHIN THE TEAM

Encourage students to reflect and share their thoughts and experiences. Respect their privacy and confidentiality. Share your own viewpoints with the students.

Instructor Notes

NURSING ASSISTANT IN ACTION

You have wheeled Mrs. Raja, a postsurgical patient who has just been discharged, to the lobby exit. As you are helping her into the car, you notice some bright red blood on the front of her dress. You suspect there may be a serious problem as the stain is getting larger. Her husband tells you. "She is fine, she wants to leave. Don't worry, I'll drive her home and we will call her doctor if necessary."

What Is Your Response/Action?

Express concern about the rate of the bleeding and tell Mrs. Raja and her husband to wait while you call for help either back to your unit or according to your institution's policy. Do not let Mrs. Raja get up out of the wheelchair because she may collapse. If other staff are near by, call to them for help. Have them get help while you stay with the patient.

Answers to Workbook Exercises

13

The following exercises will assist you to apply what you have read in Chapter 13, "Emergency Care." For each exercise, read the objective and use information you have read in Chapter 13 to answer the questions, complete the sentences, or label the diagrams.

EXERCISE 13-1

Objective: To recognize and correctly spell words related to emergency care.

Directions: Fill in the missing letters to correctly spell the 14 words listed below. The total number of letters is listed next to each word.

1. _E_MER_GEN_CY (9)
2. H_EMO_RRH_A_GE (10)
3. S_HO_CK (5)
4. F_IRS_T A_ID_ (8)
5. _S_TRO_K_E (6)
6. C_A_RDIO _PU_LMON_AR_Y (15)
7. CA_RD_I_AC_ AR_RE_S_T_ (13)
8. RES_USC_ITA_TI_ON (13)
9. _CA_RD_IO_ V_A_S_CU_LAR (14)
10. P_OI_SO_N_ (6)
11. S_EI_Z_UR_E (7)
12. _A_N_AP_HYL_AC_T_I_C (12)
13. B_IO_T_E_RR_OR_ISM (12)
14. _H_EI_ML_IC_H_ (8)

EXERCISE 13-2

Objective: To recognize the symptoms of shock.

Directions: Draw a line to connect the correct type of shock that matches the cause.

Type of Shock	Shock Causes
1. Hemorrhagic	fear
2. Respiratory	changes in body chemistry
3. Psychogenic	insufficient oxygen in the blood
4. Septic	spinal cord damage
5. Cardiogenic	insect stings
6. Neurogenic	infection
7. Anaphylactic	heart not functioning well
8. Metabolic	extreme blood loss

EXERCISE 13-3

Objective: To apply what you have learned about emergency care.

Directions: Circle the letter next to the word or statement that best completes the sentence or describes the sentence as true or false. If the sentence is false, draw a line through the incorrect part of the sentence and write the correction on the blank line.

1. Before you take any action in an emergency, you must determine all of the following *except:*
   A. What is the problem or emergency?
   B. Is there anyone available to help you?
   C. What must be done immediately to maintain life for the person in crisis?
   (D.) Which ambulance will arrive?
2. The emergency plan for home care patients should contain the telephone numbers for all of the following *except*
   A. fire rescue squads.
   (B.) emergency pedicure services.
   C. poison control center.
   D. physicians.

3. Guidelines for assisting a victim in an emergency do not include
   A. bleeding control.
   B. preventing further injury or harm.
   C. preventing shock.
   (D.) preventive care.

4. You may be called upon to perform ________ until medical help arrives.
   A. OBRA
   B. RACE
   C. PASS
   (D.) CPR

5. The ________ maneuver is used to dislodge an object and open the airway of a choking victim.
   A. karate
   B. choking
   (C.) Heimlich
   D. "last chance"

6. Placing your hands in the wrong position while doing chest compressions
   A. can improve the circulation.
   B. strengthens your hands.
   C. is not a major problem.
   (D.) can cause broken ribs and other problems for the victim.

7. Deliver 15 compressions to ~~each breath~~ during CPR.
   A. True
   (B.) False
   Correct Answer: *every two breaths*

8. Open the airway of the patient using the head-tilt/chin-lift technique.
   (A.) True
   B. False
   Correct Answer: ________________

9. A ________ is an episode, either partial or generalized, that may include alteration of consciousness, body movements, and convulsions.
   (A.) seizure
   B. stroke
   C. shock
   D. hemorrhage

10. A(n) ________ is a site where a main artery lies near the surface of the body, directly over a bone.
   A. vein
   B. airway
   C. artery
   (D.) pressure point

11. ________ can be a sign of internal bleeding.
   (A.) Dilated pupils
   B. Extreme hunger
   C. Slow pulse
   D. Headache

12. Tissue damage caused by ________ is a burn.
   A. ice
   B. snow
   (C.) heat
   D. wind

13. Complications of a burn may include
   A. infection, shock, growth.
   (B.) pain, infection, death.
   C. promotion, infection, death.
   D. tanning, sleepiness, death.

14. Pale, moist, and cold skin may be a sign of
   A. death.
   B. birth.
   C. postshower syndrome.
   (D.) internal bleeding.

15. Internal bleeding can be accompanied by vomiting of
   A. breakfast.
   (B.) blood that looks like coffee grounds.
   C. blood that is greenish.
   D. blood that resembles tea.

16. Loss of ________ and body ________ is a complication of burns.
   A. milk, image
   B. heat, temperature
   (C.) heat, fluids
   D. heat, flexibility

17. A ________ is any substance that is toxic to the body.
   A. vitamin
   B. mineral
   C. radical
   (D.) poison

18. The wrong medication or an incorrect dose of a prescribed medication may occur for all of the following reasons *except*
   (A.) the excellent eyesight of older and elderly adults.
   B. adults ignoring warning labels.
   C. teens experimenting with others' prescribed drugs.
   D. no child-proof locks on cabinets containing medications.

19. When assisting the patient who has been poisoned, you should do all of the following *except*

A. check the mouth for burns.

B. look for a container from which the poison may have come.

C. note the odors on the person's breath.

(D.) immediately induce vomiting.

20. After calling for medical assistance, a poisoning victim ~~can~~ be left alone.

A. True

(B.) False

Correct Answer: should not

21. The regional poison control center is a good source of help in situations where the patient has been ~~severely burned~~.

A. True

(B.) False

Correct Answer: poisoned.

22. If the person who has been poisoned is unconscious, ~~give fluids by mouth to minimize the effect~~.

A. True

(B.) False

Correct Answer: give nothing by mouth.

23. The interruption of the blood supply to the heart muscle is called a

A. muscle cramp.

(B.) heart attack.

C. pneumothorax.

D. Heimlich episode.

24. The most important factor in successful resuscitation is the opening of the airway.

(A.) True

B. False

Correct Answer: ______

25. If you suspect that a person has had a stroke, ~~call poison control~~.

A. True

(B.) False

Correct Answer: call 911.

26. When a person is having a seizure, you should protect him from injury and maintain a(n) ______ airway.

A. closed

(B.) patent/open

C. fluid

D. obstructed

The Human Body

14

CHAPTER OVERVIEW

Instructor Notes

I. **Anatomy and Physiology**

II. **Cells, Tissues, and Organs**
  A. Cells
    1. Structure of the Cell
    2. Cell Division
  B. Tissues
  C. Organs

III. **Body Systems**

IV. **Anatomical Position**

Instructor Notes

OBJECTIVES

When the students have completed this chapter, they will be able to:

- List the things all living cells have in common.
- Relate the parts of a cell to their functions.
- Explain the process of cellular division.
- List the basic groupings of cells that build a human body.
- Name the primary kinds of tissues, their functions, and examples of their location in the human body.
- Identify the organs and basic functions of each body system.
- Describe the body in anatomical position.

KEY TERMS

Anatomy: The study of the structure of an organism

Anterior: Located in the front; opposite of posterior

Blood and Lymph Tissue: Tissue composed of singular cells that move within a fluid to every part of the body, circulating nutrients, oxygen, and antibodies and removing waste products

Cardiac Muscle Tissue: Involuntary muscle tissue found only in the heart

Cell: The basic unit of living matter

Connective Tissue: Tissue that connects, supports, covers, lines, pads, or protects other body structures

Deep: Distant from the surface of the body

Dorsal: Refers to the back or to the back part of an organ

Epithelial Tissue: Tissue that lines, protects, secretes, absorbs, and receives sensations

Inferior: The lower portion of the body

Muscle Tissue: Tissue that ensures movement; it is capable of stretching and contracting

Nerve Tissue: Tissue that carries nervous impulses between the brain, the spinal cord, and all parts of the body

Organ: A part of the body made of several types of tissue grouped together to perform a certain function; examples are the heart, stomach, and lungs

Physiology: The study of the functions of the body dealing with the physical and chemical processes of cells, tissues, and organs of living organisms

Posterior: Located in the back or toward the rear

Superficial: On or near the surface of the body

Superior: The upper portion of the body

System: A group of organs acting together to carry out one or more body functions

Instructor Notes

Tissue: A group of cells of the same type

Ventral: On the abdominal, anterior, or front side of the body

CORE STUDENT ASSIGNMENTS

Students should:

- Read this chapter in their textbook, *Being a Nursing Assistant.*
- Underline any words or sentences they do not understand. Write down any questions they have.
- Complete the Chapter Review in their textbook.
- Read the Time Management Tip for this chapter and think about how they might use this tip in their work.
- Complete the Nursing Assistant in Action exercise.

OPTIONAL STUDENT ASSIGNMENTS

Students should:

- Complete all workbook assignments for this chapter in their copy of *Workbook for Being a Nursing Assistant.*
- Use the CD/CD-Rom disk enclosed with their textbook to hear the pronunciation of the key terms in the chapter.
- Watch the "Anatomy"section of the "Body Mechanics" video from the Care Provider Skills series.
- Use the Website address **(www.prenhall.com/wolgin)** to access the free, interactive Companion Website created for this textbook. Get hints, instant feedback, and textbook references to chapter-related multiple-choice questions. Read and react to the Nursing Assistant in Action exercise. Link to other interesting sites.

METHODOLOGY AND SUGGESTED ACTIVITIES

I. Lecture/Discussion

- Answer any questions the students may have.
- Discuss the key terms and related abbreviations. Repeat them out loud and practice using them in sentences.
- Discuss the Time Management Tip for this chapter.
- Discuss the Nursing Assistant in Action exercise.
- Discuss the Critical Thinking points for this chapter.
- Help the students to remember the terminology by matching the term to the correct definition.
- Have the students label a model or a diagram to get more familiar with structures.
- Motivate the students by offering valid reasons for studying anatomy and physiology.
- Use anatomical models, diagrams, and charts.

Instructor Notes

- Expand on the content of this chapter for advanced students.
- Discuss scenarios of patient interactions that involve complex medical terms. Discuss ways students can explain procedures they are performing using accurate, but not overwhelming medical terminology and abbreviations with patients.

II. Role Play/Lab

- Show the video for this chapter. Discuss how organs and systems work together. Watch how the muscle groups work together. Practice safe lifting techniques while envisioning the various muscle groups at work.
- Working in pairs, students can label the body areas on each other.
- Divide class into three groups. One group makes a crossword puzzle, one group makes a bingo game, and one group makes flash cards. Then the groups exchange study aids to learn the information on them.
- Have the students match each body system with body organs that are part of that particular body system.
- Write a chart on the classification of disease on the board, but omit one column and change the order. Students can fill in the blanks.
- Play "Jeopardy"-style games to promote quick recognition and responses to terminology.

III. Evaluation

- Review the answers to the Chapter Review with students.
- Review the answer to the workbook exercises with students.
- Review the students' understanding of the Time Management Tip.
- To evaluate student comprehension, give a quiz.
- Have the students visit the interactive Companion Website and take the quiz.

ANSWERS TO CHAPTER REVIEW

FILL IN THE BLANK

Read each sentence and fill in the blank line(s) with the word or words that complete the sentence. (Note: Hyphenated words get one line.)

1. The study of the structure of an organism is called *anatomy*.
2. The basic unit of living matter is called the *cell*.
3. The function of *epithelial* tissue is to protect, secrete, absorb, and receive sensations.
4. Tissues that are grouped together form *organs*.
5. A group of organs acting together to carry out one or more body functions is called a *system*.

MULTIPLE CHOICE

Instructor Notes

Choose the best answer for each question or statement.

1. Cells do all of the following *except*
   A. use food for energy.
   (B.) use carbon dioxide to break down food.
   C. grow and repair themselves.
   D. use water to transport various substances.
2. Which of the following carries impulses from a portion of the brain or spinal cord to all parts of the body?
   A. White blood cells
   B. Red blood cells
   C. Platelets
   (D.) Nerve tissue
3. Which of the following is not an organ?
   A. Stomach
   B. Liver
   (C.) Hand
   D. Brain
4. All of the activities of the body are regulated by the
   (A.) Endocrine system.
   B. Digestive system.
   C. Urinary system.
   D. Circulatory system.
5. The front side of a person is called the
   A. posterior.
   (B.) anterior.
   C. dorsal.
   D. superior.

CRITICAL THINKING

CUSTOMER SERVICE

Encourage students to reflect and share their thoughts and experiences. Respect their privacy and confidentiality. Share your own viewpoints with the students.

CULTURAL CARE

Encourage students to reflect and share their thoughts and experiences. Respect their privacy and confidentiality. Share your own viewpoints with the students.

Instructor Notes

COOPERATION WITHIN THE TEAM

Encourage students to reflect and share their thoughts and experiences. Respect their privacy and confidentiality. Share your own viewpoints with the students.

NURSING ASSISTANT IN ACTION

You are assigned to work with patients whose disease conditions are different from those you are most familiar with. How can you prepare to increase your knowledge of the most important body systems' functions and the conditions which are being treated in the unit?

What Is Your Response/Action?

Talk to the nurse/supervisor and explain your need to learn more about these particular patients' diseases. Ask questions such as "What is most important to be aware of?" and "What signs and symptoms are you looking to hear about from me?" You might also be able to learn more through unit reference material or through patient education materials.

14

Answers to Workbook Exercises

The following exercises will assist you to apply what you have read in Chapter 14, "The Human Body." For each exercise, read the objective and use information you have read in Chapter 14 to answer the questions, complete the sentences, or label the diagrams.

EXERCISE 14–1

Objective: To recognize and correctly spell words that name anatomical positions.

Directions: Unscramble the words in the Word List on the left. Then circle these same words in the Word Search at the right.

Word List

1. FORINERI *INFERIOR*
2. EPDE *DEEP*
3. LADSOR *DORSAL*
4. RECAFUSPILI *SUPERFICIAL*
5. EROSIPUR *SUPERIOR*
6. SORTERPIO *POSTERIOR*
7. TANERORI *ANTERIOR*
8. LELC *CELL*

Word Search

R	J	I	W	T	S	T	T	O	S	U	N
Q	W	T	L	D	E	E	P	S	U	T	U
D	O	R	S	A	L	W	A	I	P	R	M
I	E	D	U	N	D	A	C	T	E	V	B
P	P	O	S	T	E	R	I	O	R	J	E
P	S	U	P	E	R	F	I	C	I	A	L
I	N	F	E	R	I	O	R	A	O	K	S
D	U	M	P	I	C	E	L	L	R	O	T
I	T	I	W	O	J	A	M	M	S	T	W
O	J	O	L	R	I	T	U	V	E	Q	U

EXERCISE 14-2

Objective: To be able to apply the correct meaning of words used to name tissues of the body.

Directions: Choose the correct word(s) from the Word List to complete the sentences.

Word List

muscle tissue	nerve tissue	connective tissue
epithelial tissue	cardiac muscle tissue	blood and lymph tissue
striated muscle tissue	smooth muscle tissue	tissues

1. Skin, linings of the intestines, and linings of the glands and organs are examples of ___epithelial___ ___tissue___.
2. The function of ___connective___ ___tissue___ is to connect, support, cover or line, and pad or protect the body.
3. ___Muscle___ ___tissue___ makes body movement possible.
4. The smooth, involuntary muscles made up of ___cardiac___ ___muscle___ ___tissue___ keep the heart beating.
5. Muscles that can be moved with a conscious effort are made up of ___striated___ ___muscle___ ___tissue___.
6. ___Nerve___ ___tissue___ carries impulses to and from the brain, spinal cord, and other parts of the body.
7. The tissue that has single cells and flows through vessels is known as ___blood___ ___and___ ___lymph___ ___tissue___.
8. The dilation of such structures as the pupil of the eye and blood vessels is made possible by means of ___smooth___ ___muscle___ ___tissue___.
9. ___Tissues___ are groups of the same type of cells that work together.

EXERCISE 14-3

Objective: To be able to correctly describe cells and their functions.

Directions: Select the word(s) from the Word List to complete the sentences below.

Word List

building blocks	microscope	existed	living
oxygen	water	reproduce	

1. The cells are the fundamental ___building___ ___blocks___ of all living matter.

2. Cells can be seen only under the ___microscope___.

3. Cells use ___water___ to transport substances.

4. Most living cells grow and ___reproduce___ themselves.

5. Cells use ___oxygen___ to break down food.

6. Cells are the ___living___ parts of organisms.

7. Cells come from cells that have already ___existed___.

EXERCISE 14-4

Objective: To recognize and be able to correctly spell the names of various organs of the human body.

Directions: Label the diagram in Figure 14–1 with the correct words from the Word List below

Word List

heart	lung	kidney	large intestine	thyroid
brain	uterus	liver	small intestine	trachea
bladder	stomach	ovary	testicles	skin

FIGURE 14-1

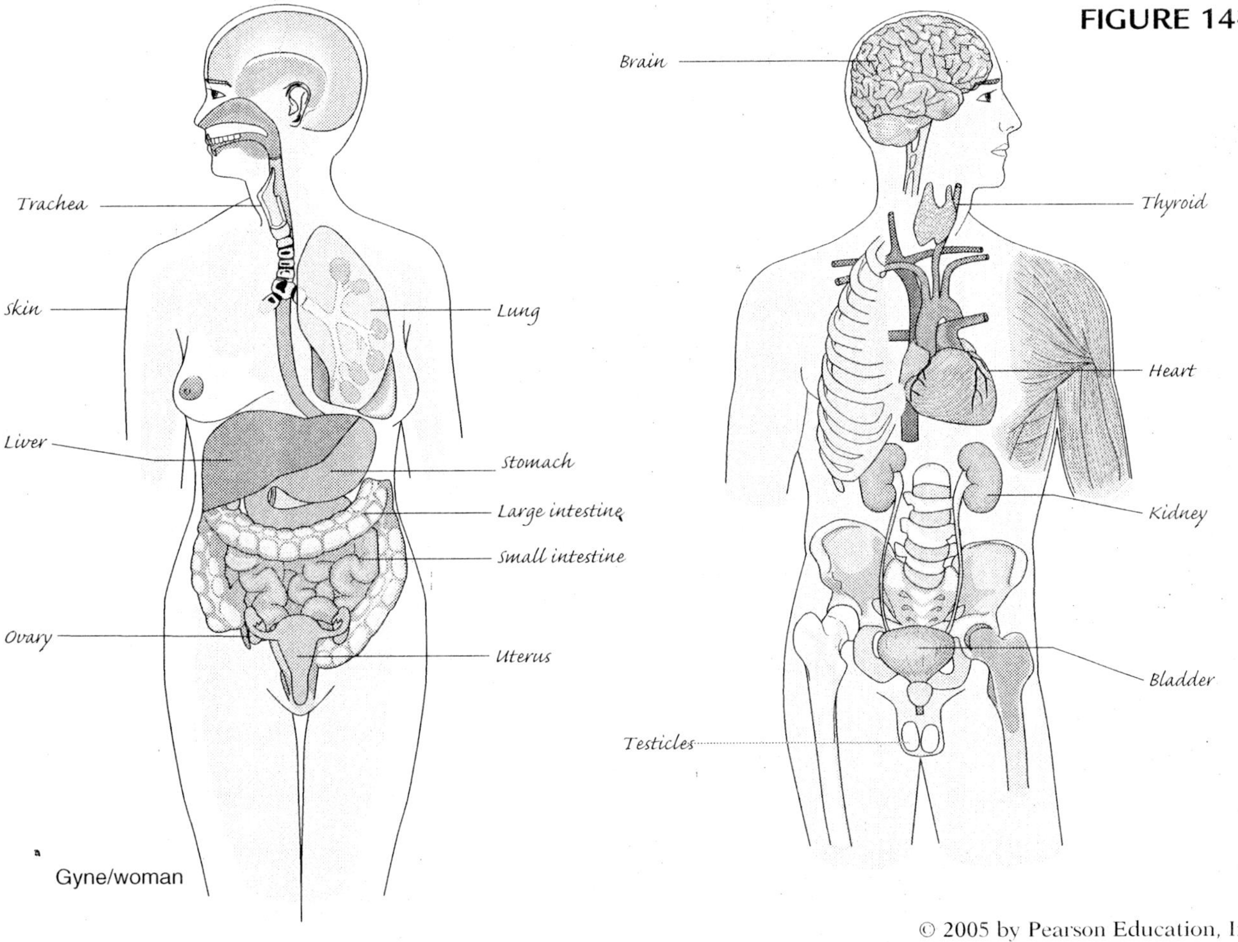

EXERCISE 14-5

Objective: To apply your understanding of how the body cells, tissues, organs, and systems relate to each other.

Directions: Label the diagram in Figure 14–2 with the correct words from the Word List. Place the words in the *order of their complexity.*

Word List

organs cells systems tissues

FIGURE 14-2

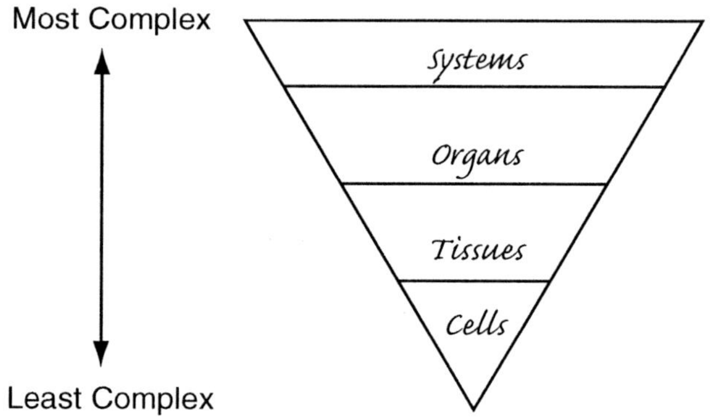

EXERCISE 14-6

Objective: To apply what you have learned about the human body.

Directions: Circle the letter next to the word or statement that best completes the sentence or describes the sentence as true or false. If the sentence is false, draw a line through the incorrect part of the sentence and write the correction on the blank line.

1. The body systems cannot work by themselves and
- (A.) are dependent on each other.
- B. so must get help from tissues.
- C. are independent of each other.
- D. let you know by complaining often.

2. The digestive system takes in and
- A. absorbs nutrients at night.
- B. absorbs daylight.
- C. absorbs nutrients as waste.
- (D.) absorbs nutrients and eliminates wastes.

3. An example of the integumentary system is
- A. the kidney.
- B. the heart.
- C. the brain.
- (D.) the skin.

4. The ~~urinary~~ system controls activities of the body.

A. True

(B.) False

Correct Answer: *nervous*

5. An organ of the respiratory system is the

(A.) larynx.

B. spleen.

B. pancreas.

B. thymus.

6. The integumentary system is the ~~second and third~~ line of defense against infection.

A. True

(B.) False

Correct Answer: *first*

7. The front side of a person is referred to as the

(A.) anterior side.

B. posterior side.

C. the frontal lobe.

D. first side.

8. Groups of cells of the same type that work together to perform a particular function are called tissues.

(A.) True

B. False

Correct Answer: ______

9. Organs that work together to perform similar tasks make up body systems.

(A.) True

B. False

Correct Answer: ______

10. The human back side, containing the spine, is called the

A. anterior or upper side.

B. posterior or under side.

C. posterior or weak side.

(D.) posterior or dorsal side.

15

Growth and Development

CHAPTER OVERVIEW

Instructor Notes

I. Growth and Development
  A. Growth
    1. Infants: Birth–1 Year
    2. Toddlers: 1–2 Years
    3. Preschoolers: 2–5 Years
    4. School-Age Children: 5–12 Years
    5. Adolescence: 12–18 Years
    6. Young, Middle, Older Adults: 18–75+ Years
    7. Old Age: 76–100+ Years
  B. Development
    1. Chronological Age
    2. Illness
    3. Injuries
  C. Chronological-Age Considerations

Instructor Notes

OBJECTIVES

When the students have completed this chapter, they will be able to:

- Describe typical growth patterns in infants, toddlers, preschoolers, school-aged children, and adolescents.
- Identify the developmental skills used to describe the various stages of development of human beings over their life spans.
- Describe the developmental tasks characteristic of each stage of development.
- Describe age-based factors, or situations, that must be kept in mind as care is given for the patient: infant, toddler, preschooler, school-age child, adolescent, young adult, middle-aged adult, or older adult.

KEY TERMS

Chronological Age: Actual age in years and months

Circumference: The distance around an object or body part, such as the head

Cognitive: The mental processes by which knowledge is acquired

Development: The motor, language, cognitive, and social skills changes that occur in a person over the course of the life span

Fine Motor: Refers to the movement of small muscles, such as those in the hands and fingers

Gross Motor: Refers to the movement of large muscles, such as those used in walking or hitting a ball

Growth: The physical changes that take place in a person's body over the life span

CORE STUDENT ASSIGNMENTS

Students should:

- Read this chapter in their textbook, *Being a Nursing Assistant.*
- Underline any words or sentences they do not understand. Write down any questions they have.
- Complete the Chapter Review in their textbook.
- Read the Time Management Tip for this chapter and think about how they might use this tip in their work.
- Complete the Nursing Assistant in Action exercise.

OPTIONAL STUDENT ASSIGNMENTS

Students should:

- Complete all workbook assignments for this chapter in their copy of *Workbook for Being a Nursing Assistant.*

- Use the CD/CD-Rom disk enclosed with their textbook to hear the pronunciation of the key terms in the chapter.
- Watch the "Age-Specific Competencies" video from the Care Provider Skills series.
- Use the Website address **(www.prenhall.com/wolgin)** to access the free, interactive Companion Website created for this textbook. Get hints, instant feedback, and textbook references to chapter-related multiple-choice questions. Read and react to the Nursing Assistant in Action exercise. Link to other interesting sites.

Instructor Notes

METHODOLOGY AND SUGGESTED ACTIVITIES

I. Lecture/Discussion

- Answer any questions the students may have.
- Discuss the key terms and related abbreviations. Repeat them out loud and practice using them in sentences.
- Discuss the Time Management Tip for this chapter.
- Discuss the Nursing Assistant in Action exercise.
- Discuss the Critical Thinking points for this chapter.
- Have the students list the developmental age groups of their family members.
- Have the students define each growth period and developmental stage as a "round-robin" game.
- Have the students list the developmental tasks of their family members.
- Make a chart and have the students match the growth period with the developmental task.
- Identify examples of various age-specific patients and have the students identify the age-specific concerns in each.
- Review the importance of continually developing with age.
- Discuss what techniques make patients of each age group feel safe and secure in the health care setting.

II. Role Play/Lab

- Show the video for this chapter. Discuss how patients of different ages need different kinds of communication styles, instructions, and equipment from their caregivers. Have the students practice altering their approach to patients based on the age of the patient.
- Have the students divide into teams of two. Have each student role play providing age-specific care. While one student role plays the patient, the other student role plays the nursing assistant. Then the students change roles and complete the exercise again.
- Role play situations that entail inaccurate age-specific assumptions. Have students point these out and suggest alternative communications, materials, and/or pieces of equipment.

III. Evaluation

- Review the answers to the Chapter Review with students.
- Review the answer to the workbook exercises with students.

Instructor Notes

- Review the students' understanding of the Time Management Tip.
- To evaluate student comprehension, give a quiz.
- Have the students visit the interactive Companion Website and take the quiz.

ANSWERS TO CHAPTER REVIEW

FILL IN THE BLANK

Read each sentence and fill in the blank line(s) with the word or words that complete the sentence. (Note: Hyphenated words get one line.)

1. In each developmental stage, there are ___tasks___ that have to be mastered.
2. The measurement of a child's head is called its ___circumference___.
3. ___Fine___ motor control refers to the movement of small muscles, such as those in the feet and hands.
4. ___Chronological___ age is the person's actual age in years and months.
5. ___Injury___ and ___illness___ can have a profound effect on a person's ability to use skills that they have already developed.

MULTIPLE CHOICE

Choose the best answer for each question or statement.

1. Growth and development usually follow patterns and stages and
   A. are always the same in all cultures.
   B. are identical in boys and girls.
   (C.) may occur at different rates in different people.
   D. are only different in old age.
2. Growth and development of infants
   A. is not predictable.
   (B.) usually follows predictable patterns.
   C. is about 5 pounds a month.
   D. is slower than other age ranges.
3. Growth and development in adolescence is
   A. more rapid than in infancy.
   B. unpredictable.
   C. faster for boys than for girls.
   (D.) characterized by development of secondary sex changes.
4. Development in a person includes learning skills such as
   A. cognitive skills.
   B. language skills.
   C. gross motor and fine motor skills.
   (D.) All of the above.

Instructor Notes

5. A developmental task of old age is
   A. coping with the death of parents.
   B. selecting a career.
   (C.) coping with the loss of friends.
   D. building socioeconomic status.

CRITICAL THINKING

CUSTOMER SERVICE

Encourage students to reflect and share their thoughts and experiences. Respect their privacy and confidentiality. Share your own viewpoints with the students.

CULTURAL CARE

Encourage students to reflect and share their thoughts and experiences. Respect their privacy and confidentiality. Share your own viewpoints with the students.

COOPERATION WITHIN THE TEAM

Encourage students to reflect and share their thoughts and experiences. Respect their privacy and confidentiality. Share your own viewpoints with the students.

NURSING ASSISTANT IN ACTION

You are working with a colleague who appears disrespectful when she talks to her patients. Her answers are short and curt. Sometimes she speaks to teenagers or older adults like they are small children. So far you have not said anything. Today your patient complains to you about your coworker's attitude.

What Is your Response/Action?

Apologize to the patient. Then go talk directly to your coworker to inform her of the problem. Tell her that the patient feels that she is not respectful of her age. If your coworker is not open to suggestion, you may consider talking to your nurse/supervisor. Your coworker may not be aware of how her communication style is perceived by patients.

Instructor Notes

15

Answers to Workbook Exercises

The following exercises will assist you to apply what you have read in Chapter 15, "Growth and Development." For each exercise, read the objective and use information you have read in Chapter 15 to answer the questions, complete the sentences, or label the diagrams.

EXERCISE 15-1

Objective: To be able to correctly match the chronological stage to the developmental stage of human growth and development.

Directions: From the Word List below, select and write the name of the developmental stage next to the matching time period on the Age List.

Word List

preschool	adolescent	toddler	older adult
school-age	young adult	infant	middle adult

Age List

5–12 years	*school-age*	1–2 year(s)	*toddler*
12–18 years	*adolescent*	18–40 years	*young adult*
65+ years	*older adult*	2–5 years	*preschool*
Birth–1 year	*infant*	40–65 years	*middle adult*

EXERCISE 15-2

Objective: To be able to recognize developmental skills and the tasks that illustrate them.

Directions: Place the correct letters next to the matching phrase.

CS = cognitive skill	GMS = gross motor skill
SS = social skill	FMS = fine motor skill
LS = language skill	

__CS__ **1.** A preschool child recognizes colors.

__LS__ **2.** The school-age child defines words.

__SS__ **3.** The older adult adjusts to retirement.

__SS__ **4.** The young adult selects a career.

__LS__ **5.** The infant vocalizes, squeals, and imitates sounds.

__GMS__ **6.** The toddler throws balls.

__GMS__ **7.** The infant rolls over, pulls to sit, crawls, and stands alone.

__FMS__ **8.** The school-age child draws a man having six parts.

__FMS__ **9.** The infant feeds himself crackers.

__SS__ **10.** The toddler expresses needs or indicates wants without crying.

EXERCISE 15-3

Objective: To apply what you have learned about nursing assistant behaviors and patient age-specific considerations.

Directions: Match the letter of the developmental stage with the correct age-specific consideration. Select only one answer for each statement.

Developmental Stages List

A. Infant: Birth–1 year.	E. Adolescent: 12–18 years
B. Toddler: 1–2 year(s)	F. Young adult: 18–40 years
C. Preschool: 2–5 years	G. Middle adult: 40–65 years
D. School-age: 5–12 years	H. Older adult: 65+ years

Age-specific Consideration

__A__ **1.** Place visually interesting objects where the child can observe them.

__C__ **2.** Explain procedures in simple words, describing only what the patient will see.

__D__ **3.** Describe how long children will have to undergo a painful procedure.

__B__ **4.** Keep small objects, which may cause choking, out of child's reach.

__H__ **5.** Patient may request that a family member be present to provide support in making a health care decision.

E 6. Remember that body image is very important at this stage.

G 7. Remember that they have many obligations, such as parenthood and the care of their parents.

F 8. They are often concerned about how illness will affect their lifelong goals.

EXERCISE 15-4

Objectives: To apply what you have learned about your role as a nursing assistant.

Directions: Circle the letter next to the statement that best completes the sentence or describes the sentence as true or false. If the sentence is false, draw a line through the incorrect part of the sentence and write the correction on the blank line.

1. Growth refers to the measurable physical changes human beings experience throughout their lives.
   (A.) True
   B. False
   Correct Answer: ____________________
2. Development refers to the accomplishment of, and the increase in, the ability to use skills that people acquire over their life span.
   (A.) True
   B. False
   Correct Answer: ____________________
3. Growth and development usually follow
   A. growth spurts.
   B. each other.
   (C.) stages.
   D. death.
4. Growth continues through all the stages of life, but it begins
   A. at the beginning.
   (B.) at conception.
   C. at birth.
   D. with life skills.
5. The gain in weight of infants from birth to 1 year
   (A.) is predictable within parameters.
   B. helps the mother feel better.
   C. is a sign of problems.
   D. is not measurable.

6. One indicator of proper growth is detected by
- A. measuring the baby's feet.
- B. measuring the mother's feet.
- C. measuring the umbilical cord.
- (D.) measuring the circumference of the baby's head periodically.

7. Humans build on skills they have developed
- (A.) at a previous stage of development.
- B. while sleeping.
- C. from observing their parents.
- D. through a nursing assistant course.

8. Injuries such as strokes make it necessary to relearn skills from earlier stages of development.
- (A.) True
- B. False

Correct Answer: ______________________

9. When people are ~~happy~~, they often behave at a lower developmental stage than their chronological age would indicate.
- A. True
- (B.) False

Correct Answer: *ill (or injured)*

10. The nursing assistant's ability to relate appropriately to patients is dependent on
- (A.) their awareness of the impact illness can have on patients at each stage of growth and development.
- B. the patient's attitude.
- C. whether they study this chapter.
- D. their immediate supervisor.

16

The Musculoskeletal System and Related Care

CHAPTER OVERVIEW

Instructor Notes

Instructor Notes

OBJECTIVES

When the students have completed this chapter, they will be able to:

- Identify the functions of the muscular system.
- Explain how groups of muscles work together to perform body motion.
- List the functions of the skeletal system.
- List the four general types of bones and give examples of each.
- Name three major types of joints and give examples of each.
- Label a diagram of the skeletal and surface muscles.
- Describe how aging affects the musculoskeletal system.
- List common diseases and disorders of the musculoskeletal system.
- Describe the scope of orthopedic nursing care and the purposes of orthopedic equipment.
- Describe and explain the reasons for special skin care for the orthopedic patient.
- List important points to observe while performing any nursing task involving patients in traction.
- List important points to observe while performing any nursing task involving patients in plaster casts.
- Identify several types of supportive devices and the nursing assistant's role in caring for patients who use such devices.

KEY TERMS

Abduction: Movement of an arm or leg away from the center of the body

Adduction: Movement of an arm or leg toward the center of the body

Arthritis: Chronic condition of inflammation of the joints

Atrophy: Wasting away of muscles; decrease in muscle size

Contract: Get smaller; shortening the length of muscle, thereby making the angle formed by bones and muscles smaller

Contracture: An abnormal shortening of a muscle

Extension: Straightening or lengthening a muscle, thereby making the angle formed by bones and muscles greater

Flex: To bend; the act of bending a body part

Flexion: Bending of a joint (elbow, wrist, knee)

Fracture: A break in a bone

Joint: A part of the body where two bones come together

Ligament: Tough, white fibrous cord that connects bone to bone

Orthopedics: The medical specialty that covers the treatment of broken bones, deformities, or diseases that attack the bones, joints, and muscles

Osteoarthritis: A degenerative, painful bone disease affecting the spine, hips, finger joints, or knees

Instructor Notes

Relax: To place in a resting position, in which muscle tension decreases and fibers lengthen

Rheumatoid Arthritis: A chronic disease condition affecting the connective tissue of the body, especially the joints

Traction: Exertion of pull by means of weights or pulleys, often used for realignment of bones or other limb tissues

Trapeze: A triangle-shaped bar attached to the overbed frame of a traction setup that enables the patient to pull himself up in bed

Walker: A metal frame device with handgrips and four legs that is open on one side; provides stability and security for the patient who is weak on one side or restricted in the amount of weight he can put on one foot

CORE STUDENT ASSIGNMENTS

Students should:

- Read this chapter in their textbook, *Being a Nursing Assistant*.
- Underline any words or sentences they do not understand. Write down any questions they have.
- Complete the Chapter Review in their textbook.
- Read the Time Management Tip for this chapter and think about how they might use this tip in their work.
- Complete the Nursing Assistant in Action exercise.

OPTIONAL STUDENT ASSIGNMENTS

Students should:

- Complete all workbook assignments for this chapter in their copy of *Workbook for Being a Nursing Assistant*.
- Use the CD/CD-Rom disk enclosed with their textbook to hear the pronunciation of the key terms in the chapter.
- Watch the "Body Mechanics" video from the Care Provider Skills series.
- Use the Website address **(www.prenhall.com/wolgin)** to access the free, interactive Companion Website created for this textbook. Get hints, instant feedback, and textbook references to chapter-related multiple-choice questions. Read and react to the Nursing Assistant in Action exercise. Link to other interesting sites.

METHODOLOGY AND SUGGESTED ACTIVITIES

I. Lecture/Discussion

- Answer any questions the students may have.
- Discuss the key terms and related abbreviations. Repeat them out loud and practice using them in sentences.
- Discuss the Time Management Tip for this chapter.
- Discuss the Nursing Assistant in Action exercise.

Instructor Notes

- Discuss the Critical Thinking points for this chapter.
- Discuss personal safety and protection. Emphasize the importance of following Universal Precautions.
- Use a model skeleton to enhance this lesson. Identify examples of each type of bone on the skeleton. Use the skeleton to demonstrate the movements of different types of joints.
- Review and discuss the diseases and conditions affecting bones, joints, and connective tissue.
- Consider arranging a visit from a physical therapist.
- Ask the students if they have ever broken an arm or leg. Have them share their experiences.

II. Role Play/Lab

- Show the video for this chapter. Watch how the muscle groups work together. Have the students practice moving and bending as they note the flexion and extension of their muscles. Practice exercises that can reduce stress and strain to muscles groups. Encourage students to "warm up" prior to lifting.
- Pass around a model of a skull so the students can familiarize themselves with the bones in the diagram. Plastic "skeletons" are also helpful for student learning.
- Display and demonstrate supportive and prosthetic devices, as appropriate.
- As a class project, have the students write a checklist for observing a patient in traction.
- Display the equipment for caring for musculoskeletal systems and have students practice using it.
- Have students practice placing each other in total hip precautions.
- Have the student practice active range-of motion and, passive range-of motion exercises.

III. Evaluation

- Review the answers to the Chapter Review with students.
- Review the answer to the workbook exercises with students.
- Review the students' understanding of the Time Management Tip.
- To evaluate student comprehension, give a quiz.
- Have the students visit the interactive Companion Website and take the quiz.

ANSWERS TO CHAPTER REVIEW

FILL IN THE BLANK

Read each sentence and fill in the blank line(s) with the word or words that complete the sentence. (Note: Hyphenated words get one line.)

1. ___Traction___ is the exertion of pull by weights or pulleys, often used for realignment of bones or other limb tissues.

Instructor Notes

2. The wasting away of or decrease in muscle size is called ___atrophy___.

3. ___Ligaments___ connect bone to bone.

4. ___Tendons___ connect muscle to bone.

5. ___Casts___ are used as a support to hold injured bones in alignment while they are healing.

MULTIPLE CHOICE

Choose the best answer for each question or statement.

1. Flexion refers to
   (A.) bending a part of the body.
   B. straightening a part of the body.
   C. relaxing a part of the body.
   D. All of the above.

2. Which of the following is not true about bones?
   A. There are 206 bones in the body.
   B. Bones are the framework of the body.
   (C.) Bones work together to provide body motion.
   D. Bones store vital minerals.

3. Which of the following is not true about muscles?
   A. Muscles provide the motion for our bodies.
   B. Muscles provide the motion for structures within our bodies.
   C. Muscles have an exceptionally rich blood supply.
   (D.) Muscles are joined by sutures

4. All of the following are diseases and disorders of the musculoskeletal system *except*
   A. bursitis.
   (B.) dermatitis.
   C. arthritis.
   D. osteoporosis.

5. Care for the total hip replacement patient may include all of the following *except*
   A. keeping a wedge-shaped pillow between the legs.
   B. turning the patient to the back and to the unoperated side.
   (C.) the patient will bear full weight on the operative leg.
   D. the patient cannot bend more than 60 degrees for 10 days after surgery.

Instructor Notes

CRITICAL THINKING

CUSTOMER SERVICE

Encourage students to reflect and share their thoughts and experiences. Respect their privacy and confidentiality. Share your own viewpoints with the students.

CULTURAL CARE

Encourage students to reflect and share their thoughts and experiences. Respect their privacy and confidentiality. Share your own viewpoints with the students.

COOPERATION WITHIN THE TEAM

Encourage students to reflect and share their thoughts and experiences. Respect their privacy and confidentiality. Share your own viewpoints with the students.

NURSING ASSISTANT IN ACTION

You are assigned to care for a frail elderly woman who has difficulty walking. She has stooped posture and osteoporosis. The slippers she is wearing do not seem to be staying on her feet very well. You are concerned she may trip or fall as she is making her way to the dining room to eat. You offer her your arm and say, "Let me escort you to your table, Ms. Sanford." She refuses your help and tells you she is perfectly capable of walking on her own. Your coworker overhears her remark and comments that if she falls it is her own fault.

What Is Your Response/Action?

First, you could walk next to Ms. Sanford without holding her to ensure her safety. Next, you could talk to your coworker and mention that Ms. Sanford is most likely trying to maintain her independence and her dignity by walking alone. Ms. Sanford's feelings may have been hurt by this remark or it may have spurred her to try and be even more independent and risk her safety. Finding better slippers may solve the safety problem as well as maintain Ms. Sanford's independence.

16

Answers to Workbook Exercises

The following exercises will assist you to apply what you have read in Chapter 16, "The Musculoskeletal System and Related Care." For each exercise, read the objective and use information you have read in Chapter 16 to answer the questions, complete the sentences, or label the diagrams.

EXERCISE 16-1

Objective: To recognize and be able to correctly spell the parts of the musculoskeletal system.

Directions: Label the diagram in Figure 16-1 with the correct words from the Word List below.

Word List

Muscles:

tibialis anterior	gastrocnemius	sartorius
rectus abdominus	quadriceps femoris	deltoid
pectoralis major	sternocleidomastoidius	biceps
tensor facia latae	peroneus longus	
abdominal muscle	intercostals	

Bones:

Humerus	fibula	clavicle	metacarpals
metatarsals	scapula	tibia	ribs
vertebrae	maxilla	radius	femur
sternum	frontal bone	pelvic bone	
cervical vertebrae	patella	ulna	
parietal	phalanges	mandible	

FIGURE 16.1

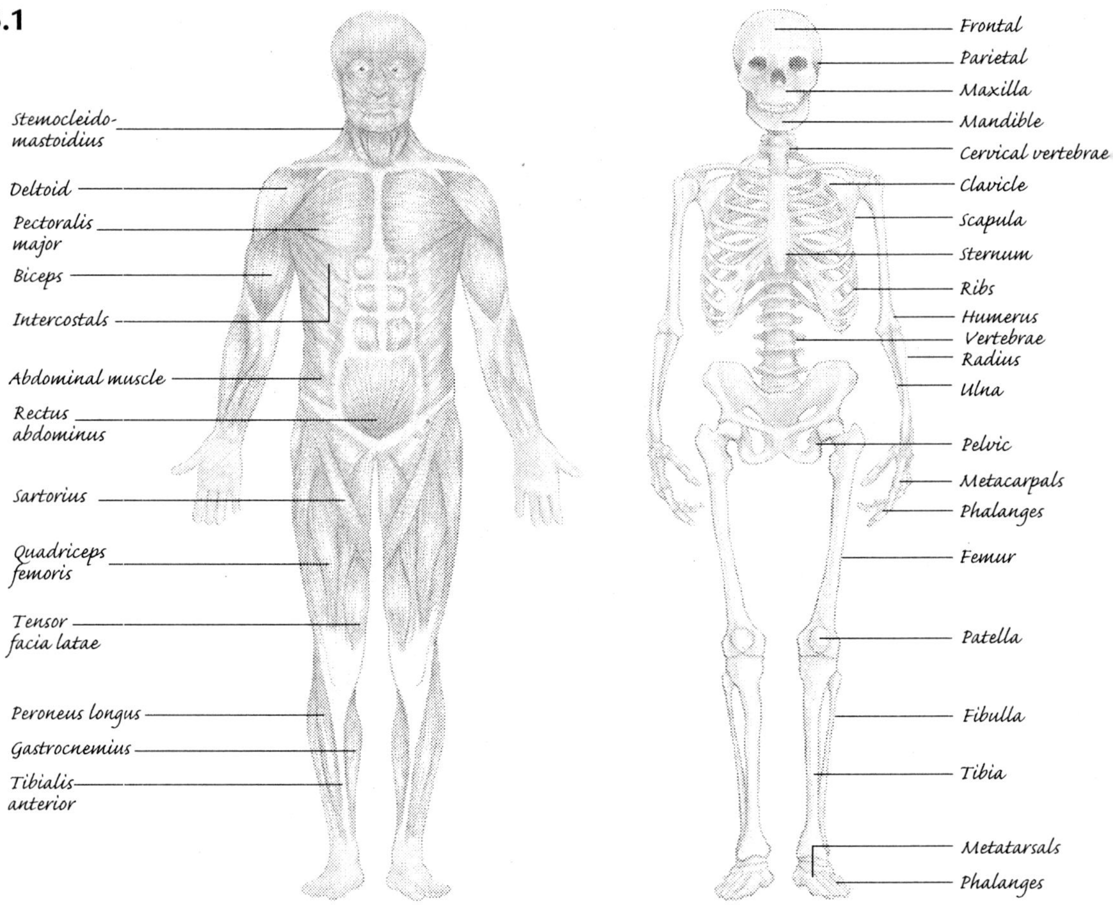

EXERCISE 16-2

Objective: To be able to name the category to which bones belong.

Directions: Draw a line to connect the bone with the correct category.

Category	Bone
Long bones	Vertebrae
Short bones	Ribs
Irregular bones	Phalanges
Flat bones	Femurs

EXERCISE 16-3

Objective: To correctly identify the types of joints of the human body.

Directions: Circle the words in the Word List below that identify the major types of joints of the human body.

Word List

(shoulder) metatarsals (elbow) femur (wrist) mandible
radius (ankle) scapula (hip) radius tibia
(hinge) (ball-and-socket) (pivot) (irregular joints of the spine)
(knee)

EXERCISE 16-4

Objective: To recognize and correctly spell words that name the muscles of the body.

Directions: Unscramble the words in the Word List on the left. Then circle the same words in the Word Search at the right.

Word List

1. TIDOLED ___DELTOID___
2. SUTSAV ___VASTUS___
3. ROTRASSUI ___SARTORIUS___
4. SEPCIB ___BICEPS___
5. LORTINCESTA ___INTERCOSTAL___
6. MIUSENROTSAGC ___GASTROCNEMIUS___
7. CURTES ___RECTUS___
8. LABITISI ___TIBIALIS___
9. TERBEREVA ___VERTEBRAE___

Word Search

D	A	B	D	O	M	U	N	I	L	U	Y	P	O	V	A	R
E	S	B	V	R	E	N	N	N	U	M	E	Q	H	A	A	E
L	A	K	O	P	M	Y	W	T	X	U	P	I	J	S	A	C
T	R	B	I	C	E	P	S	E	U	P	P	E	R	T	Q	T
O	T	H	G	A	S	R	R	R	C	N	E	M	I	U	S	U
I	O	W	N	I	M	C	I	C	E	R	H	I	V	S	Z	S
D	R	O	G	A	S	T	R	O	C	N	E	M	I	U	S	O
D	I	T	I	B	I	A	L	S	T	O	F	W	O	R	D	S
P	U	L	L	I	V	E	R	T	E	B	R	A	E	R	T	Y
H	S	H	U	M	P	A	A	A	A	D	A	F	A	L	L	X
M	A	H	T	I	B	I	A	L	I	S	T	T	L	E	L	A

EXERCISE 16-5

Objective: To recall common diseases and disorders of the orthopedic patient.

Directions: Complete the sentences with the correct words from the Word List below.

Word List

sprain	bone	simple fracture	joint dislocation
compound	Guillain-Barré	tuberculosis	muscular dystrophy
arthritis	spinal cord	poliomyelitis	trauma to spinal cord
atrophy	contracture		

1. An injury in which ligaments are partially torn is a(n) ___sprain___.
2. A fracture of a bone with no bone sticking out through the skin is called a(n) ___simple___ ___fracture___.
3. ___Tuberculosis___ can be a disease of the bone; usually affects the lungs.
4. ___Arthritis___ is known as a joint disease.
5. A(n) ___joint___ ___dislocation___ is the pulling out (displacement) of a bone end that forms part of a joint.
6. ___Trauma to spinal cord___ can result in damage to the ___spinal___ ___cord___, causing paralysis of some area of the body.
7. A nervous system disease is the ___Guillain-Barré___ syndrome.
8. ___Poliomyelitis___ is a disease that is not often seen due to the use of preventive vaccines in babies and young children.
9. A disorder that can occur when muscles are immobile for several weeks or months is ___muscular___ ___dystrophy___.
10. A(n) ___compound___ fracture is when the ___bone___ is broken and there is an external wound or bone protruding through the skin.
11. Wasting away of muscles is called ___atrophy___.
12. A ___contracture___ is the abnormal shortening of a muscle.

EXERCISE 16-6

Objective: To apply what you have learned about the musculoskeletal system and related care.

Directions: Circle the letter next to the statement that best completes the sentence or describes the sentence as true or false. If the sentence is false, draw a line through the incorrect part of the sentence and write the correction on the blank line.

1. The healing of broken bones is a gradual process in which ________ is deposited at the fracture site.

A. iron
(B.) calcium
C. glue
D. blood

2. During each body movement, the skeletal system, the muscular system, the circulatory system, and the ~~reproductive system~~ are all interacting.

A. True
(B.) False
Correct Answer: nervous system

3. Which of the following is a condition/disease of the bone?

A. Arthritis
B. Osteoporosis
C. Rheumatoid arthritis
(D.) All of the above

4. The knee is an example of a ________ joint.

A. rapid
B. stiff
C. painful
(D.) hinge

5. The use of a continuous passive range-of-motion machine (CPM) promotes ________ of the knee joint after total knee replacement surgery.

A. strength
B. rigidity
(C.) flexibility
D. tenderness

6. The ________ connect muscle to bone.

(A.) tendons
B. tenderloins
C. nerves
D. synapses

7. Nursing assistants need to be familiar with orthopedic equipment such as
   A. splints, nasogastric tubes, and casts.
   B. casts, walkers, and thermometers.
   C. walkers, casts, and zippers.
   (D.) splints, casts, and walkers.

8. In the past, traction and bedrest were the methods of treatment for fractures, but today the emphasis is on
   A. low-fat diets.
   B. improved methods of surgery and extended hospital stays.
   (C.) lighter casting materials and early ambulation.
   D. shortened hospital stays and low-fat diets.

9. When ambulating a total hip replacement (THR) patient, it is important to know how much weight bearing is allowed on the affected leg.
   (A.) True
   B. False
   Correct Answer: ______________________________

10. One of the benefits of early ambulation is fewer circulatory side effects.
    (A.) True
    B. False
    Correct Answer: ______________________________

11. A device that replaces a bone or a joint is called a
    A. protrusion.
    (B.) prosthesis.
    C. proboscis.
    D. partition.

12. Some braces must be worn continually, and some are worn only when the patient is out of bed. Therefore, it is important to check the plan of care or ask your immediate supervisor for instructions if your patient is using a brace.
    (A.) True
    B. False
    Correct Answer: ______________________________

13. Restricted __________ means that an orthopedic patient will need special skin care.
    A. permission
    (B.) mobility
    C. diet
    D. tolerance

14. The type of surgery a patient has will determine what kind of walker he should use.
    (A.) True
    B. False
    Correct Answer: ______________________________

15. You should change the position of an immobile patient at least every ~~4~~ hours.

A. True

(B.) False

Correct Answer: 2

16. A trapeze is a device that is suspended from an over-the-bed frame and allows the patient to

A. receive better television reception.

B. summon the nurse.

C. swing forward and backward.

(D.) move or lift himself more easily.

17. In the past, casts were made only out of plaster, a heavy material. Now casts are more often made of plastic or fiberglass. These modern casts are lighter, allowing the patient to move more easily.

(A.) True

B. False

Correct Answer: __________

18. Casts can become too tight after they are applied, causing the skin on either side of the cast edge to become blue or pale in color or ~~hot~~ to the touch.

A. True

(B.) False

Correct Answer: cool

19. Any complaint of pain around, under, or near the cast must be reported immediately to the nurse or your immediate supervisor.

(A.) True

B. False

Correct Answer: __________

20. Cast are made of which of the following materials?

A. Gortey

B. Plaster

C. Fiberglass

(D.) All of the above

21. Casted extremities should be compared to uncasted extremities for

A. changes in length.

B. changes in flexibility.

(C.) changes in size, color, and warmth.

D. the presence of nodules.

22. An unusual odor coming from a cast could mean that

A. fiber in the diet has been increased.

B. it is ready to be removed.

C. the extremity has healed.

(D.) a pressure ulcer or infection is developing under the cast.

17

The Integumentary System and Related Care

CHAPTER OVERVIEW

Instructor Notes

I. **The Skin (Integumentary System)**
   A. Appendages of the Skin
   B. Primary Functions of the Skin
   C. Inspecting the Skin
   D. Common Disorders of the Skin

II. **Care of the Patient with Potential Skin Problems**
   A. Pressure Ulcers
   B. Risk Factors for Pressure Ulcer Development
   C. Signs of a Pressure Ulcer
   D. Preventing Pressure Ulcers
   E. Foot Care

III. **Equipment and Devices That Reduce Pressure on the Skin**
   A. Mattresses, Overlays, and Beds
      1. Foam Mattresses
      2. Four-Inch High-Density Foam
      3. Static Air Mattress
      4. Alternating Air Mattress
      5. Specialty Bed
      6. Eggcrate Mattress
   B. Chair Cushions
   C. Extremities: Foot, Heel, Arms
      1. Protective Boots
      2. Orthotic Devices
      3. Foot Elevators ("Donuts")
      4. Foot Cradle
      5. Footboard
      6. Sheepskin Pad
      7. Heel or Elbow Protectors
   D. Other Devices

Instructor Notes

OBJECTIVES

When the students have completed this chapter, they will be able to:

- Describe the functions of the skin, including how heat is conserved and dispersed.
- List the conditions to take note of or report when examining a person's skin.
- Describe the common disorders of the skin.
- Describe age-related changes in the skin.
- Describe pressure ulcers and list the factors that contribute to their development.
- Discuss how to prevent pressure ulcers.
- Discuss guidelines for foot care.
- Describe the equipment and devices that reduce pressure on the skin.
- Describe the procedure for safe skin cleansing and moisturizing.

KEY TERMS

Atrophic Skin: Thin, fragile, less elastic skin frequently associated with aging

Bony Prominences: Places where bones are close to the surface of the skin

Dermis: The inner layer of skin

Epidermis: The outer layer or surface of the skin

Friction Injuries: Injuries resulting from the patient sliding against hard surfaces

Incontinent: Unable to control urine or feces

Integumentary System: The body system that includes the skin, hair, nails, and sweat and oil glands, that provides the first line of defense against infection, maintains body temperature, provides fluids, and eliminates wastes

Lesion: An abnormality, either benign or cancerous, of the tissues of the body, such as a wound, sore, rash, boil, tumors, or growths

Obese: Very overweight

Perineum: The body area between the thighs (external genitalia and rectal area)

Pressure Ulcers: Also called bedsores; areas of the skin that become broken and painful; caused by continuous pressure on a body part and usually occurring when a patient is kept in one position for a long period of time

Shear Injuries: Result from the skin remaining in place on top of a surface while the underlying structures, such as the bone, slide downward

CORE STUDENT ASSIGNMENTS

Instructor Notes

Students should:

- Read this chapter in their textbook, *Being a Nursing Assistant.*
- Underline any words or sentences they do not understand. Write down any questions they have.
- Complete the Chapter Review in their textbook.
- Read the Time Management Tip for this chapter and think about how they might use this tip in their work.
- Complete the Nursing Assistant in Action exercise.

OPTIONAL STUDENT ASSIGNMENTS

Students should:

- Complete all workbook assignments for this chapter in their copy of *Workbook for Being a Nursing Assistant.*
- Use the CD/CD-Rom disk enclosed with their textbook to hear the pronunciation of the key terms in the chapter.
- Watch the "Bed Bath" video from the Care Provider Skills series to learn about how to take good care of skin.
- Use the Website address **(www.prenhall.com/wolgin)** to access the free, interactive Companion Website created for this textbook. Get hints, instant feedback, and textbook references to chapter-related multiple-choice questions. Read and react to the Nursing Assistant in Action exercise. Link to other interesting sites.

METHODOLOGY AND SUGGESTED ACTIVITIES

I. Lecture/Discussion

- Answer any questions the students may have.
- Discuss the key terms and related abbreviations. Repeat them out loud and practice using them in sentences.
- Discuss the Time Management Tip for this chapter.
- Discuss the Nursing Assistant in Action exercise.
- Discuss the Critical Thinking points for this chapter.
- Discuss personal safety and protection. Emphasize the importance of following Universal Precautions.
- Offer examples of case studies of common diseases and disorders of the integumentary system.
- Explain the role of the skin in regulating body temperature.
- Discuss the function of the epidermis and the dermis as the protective covering of the body.
- Consider inviting a wound care specialist to talk to the students about skin care and pressure reduction strategies.

Instructor Notes

II. Role Play/Lab
- Show the videos for this chapter. Discuss how soap can dry the skin. Review and demonstrate how various skin care products help the skin. Have the students select skin care products for best use with patients of various cultural backgrounds.
- Have the students practice applying some pressure-reducing equipment to each other.
- Arrange a field trip to a local burn center.
- Invite a dermatologist to speak to the class.
- Display and demonstrate the skin care products used in your institution.
- Have the students stay absolutely still to experience immobility and pressure sensations.

III. Evaluation
- Review the answers to the Chapter Review with students.
- Review the answers to the workbook exercises with students.
- Review the students' understanding of the Time Management Tip.
- To evaluate student comprehension, give a quiz.
- To evaluate student skills, administer the competency checklist.
- Have the students visit the interactive Companion Website and take the quiz.

ANSWERS TO CHAPTER REVIEW

FILL IN THE BLANK

Read each sentence and fill in the blank line(s) with the word or words that complete the sentence. (Note: Hyphenated words get one line.)

1. ____Epidermis____ is the outer layer or surface of the skin.
2. ____Dermis____ is the inner layer of skin.
3. A ____pressure____ ____ulcer____ is an area of tissue destruction or lesion resulting from prolonged, unrelieved pressure.
4. When the head of the bed is elevated too high, and the patient slides down in bed, it can result in a ____friction____ or ____shear____ injury.
5. Pressure sores on the feet can be serious, sometimes leading to ____amputation____ and even death.

MULTIPLE CHOICE

Choose the best answer for each question or statement.

1. Which of the following is not a function of the integumentary system?
   A. The skin is the first line of defense against infection.
   B. The skin maintains body temperature.
   C. The skin covers and protects underlying structures from injury.
   (D.) The skin provides movement for the body.

Instructor Notes

2. Which of the following is not an observation about skin?
   A. Color
   (B.) Pressure
   C. Rashes
   D. Reddened, darkened areas
3. Which of the following is not a common disorder of the skin?
   (A.) Arthritis
   B. Excoriations
   C. Impetigo
   D. Herpes zoster
4. As patients age, their skin may experience all of these changes *except*
   A. thinning of skin.
   B. atrophy of skin.
   C. development of brown spots.
   (D.) reddening of skin.
5. Which of these following conditions should you report to the nurse?
   A. Reddening of skin
   B. Cyanosis
   C. A black "scablike" skin (eschar)
   (D.) All of the above.

CRITICAL THINKING

CUSTOMER SERVICE

Encourage students to reflect and share their thoughts and experiences. Respect their privacy and confidentiality. Share your own viewpoints with the students.

CULTURAL CARE

Encourage students to reflect and share their thoughts and experiences. Respect their privacy and confidentiality. Share your own viewpoints with the students.

COOPERATION WITHIN THE TEAM

Encourage students to reflect and share their thoughts and experiences. Respect their privacy and confidentiality. Share your own viewpoints with the students.

NURSING ASSISTANT IN ACTION

You are caring for an elderly woman who is diabetic. The skin on both of her swollen legs is red. You see she has new sores on both legs. Ms. Francis tells you that the skin on her legs feels like it is burning. She applied some lotion on them and that only made it worse.

Instructor Notes

What Is Your Response/Action?

You should report your observations to the nurse immediately. Then you would most likely wash the lotion off Ms. Francis's legs. She may be having a reaction to the lotion that is causing her skin to turn red and create sores. As a diabetic, Ms. Francis may have a harder time healing skin compared to a nondiabetic patient.

Answers to Workbook Exercises

17

The following exercises will assist you to apply what you have read in Chapter 17, "The Integumentary System and Related Care." For each exercise, read the objective and use information you have read in Chapter 17 to answer the questions, complete the sentences, or label the diagrams.

EXERCISE 17-1

Objective: To recognize the definitions of words related to the integumentary system and related care.

Directions: Place the letter of the correct definition next to the matching word(s) from the Word List below.

Word List

__K__ **1.** epidermis

__H__ **2.** atrophic skin

__L__ **3.** bony prominences

__G__ **4.** shear injuries

__B__ **5.** lesion

__C__ **6.** incontinent

__J__ **7.** perineum

__D__ **8.** integumentary system

__F__ **9.** dermis

__A__ **10.** friction injuries

__E__ **11.** pressure ulcers

__I__ **12.** obese

Definitions

A. Injuries resulting from the patient sliding against hard surfaces

B. An abnormality, either benign or cancerous, of the tissues of the body, such as a wound, sore, rash, boil, tumors, or growths

C. Unable to control urine or feces

D. The body system that includes the skin, hair, nails, and sweat and oil glands, that provides the first line of defense against infection, maintains body temperature, provides fluids, and eliminates wastes

E. Also called bedsores; areas of the skin that become broken and painful; caused by continuous pressure on a body part and usually occurring when a patient is kept in one position for a long period of time

F. The inner layer of skin

G. Result from the skin remaining in place on top of a surface while the underlying structures, such as bone, slide downward

H. Thin, fragile, less elastic skin frequently associated with aging

I. Very overweight

J. The body area between the thighs (external genitalia and rectal area)

K. The outer layer or surface of the skin

L. Places where bones are close to the surface of the skin

EXERCISE 17-2

Objective: To identify important protective devices for the skin.

Directions: Read the following riddles carefully before writing the correct answer on the blank line.

1. This device helps to elevate an extremity off the bed. What is it? *Hint:* An alternative meaning goes well with coffee in the morning.
   ______donut______

2. This item is used to keep blankets off the legs and feet. What is it? *Hint:* An alternative meaning is a small bed for a baby. ______cradle______

3. This device prevents a serious deformity to the foot. What is it? *Hint:* An alternative meaning is something you would want to wear in the snow or rain. ______boot______

EXERCISE 17-3

Objective: To recognize and correctly spell the structures of the skin.

Directions: Label the diagram in Figure 17-1 with the correct words from the Word List below.

Word List

sweat gland	epidermis	hair
sebaceous gland	dermis	fat
pores	blood vessel	nerve

FIGURE 17-1

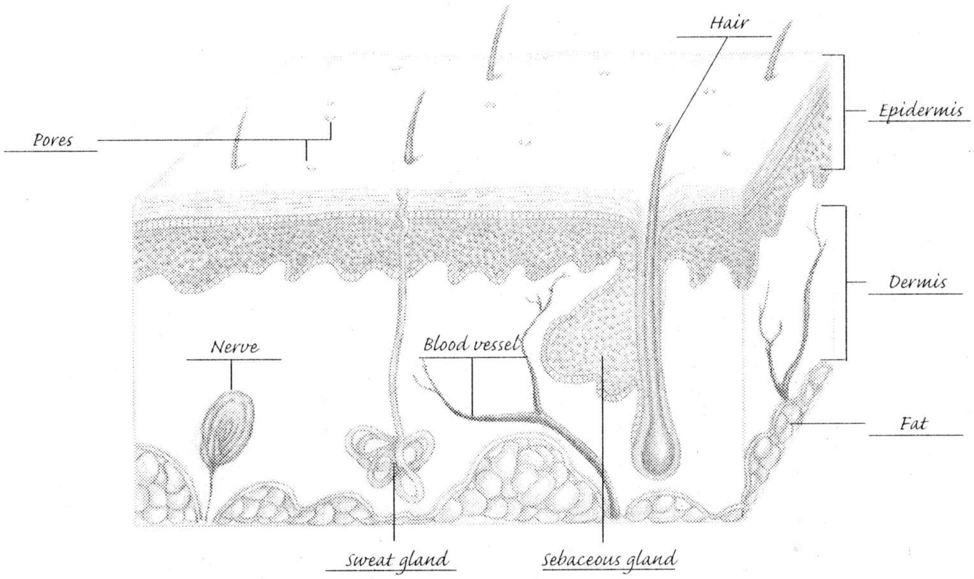

EXERCISE 17-4

Objective: To apply what you have learned about the integumentary system and related care.

Directions: Circle the letter of the word or phrase that best completes the sentence or describes the sentence as true or false. If the sentence is false, draw a line through the incorrect part of the sentence and write the correction on the blank line.

1. The ________ covers the entire body.
   A. dermis
   B. epidermis
   C. skin
   (D.) all of the above

2. ________ is responsible for the color of the skin.
   A. Dermis
   B. Epidermis
   C. Toner
   (D.) Pigment

3. The primary function of the skin is all of the following *except* to
   A. cover and protect underlying body structures from injury and invasion by microorganisms.
   (B.) provide an area for exchange of oxygen.
   C. help regulate body temperature.
   D. eliminate wastes through perspiration.

4. Serious health problems can cause ________ in the skin.
   (A.) changes
   B. improvement
   C. illumination
   D. healthy growth

5. Fungus is caused by ________ organisms.
   A. animal-like
   (B.) plant-like
   C. child-like
   D. solar-like

6. Chicken pox viruses can cause another painful skin disease called
   A. athlete's foot.
   B. pediculisis pedis.
   (C.) shingles.
   D. psoriasis.

7. As people age, the skin
   A. becomes more elastic.
   B. flakes away.
   C. grows thicker and tougher.
   (D.) becomes less elastic and more fragile.

8. People who are in shock will have skin that is more pale than usual.
   (A.) True
   B. False
   Correct Answer: ________________________________

9. Loss of fat cells in the skin can make a person feel ________ even when room temperatures feel warm to others.
   A. thinner
   B. warmer
   (C.) cold
   D. sweaty

10. Decreased ______ caused by prolonged pressure in an area can lead to pressure ulcers.
    A. digestion
    (B.) circulation
    C. exercise
    D. posture

11. In addition to prolonged pressure, other reasons for decubitus ulcer formation are all of the following *except*
    A. a lack of cleanliness.
    B. moisture.
    C. material from wound drainage.
    (D.) body lotion applied in a circular motion after the bath.

12. All patients need to be observed to prevent pressure ulcer formation. All of the following are risk factors for pressure ulcers *except*

A. moist skin.
B. mobility problems.
(C.) good nutrition.
D. numbness in a body part.

13. The pressure ulcer visible on the surface is often much smaller than the skin damage below the surface.

(A.) True
B. False
Correct Answer: ______________________________

14. The best place to check for signs of pressure are all of the following *except*

(A.) the abdomen.
B. the elbows.
C. the hips.
D. the sacrum.

15. The nursing assistant should report the first signs (redness) of a pressure ulcer formation to the immediate supervisor.

(A.) True
B. False
Correct Answer: ______________________________

16. A type of pressure ulcer that is difficult to heal is

A. a small ulcer.
B. a moderate-sized ulcer.
C. a large ulcer.
(D.) all of the above.

17. Friction/shear injuries can occur if

A. the side rails are too high.
B. the patient ambulates often.
C. the gown is not tied tightly.
(D.) the head of the bed is elevated too high.

18. To prevent friction/shear injuries,

A. use a restraint on active patients.
B. restrict bed movement.
(C.) use a draw sheet to pull patients up in bed and for turning them.
D. leave the patient on the bedpan for more than 20 minutes.

19. To prevent pressure between the legs when positioning the patient, use pillows.

(A.) True
B. False
Correct Answer: ______________________________

20. A patient using an eggcrate mattress ~~will not~~ develop a pressure ulcer.
    A. True
    (B.) False
    Correct Answer: *may still*

21. The feet must be kept in good alignment to prevent a serious deformity called
    A. alignment pox.
    B. athlete's foot.
    C. chin drop.
    (D.) foot drop.

22. Do not place an incontinent patient
    (A.) directly on the plastic side of the bed protector.
    B. directly on an incontinent pad.
    C. on a clean dry sheet.
    D. into a disposable diaper before sitting them in a chair.

23. The patient's position should be changed at least every 2 hours
    A. unless you are busy.
    B. unless they refuse to be repositioned.
    (C.) or less.
    D. during the day only.

24. If the patient's toenails need to be trimmed, the nursing assistant should
    A. trim them immediately.
    B. soak them before trimming them.
    (C.) notify the nurse.
    D. call the doctor.

25. In order to provide all the care a patient needs within a limited time frame, you must
    A. stop when tired.
    B. arrive earlier or work later than assigned.
    C. skip some of the work.
    (D.) plan the day efficiently

COMPETENCY CHECKLIST 17-1: SKIN CARE

ACTIVITY	S	U	COMMENTS
Student will demonstrate the correct method of providing safe skin cleansing for the incontinent patient.			

18

The Circulatory and Respiratory Systems and Related Care

CHAPTER OVERVIEW

Instructor Notes

I. **The Circulatory System: Anatomy and Physiology**
   A. The Heart
   B. The Blood
   C. The Blood Vessels
   D. Inactivity and Blood Circulation

II. **The Circulatory System and the Normal Aging Process**

III. **Common Diseases and Disorders of the Circulatory System**

IV. **The Respiratory System: Anatomy and Physiology**
   A. Oxygen and Carbon Dioxide Exchange
   B. Respiratory Care after Surgery

V. **The Respiratory System and the Normal Aging Process**

VI. **Common Diseases and Disorders of the Respiratory System**
   A. Tuberculosis
   B. Chronic Obstructive Pulmonary Disease
   C. Indications a Patient May Require Supplemental Oxygen
   D. Therapies Related to Respiratory Disease

Instructor Notes

OBJECTIVES

When the students have completed this chapter, they will be able to:

- Describe the functions of the heart and blood.
- Label a diagram with the organs of the circulatory and respiratory systems.
- Describe the functions of the respiratory system.
- Summarize how the circulatory and respiratory systems change with age.
- Identify common diseases and disorders of the respiratory and circulatory systems.
- List important precautions for patients with tuberculosis.
- List important precautions for patients receiving oxygen therapy.

KEY TERMS

Anemia: A shortage of red blood cells

Artery: Blood vessel that carries oxygenated blood away from the heart

Blood Pressure: The force of the blood pushing against the walls of the blood vessels

Cardiac: Pertaining to the heart

Circulation: The continuous movement of blood through the heart and blood vessels to all parts of the body

Circulatory System: The heart, blood vessels, blood, and all organs that pump and carry blood and other fluids throughout the body

Heart: A four-chambered, hollow, muscular organ that lies in the chest cavity and pumps the blood through the lungs and into all parts of the body

Plasma: The liquid portion of the blood

Pulmonary: Pertaining to the lungs

Respiratory System: The group of body organs that carries on the body function of respiration; the system brings oxygen into the body and eliminates carbon dioxide

Tuberculosis (TB): A highly infectious disease that usually affects the lungs

Vein: Blood vessel that carries blood from parts of the body back to the heart

CORE STUDENT ASSIGNMENTS

Students should:

- Read this chapter in their textbook, *Being a Nursing Assistant*.
- Underline any words or sentences they do not understand. Write down any questions they have.
- Complete the Chapter Review in their textbook.
- Read the Time Management Tip for this chapter and think about how they might use this tip in their work.
- Complete the Nursing Assistant in Action exercise.

OPTIONAL STUDENT ASSIGNMENTS

Instructor Notes

Students should:

- Complete all workbook assignments for this chapter in their copy of *Workbook for Being a Nursing Assistant*.
- Use the CD/CD-Rom disk enclosed with their textbook to hear the pronunciation of the key terms in the chapter.
- Watch the "Measuring Vital Signs" video from the Care Provider Skills series.
- Use the Website address **(www.prenhall.com/wolgin)** to access the free, interactive Companion Website created for this textbook. Get hints, instant feedback, and textbook references to chapter-related multiple-choice questions. Read and react to the Nursing Assistant in Action exercise. Link to other interesting sites.

METHODOLOGY AND SUGGESTED ACTIVITIES

I. Lecture/Discussion

- Answer any questions the students may have.
- Discuss the key terms and related abbreviations. Repeat them out loud and practice using them in sentences.
- Discuss the Time Management Tip for this chapter.
- Discuss the Nursing Assistant in Action exercise.
- Discuss the Critical Thinking points for this chapter.
- Discuss personal safety and protection. Emphasize the importance of following Universal Precautions. Stress the need to wear protective equipment.
- Describe the flow of blood through the body. Play matching games to learn the parts of the heart and lungs.
- Offer examples of case studies of common diseases and disorders of the circulatory system. Review CPR themes.
- Offer examples of case studies of common diseases and disorders of the respiratory system.
- Explain the necessity for memorizing adult normal rates and the policy for reporting abnormal findings.
- Arrange for a respiratory therapist to talk with the students.
- Visit a cardiac rehabilitation center.
- Discuss the impact of smoking on the body.

II. Role Play/Lab

- Show the video for this chapter. Discuss the importance of accuracy of vital signs to patient treatment decisions.
- Play a bingo-style game with the diseases of the circulatory and respiratory system.
- Use flash cards to help the students learn the diseases and body systems.
- Review and demonstrate the use of personal protective equipment for tuberculosis.
- Have the students practice coughing and deep breathing and using an incentive spirometer.

Instructor Notes

- Have the students practice applying nasal cannula tubing and checking for skin breakdown or irritation.

III. Evaluation

- Review the answers to the Chapter Review with students.
- Review the answer to the workbook exercises with students.
- Review the students' understanding of the Time Management Tip.
- To evaluate student comprehension, give a quiz.
- Have the students visit the interactive Companion Website and take the quiz.

ANSWERS TO CHAPTER REVIEW

FILL IN THE BLANK

Read each sentence and fill in the blank line(s) with the word or words that complete the sentence. (Note: Hyphenated words get one line.)

1. The ____heart____ is a four-chambered, hollow, muscular organ that lies in the chest cavity and pumps blood through the lungs and into all parts of the body.
2. ____Plasma____ is the liquid portion of the blood.
3. The structures that carry oxygenated blood from the heart are called ____arteries____.
4. If food gets into the trachea or in the lungs, it is known as ____aspiration____.
5. ____Peripheral____ ____vascular____ disease results from restricted or poor functioning of the valves of the veins.

MULTIPLE CHOICE

Choose the best answer for each question or statement.

1. Functions of the blood include all of the following *except*
   A. carries oxygen from the lungs to the cells.
   (B.) protects underlying structures.
   C. carries carbon dioxide from the cells to the lungs.
   D. carries waste products from the cells to the kidneys.
2. Which of the following is not true about the heart?
   A. It acts as a pump for the body.
   B. It is made up of four chambers.
   C. It is a muscular organ.
   (D.) It is the primary defense against infection for the body.

Instructor Notes

3. Blood pressure is
   (A.) the force of the blood pushing against the walls of the blood vessels.
   B. the force of the blood pushing against the valves of the heart.
   C. the force of the blood pushing against the lungs.
   D. the ability of the heart to pump blood.

4. Common diseases and disorders of the circulatory system include all of the following *except*
   A. arteriosclerosis.
   (B.) psoriasis.
   C. myocardial infarction.
   D. congestive heart failure.

5. Common diseases and disorders of the respiratory system include all of the following *except*
   A. sinusitis.
   B. pneumonia.
   (C.) anemia.
   D. bronchitis.

CRITICAL THINKING

CUSTOMER SERVICE

Encourage students to reflect and share their thoughts and experiences. Respect their privacy and confidentiality. Share your own viewpoints with the students.

CULTURAL CARE

Encourage students to reflect and share their thoughts and experiences. Respect their privacy and confidentiality. Share your own viewpoints with the students.

COOPERATION WITHIN THE TEAM

Encourage students to reflect and share their thoughts and experiences. Respect their privacy and confidentiality. Share your own viewpoints with the students.

NURSING ASSISTANT IN ACTION

You are caring for a 57-year-old patient who has chronic emphysema and COPD. He was smoking two to three packs of cigarettes a day before being admitted to the hospital. He has difficulty breathing, coughs, and spits up lots of thick secretions. He is asking for you to give him his cigarettes. He is too sick to leave his room to go smoke outside. Your facility has a no smoking policy. You think maybe some nicotine patches might be helpful, but are unsure if his doctor would order these.

Instructor Notes

What Is Your Response/Action?

Due to the increased fire potential of smoking in a hospital, where oxygen and other flammable materials are commonly used, you should follow your instinct by not giving him the cigarettes. Not only is this bad for his health, it also puts other patients and staff at risk due to the fire potential of smoking in a hospital. The nicotine patches are a good idea to suggest to the nurse. She can talk to the physician about an order for the patches.

Answers to Workbook Exercises

18

The following exercises will assist you to apply what you have read in Chapter 18, "The Circulatory and Respiratory Systems and Related Care." For each exercise, read the objective and use information you have read in Chapter 18 to answer the questions, complete the sentences, or label the diagram.

EXERCISE 18-1

Objective: To recognize definitions of words related to the circulatory system and patient care.

Directions: Place the letter of the correct definition next to the matching word(s) from the Word List.

Word List

B **1.** anemia

I **2.** heart

E **3.** blood pressure

A **4.** circulation

L **5.** vein

C **6.** tuberculosis

J **7.** pulmonary

K **8.** respiratory system

D **9.** artery

F **10.** circulatory system

H **11.** plasma

G **12.** cardiac

Definitions

A. The continuous movement of blood through the heart and blood vessels to all parts of the body

B. A shortage of red blood cells

C. A highly infectious disease that usually affects the lungs

D. Blood vessel that carries oxygenated blood away from the heart

E. The force of the blood pushing against the walls of the blood vessels

F. The heart, blood vessels, blood, and all organs that pump and carry blood and other fluids throughout the body

G. Pertaining to the heart

H. The liquid portion of the blood

I. A four-chambered, hollow, muscular organ that lies in the chest cavity and pumps the blood through the lungs and into all parts of the body

J. Pertaining to the lungs

K. The group of body organs that carries on the body function of respiration; the system brings oxygen into the body and eliminates carbon dioxide

L. Blood vessel that carries blood from parts of the body back to the heart

EXERCISE 18-2

Objective: To recognize and be able to correctly spell the names of various parts of the circulatory system.

Directions: Label the diagram in Figure 18-1 with the correct words from the word list below.

Word List

pulmonary capillaries	pulmonary veins	aorta (artery)
pulmonary arteries	systemic capillaries	venule
arteriole	capillaries	vena cavae (vein)

FIGURE 18-1

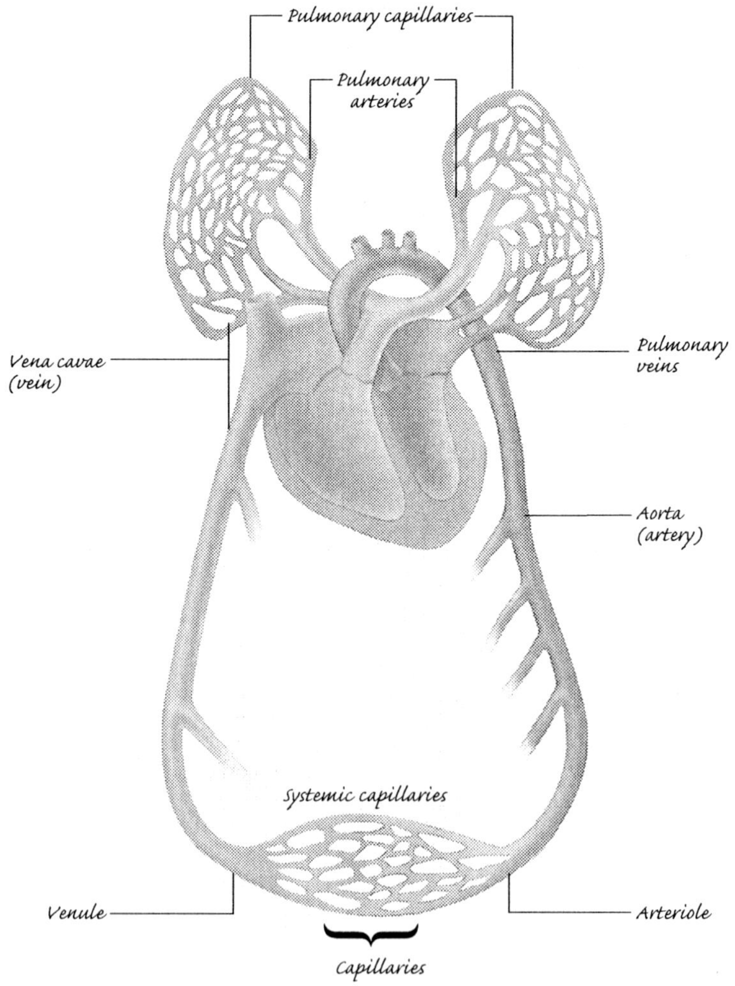

EXERCISE 18-3

Objective: To recognize and be able to correctly spell the names of various parts of the heart.

Directions: Label the diagram in Figure 18-2 with the correct words from the word list below.

Word List

superior vena cava	pulmonary veins
pulmonary artery	left ventricle
inferior vena cava	right ventricle
myocardium (muscle)	pulmonary artery
aorta	epicardium (outer covering)
left atrium	pulmonary veins
right atrium	

FIGURE 18-2

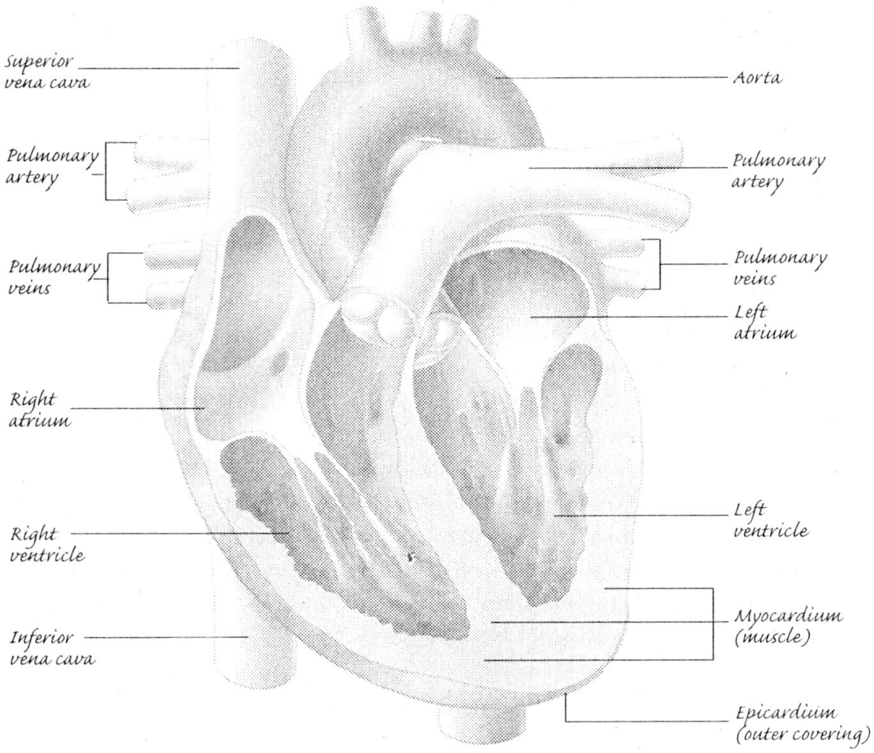

EXERCISE 18-4

Objective: To recognize and be able to correctly spell the names of various parts of the system of arteries.

Directions: Label the diagram in Figure 18-3 with the correct words from the word list below.

Word List

right common carotid	innominate artery	aortic arch
pulmonary artery	right subclavian artery	common iliac
descending aorta	left subclavian artery	femoral artery
left common carotid	right and left coronary arteries	ascending aorta

FIGURE 18-3

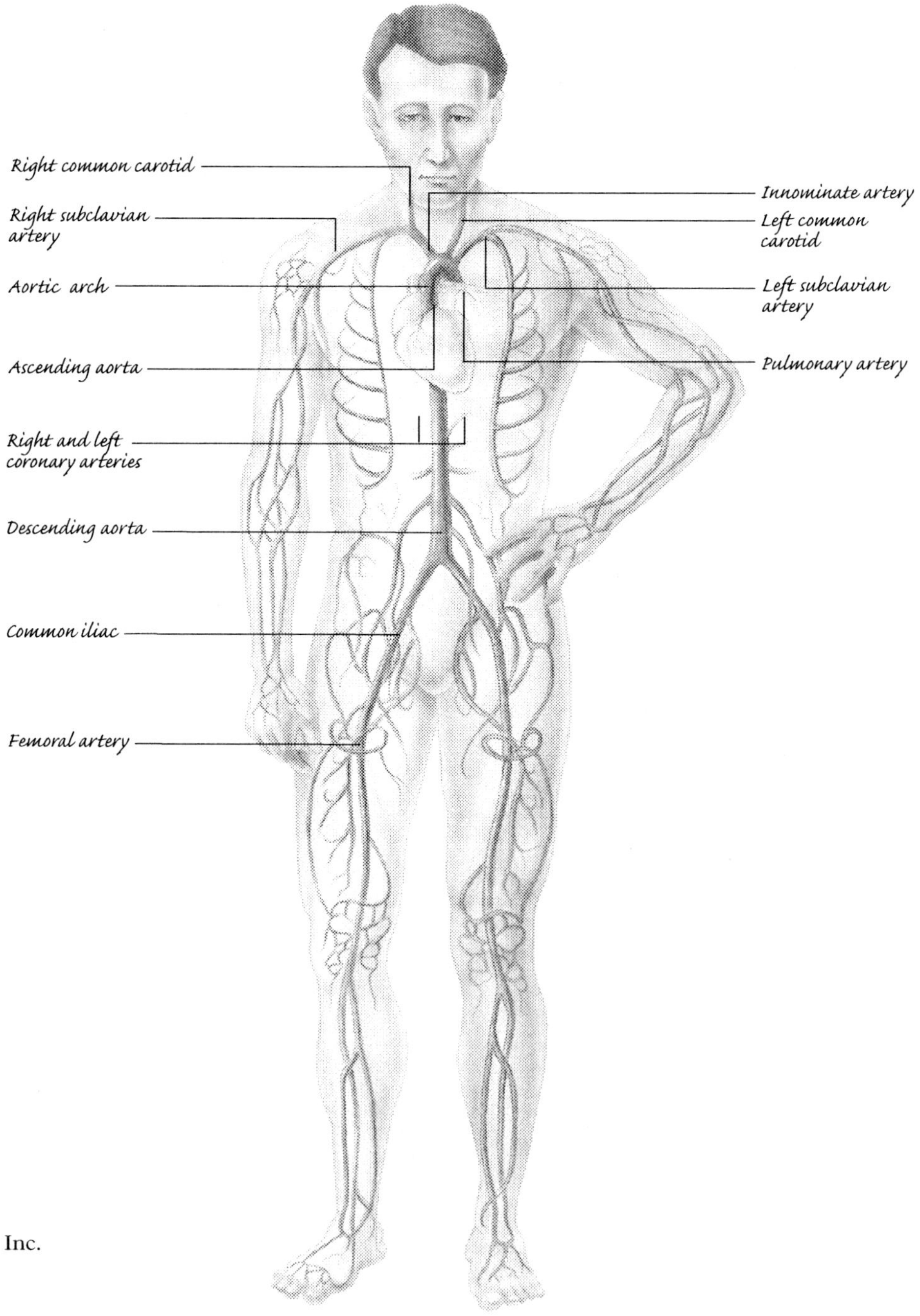

EXERCISE 18-5

Objective: To recognize and be able to correctly spell the names of various parts of the system of veins.

Directions: Label the diagram in Figure 18-4 with the correct words from the word list below.

Word List

internal jugular vein	external jugular vein	femoral vein
iliac vein	inferior vena cava	innominate vein
subclavian vein	superior vena cava	

FIGURE 18-4

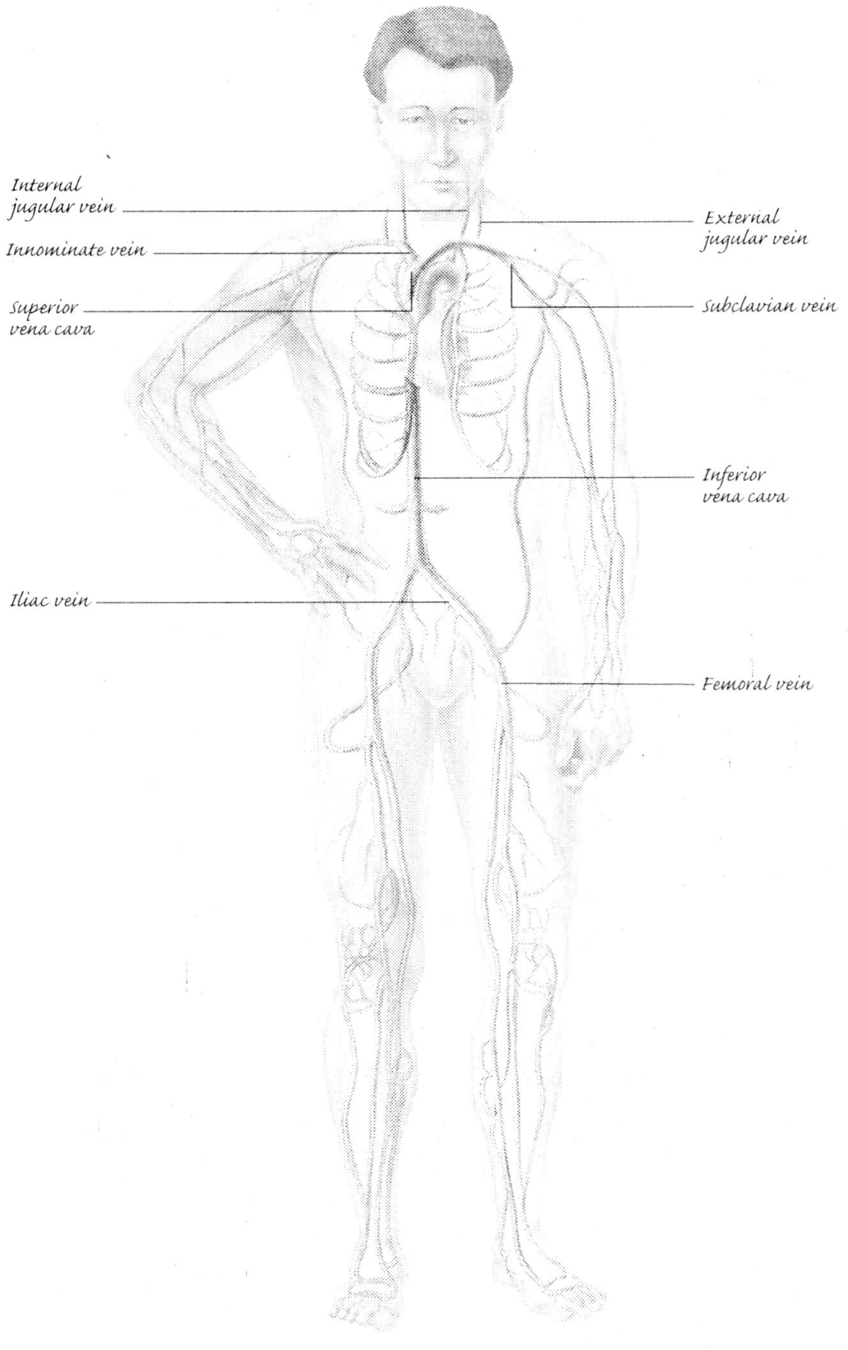

EXERCISE 18-6

Objective: To recognize and be able to correctly spell the names of various parts of the respiratory system.

Directions: Label the diagram in Figure 18-5 with the correct words from the word list below.

Word List

adenoids	epiglottis	pleura	diaphragm
cells	ribs	tongue	pharynx
pulmonary artery	bronchiole	frontal sinus	tonsils
left main bronchus	pleural space	trachea	esophagus
pulmonary vein	alveolus (air sac)	capillaries	nasal cavity
bronchial cilia	oral cavity	mucus	
right main bronchus	larynx		

FIGURE 18-5

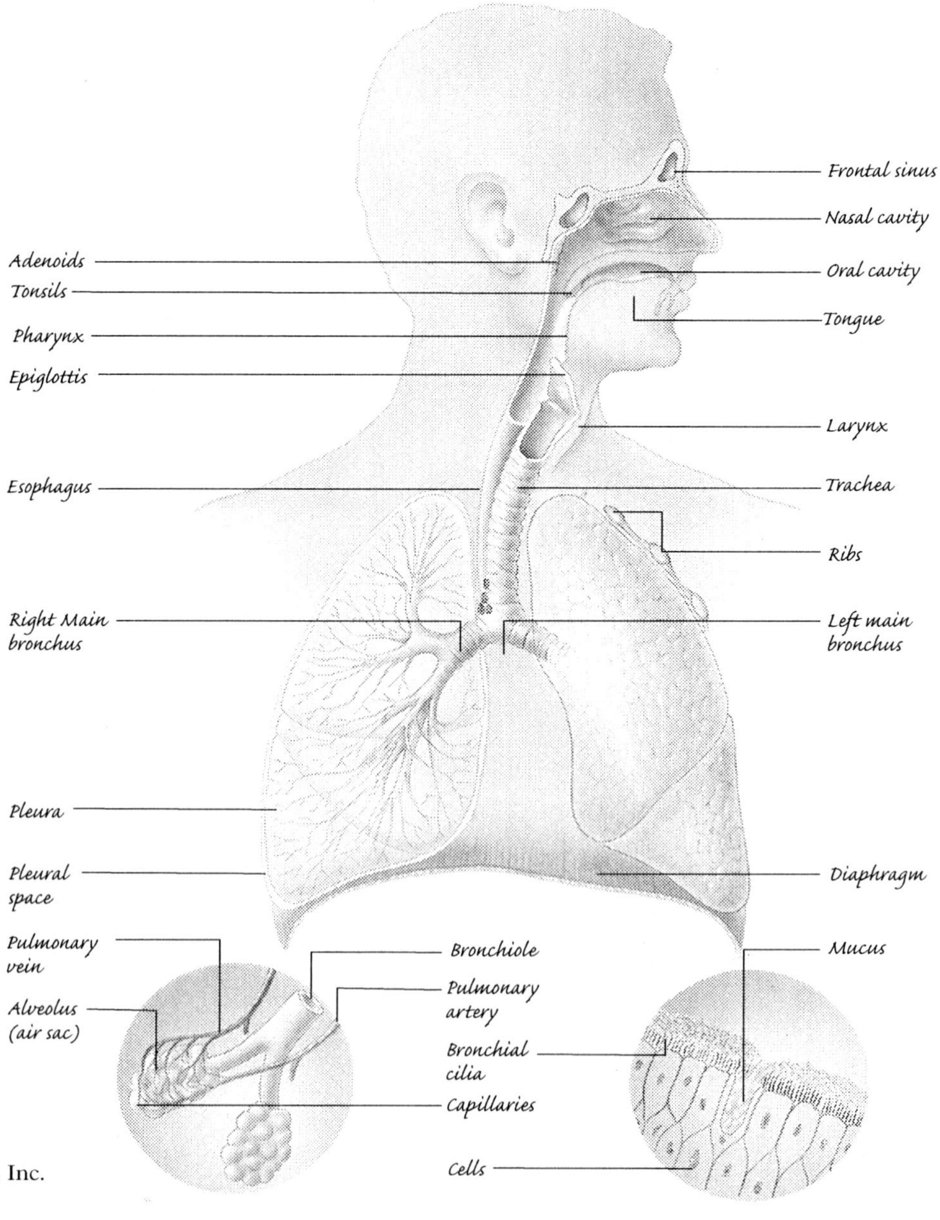

EXERCISE 18-7

Objective: To apply what you have learned about the circulatory system and related care.

Directions: Circle the letter next to the word or statement that best completes the sentence or describes the sentence as true or false. If the sentence is false, draw a line through the incorrect part of the sentence and write the correction on the blank line.

1. The ________ blood cells fight infection.
- A. red
- (B.) white
- C. plasma
- D. new

2. The heart is located in the chest cavity,
- (A.) pointing slightly to the patient's left.
- B. hanging low in the abdomen.
- C. pointing slightly to the patient's right.
- D. behind the large intestine.

3. The heart muscle must be supplied with blood
- A. carrying carbon dioxide.
- (B.) carrying oxygen.
- C. that is thick and slow.
- D. once every hour.

4. A pulmonary embolism is a blood clot that lodges in the
- A. feet.
- B. heart.
- C. brain.
- (D.) lungs.

5. A pulmonary embolism causes chest pain, difficulty in breathing, and
- A. is not serious.
- B. is treated with bed rest.
- (C.) is life threatening.
- D. all of the above.

6. One reason older adults tire easily is that
- A. they are lazy.
- B. they do not get enough sleep.
- C. the brain has become smaller.
- (D.) the heart has reduced output because of weaker heart muscle.

7. The respiratory system's function is to allow
- A. urine to leave the blood.
- (B.) oxygen to move from the air into the blood.
- C. urine to enter the kidneys.
- D. blood to enter the brain.

8. Because we need oxygen to live, it is necessary to keep the respiratory system pathway (trachea, larynx, bronchi, lungs) open and functioning.
   (A.) True
   B. False
   Correct Answer: ______________________

9. If the epiglottis is not functioning, then ________ may occur in the lungs.
   A. stomatitis
   B. epiglottitis
   (C.) aspiration
   D. hypertension

10. In the lungs, the oxygen molecules get exchanged for carbon dioxide in the alveolar sacs.
   (A.) True
   B. False
   Correct Answer: ______________________

11. Chronic obstructive pulmonary disease (COPD) refers to a group of respiratory disorders, including all of the following *except*
   A. asthma.
   B. bronchitis.
   C. emphysema.
   (D.) tuberculosis.

12. The incidence of tuberculosis (TB) has been ~~decreasing~~ in recent years.
   A. True
   (B.) False
   Correct Answer: *increasing*

13. A patient with COPD will have difficulty
   A. swimming
   B. running.
   C. breathing.
   (D.) all of the above.

14. A person with obstructed breathing may mouth-breathe and require
   (A.) more frequent mouth care.
   B. more back rubs.
   C. more steaming showers.
   D. more sleep.

15. Oxygen and carbon dioxide are exchanged at the cellular level as well as in the lungs.
   (A.) True
   B. False
   Correct Answer: ______________________

16. The circulatory and respiratory systems
- A. are separate, and one is not affected by the other.
- B. are the same system.
- C. can take the place of the endocrine system.
- (D.) work closely together, and a condition that affects one may affect the other.

17. Patients who have diseases or limiting conditions of the circulatory or respiratory system will often find the activities of daily living difficult.
- (A.) True
- B. False

Correct Answer: ______________________________

18. After surgery, patients are encouraged to cough and deep-breathe to
- A. give them exercise.
- B. keep them oriented.
- (C.) expand the alveolar sacs and promote the exchange of oxygen.
- D. improve their coughing skills.

19. Tuberculosis is transmitted by which of the following?
- A. Coughing.
- B. Sneezing.
- C. Speaking.
- (D.) All of the above.

20. As a nursing assistant, which of the following observations would you report immediately to the nurse?
- A. The patient is tired after walking in the hall.
- (B.) The patient is short of breath in bed.
- C. The patient is tired of TV.
- D. The patient is hungry for a snack.

19

Measuring Vital Signs

CHAPTER OVERVIEW

Instructor Notes

I. **Vital Signs**

II. **Body Temperature**
   A. Types of Thermometers
   B. Recording the Patient's Temperature
   C. Measuring Rectal Temperature

III. **Pulse**
   A. Radial Pulse
   B. The Apical Pulse and Pulse Deficit

IV. **Respirations**
   A. Abnormal Respiration

V. **Blood Pressure**
   A. Instruments for Measuring Blood Pressure
   B. Electronic Blood Pressure Monitoring Apparatus

VI. **Pain—The Fifth Vital Sign**

Instructor Notes

OBJECTIVES

When the students have completed this chapter, they will be able to:

- List and describe the different types of thermometers.
- Read a Fahrenheit and centigrade (Celsius) thermometer accurately.
- Demonstrate the procedure for measuring oral temperatures.
- Demonstrate the procedure for measuring rectal temperatures.
- Demonstrate the procedure for measuring axillary temperatures.
- Demonstrate the proper use of a battery-operated electronic thermometer.
- Count the radial and apical pulse.
- Report the rate and rhythm of the pulse accurately.
- Count a patient's respirations accurately.
- Determine if the patient's breathing is labored or abnormal.
- Explain systolic pressure.
- Explain diastolic pressure.
- Demonstrate the use of aneroid and mercury types of blood pressure equipment accurately and efficiently.
- Demonstrate how to use a stethoscope.
- Measure a patient's blood pressure accurately.
- Use a pain measurement scale to evaluate the intensity of a patient's pain.

KEY TERMS

Abdominal Respiration: Breathing in which the patient is using mostly the abdominal muscles

Aneroid Sphygmomanometer: Dial-type blood pressure equipment

Apical Pulse: A measurement of heartbeats at the apex of the heart, located just under the left breast

Apnea: Periods of not breathing

Axillary: The area under the arms; the armpits

Blood Pressure: The force of the blood exerted on the inner walls of the arteries, veins, and chambers of the heart as blood flows or circulates through the structures

Bradycardia: Heart rate below 60 beats per minute

Centigrade: A system for measurement of temperature using a scale divided into 100 units or degrees; in this system, the freezing temperature of water is 0°C and water boils at 100°C; often referred to as *Celsius*

Cheyne-Stokes Respiration: One kind of irregular breathing. At first the breathing is slow and shallow; then the respiration becomes faster and deeper until it reaches a peak. The respiration then slows down and becomes shallow again. The breathing may then stop completely for 10 seconds and then begin the pattern again. This type of respiration may be caused by certain cerebral (brain), cardiac (heart), or pulmonary (lung) diseases or conditions

Instructor Notes

Diastolic Blood Pressure: In taking a patient's blood pressure, one records the bottom number as the reading for the diastolic pressure; this is the relaxing phase of the heartbeat

Dyspnea: Insufficient oxygenation of the blood resulting in labored or difficult breathing

Exhaling: The process of breathing out air in respiration

Fahrenheit: A system for measuring temperature. In the Fahrenheit system, the temperature of water at boiling is 212°. At freezing, it is 32°. These temperatures are usually written 212°F and 32°F

Force: Strength or power; used to describe the beat of the pulse

Hypertension: High blood pressure

Hypotension: Low blood pressure

Inhaling: The process of breathing in air in respiration

Irregular Respiration: The depth of breathing changes and the rate of the rise and fall of the chest is not steady

Labored Respiration: Working hard to breathe

Mercury Sphygmomanometer: Blood pressure equipment containing a column of mercury

Oral: Anything to do with the mouth; examples are eating and speaking

Pulse: The rhythmic expansion and contraction of the arteries caused by the beating of the heart; the expansion and contraction show how fast, how regular, and with what force the heart is beating

Pulse Deficit: A difference between the apical heartbeat and the radial pulse rate

Radial Pulse: This is the pulse felt at a person's wrist at the radial artery

Rate: Used to describe the number of pulse beats per minute

Rectal: Pertaining to the rectum

Rhythm: Used to describe the regularity of the pulse beats

Shallow Respiration: Breathing with only the upper part of the lungs

Sphygmomanometer: An apparatus for measuring blood pressure

Stertorous Respiration: The patient makes abnormal noises like snoring sounds when breathing

Stethoscope: An instrument that allows one to listen to various sounds in the patient's body, such as the heartbeat or breathing sounds

Systolic Blood Pressure: The force with which blood is pumped when the heart muscle is contracting; when taking a patient's blood pressure, the systolic blood pressure is recorded as the top number

Tachycardia: Heart rate over 100 beats per minute

Thermometer: An instrument used for measuring temperature

Vital Signs: Measurements reflecting the patient's physical well-being and condition

Instructor Notes

CORE STUDENT ASSIGNMENTS

Students should:

- Read this chapter in their textbook, *Being a Nursing Assistant.*
- Underline any words or sentences they do not understand. Write down any questions they have.
- Complete the Chapter Review in their textbook.
- Read the Time Management Tip for this chapter and think about how they might use this tip in their work.
- Complete the Nursing Assistant in Action exercise.

OPTIONAL STUDENT ASSIGNMENTS

Students should:

- Complete all workbook assignments for this chapter in their copy of *Workbook for Being a Nursing Assistant.*
- Use the CD/CD-Rom disk enclosed with their textbook to hear the pronunciation of the key terms in the chapter.
- Watch the "Measuring Vital Signs" video from the Care Provider Skills series.
- Use the Website address **(www.prenhall.com/wolgin)** to access the free, interactive Companion Website created for this textbook. Get hints, instant feedback, and textbook references to chapter-related multiple-choice questions. Read and react to the Nursing Assistant in Action exercise. Link to other interesting sites.

METHODOLOGY AND SUGGESTED ACTIVITIES

I. Lecture/Discussion

- Answer any questions the students may have.
- Discuss the key terms and related abbreviations. Repeat them out loud and practice using them in sentences.
- Discuss the Time Management Tip for this chapter.
- Discuss the Nursing Assistant in Action exercise.
- Discuss the Critical Thinking points for this chapter.
- Discuss personal safety and protection. Emphasize the importance of following Universal Precautions. Stress the need to wear protective equipment, when appropriate.
- Discuss the care of thermometers and guidelines to follow.
- Discuss the various methods for obtaining vital signs and reasons to use one versus another.
- Discuss how to calculate Fahrenheit and centigrade temperatures.
- Emphasize the importance of accuracy and the serious medical decisions made based on the results of vital signs.
- Explain that it is almost impossible to breathe normally when you are aware that the rate is being observed.
- Demonstrate all five types of abnormal respiration.

Instructor Notes

- Emphasize proper placement of the thermometer and of the blood pressure cuff for accurate results.
- Review and discuss the role of pain related to vital signs. Discuss the role of culture and generational thoughts on pain.

II. Role Play/Lab

- Show the video for this chapter. Discuss limitations of the different types of thermometers and blood pressure equipment. Reinforce that using the proper size equipment is essential for accuracy.
- Demonstrate all procedures and review tips for accuracy.
- Divide the students into teams to practice the skills. Have them validate blood pressures with a double stethoscope so that they can hear the sounds.
- Show and demonstrate the different types of thermometers and blood pressure machines.
- Have the students take their own vital signs on each other.
- As students are proficient, have them take vital signs for a clinic.
- Have the students practice asking patients (other students) to rate their pain. Practice reporting these findings to the nurse.

III. Evaluation

- Review the answers to the Chapter Review with students.
- Review the answers to the workbook exercises with students.
- Review the students' understanding of the Time Management Tip.
- To evaluate student comprehension, give a quiz.
- Have the students visit the interactive Companion Website and take the quiz.

ANSWERS TO CHAPTER REVIEW

FILL IN THE BLANK

Read each sentence and fill in the blank line(s) with the word or words that complete the sentence. (Note: Hyphenated words get one line.)

1. Body ___*temperature*___ is the measurement of the amount of heat in the body.
2. ___*Axillary*___ temperatures are measured under the armpit of the patient.
3. Glass thermometers often contain a dangerous element called ___*mercury*___.
4. One of the easiest and most common places to take a pulse is the ___*radial*___ pulse.
5. The ___*systolic*___ pressure heard when taking a blood pressure represents the contraction of the heart.

Instructor Notes

MULTIPLE CHOICE

Choose the best answer for each question or statement.

1. When using a glass thermometer, do all of the following *except*
   A. wash your hands.
   (B.) hold the mercury tip end and shake.
   C. stand back from any hard surfaces to avoid breaking the thermometer.
   D. shake the thermometer down after use.
2. If a patient cannot read, which pain measurement scale could you use?
   A. One with words
   B. One with numbers
   (C.) One with sad and happy faces
   D. One with birds and flowers
3. When taking a patient's pulse, it is important to note
   A. the rate.
   B. the rhythm.
   C. the force.
   (D.) All of the above.
4. Apnea is
   A. difficult breathing.
   B. when the patient uses his abdominal muscles to breathe.
   (C.) not breathing.
   D. fast breathing followed by slow, shallow breaths.
5. Do not take a blood pressure in an arm with
   A. an IV.
   B. a surgical site.
   C. an AV shunt.
   (D.) All of the above.

CRITICAL THINKING

CUSTOMER SERVICE

Encourage students to reflect and share their thoughts and experiences. Respect their privacy and confidentiality. Share your own viewpoints with the students.

CULTURAL CARE

Encourage students to reflect and share their thoughts and experiences. Respect their privacy and confidentiality. Share your own viewpoints with the students.

Instructor Notes

COOPERATION WITHIN THE TEAM

Encourage students to reflect and share their thoughts and experiences. Respect their privacy and confidentiality. Share your own viewpoints with the students.

NURSING ASSISTANT IN ACTION

You are assigned to take Mr. Powers' blood pressure. He tells you to come back later because he just got off his cell phone talking with his wife. He says, "Every time I talk to her, I see red. If you take my blood pressure now, it will be really high. One look at that number and my doctor will order me back on the anti-hypertensive medications. Go away or make one up!"

What Is Your Response/Action?

Mr. Powers has a good point. If he is upset, his blood pressure may be elevated. Unless given directions from the nurse, give Mr. Powers about 5 minutes to calm down. Then return to check his vital signs. Do not be tempted to make up a set of vital signs! It would be a good idea to tell the nurse that Mr. Powers has had an upsetting phone call; that way she will know what kind of day he has had.

Instructor Notes

19

Answers to Workbook Exercises

The following exercises will assist you to apply what you have read in Chapter 19, "Measuring Vital Signs." For each exercise, read the objective and use information you have read in Chapter 19 to answer the questions, complete the sentences, or label the diagrams.

EXERCISE 19-1

Objective: To recognize the names of equipment commonly used to measure vital signs.

Directions: Label the pictures in Figure 19-1 with the number of the correctly matching name from the Word List below.

Word List

1. electronic oral/rectal thermometer
2. glass thermometer
3. disposable thermometer
4. aneroid sphygmomanometer
5. mercury sphygmomanometer
6. bell stethoscope
7. electronic ear thermometer
8. diaphragm stethoscope

FIGURE 19-1

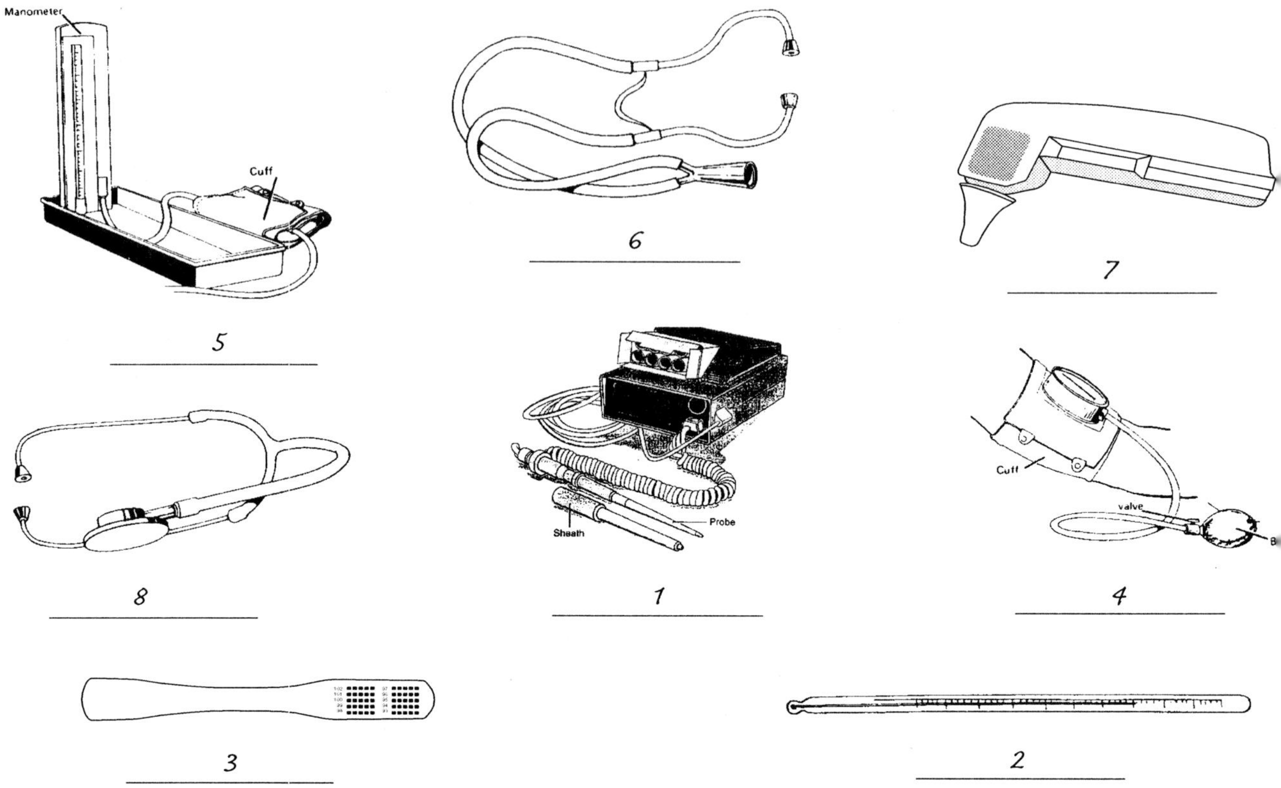

EXERCISE 19-2

Objective: To recognize the definitions of words related to measuring vital signs.

Directions: Place the letter of the correct definition next to the matching word(s) from the Word List.

Word List

N **1.** labored respiration

O **2.** mercury sphygmomanometer

P **3.** oral

Q **4.** pulse

AA **5.** systolic blood pressure

BB **6.** thermometer

F **7.** abdominal respiration

G **8.** aneroid sphygmomanometer

Y **9.** stertorous respiration

Z **10.** stethoscope

K **11.** centigrade

U **12.** rectal

V **13.** rhythm

H **14.** apical pulse

I **15.** axillary

J **16.** blood pressure

L **17.** Cheyne-Stokes respiration

R 18. pulse deficit

E 19. irregular respiration

S 20. radial pulse

T 21. rate

W 22. shallow respiration

X 23. sphygmomanometer

A 24. exhaling

B 25. Fahrenheit

M 26. diastolic blood pressure

CC 27. apnea

C 28. force

D 29. inhaling

DD 30. tachycardia

EE 31. hypertension

FF 32. Bradycardia

GG 33. hypotension

Definitions

A. The process of breathing out air in respiration

B. A system for measuring temperature; in the Fahrenheit system, the temperature of water at boiling is 212°. At freezing, it is 32°. These temperatures are usually written 212°F and 32°F.

C. Strength or power; used to describe the beat of the pulse

D. The process of breathing in air in respiration

E. The depth of breathing changes and the rate of the rise and fall of the chest is not steady

F. Breathing in which the patient is using mostly the abdominal muscles

G. Dial-type blood pressure equipment

H. A measurement of the heartbeats at the apex of the heart, located just under the left breast

I. The area under the arms; the armpits

J. The force of the blood exerted on the inner walls of the arteries, veins, and chambers of the heart as it flows or circulates through the structure

K. A system for measurement of temperature using a scale divided into 100 units or degrees; in this system, the freezing temperature of water is 0°C and water boils at 100°C; often referred to as Celsius

L. One kind of irregular breathing. At first the breathing is slow and shallow; then the respiration becomes faster and deeper until it reaches a peak. The respiration then slows down and becomes shallow again. The breathing may then stop completely for 10 seconds and then begin the pattern again; this type of respiration may be caused by certain cerebral (brain), cardiac (heart), or pulmonary (lung) diseases or conditions.

M. In taking a patient's blood pressure, one records the bottom number as the reading for the diastolic pressure; this is the relaxing phase of the heartbeat

N. Working hard to breathe

O. Blood pressure equipment containing a column of mercury

P. Anything to do with the mouth; examples are eating and speaking

Q. The rhythmic expansion and contraction of the arteries caused by the beating of the heart; the expansion and contraction show how fast, how regular, and with what force the heart is beating

R. A difference between the apical heartbeat and the radial pulse rate

S. This is the pulse felt at a person's wrist at the radial artery

T. Used to describe the number of pulse beats per minute

U. Pertaining to the rectum

V. Used to describe the regularity of the pulse beats

W. Breathing with only the upper part of the lungs

X. An apparatus for measuring blood pressure

Y. The patient makes abnormal noises like snoring sounds when breathing

Z. An instrument that allows one to listen to various sounds in the patient's body, such as the heartbeat or breathing sounds

AA. The force with which blood is pumped when the heart muscle is contracting; when taking a patient's blood pressure, the systolic blood pressure is recorded as the top number

BB. An instrument used for measuring temperature

CC. Periods of not breathing

DD. Heart rate over 100 beats per minute

EE. High blood pressure

FF. Heart rate below 60 beats per minute

GG. Low blood pressure

EXERCISE 19-3

Objective: To identify the common areas of the body where a pulse can be measured.

Directions: Label the diagram in Figure 19-2 with the correct words from the Word List below.

Word List

femoral pulse	temporal pulse	apical pulse	popliteal pulse
radial pulse	brachial pulse	pedal pulse	carotid pulse

FIGURE 19-2

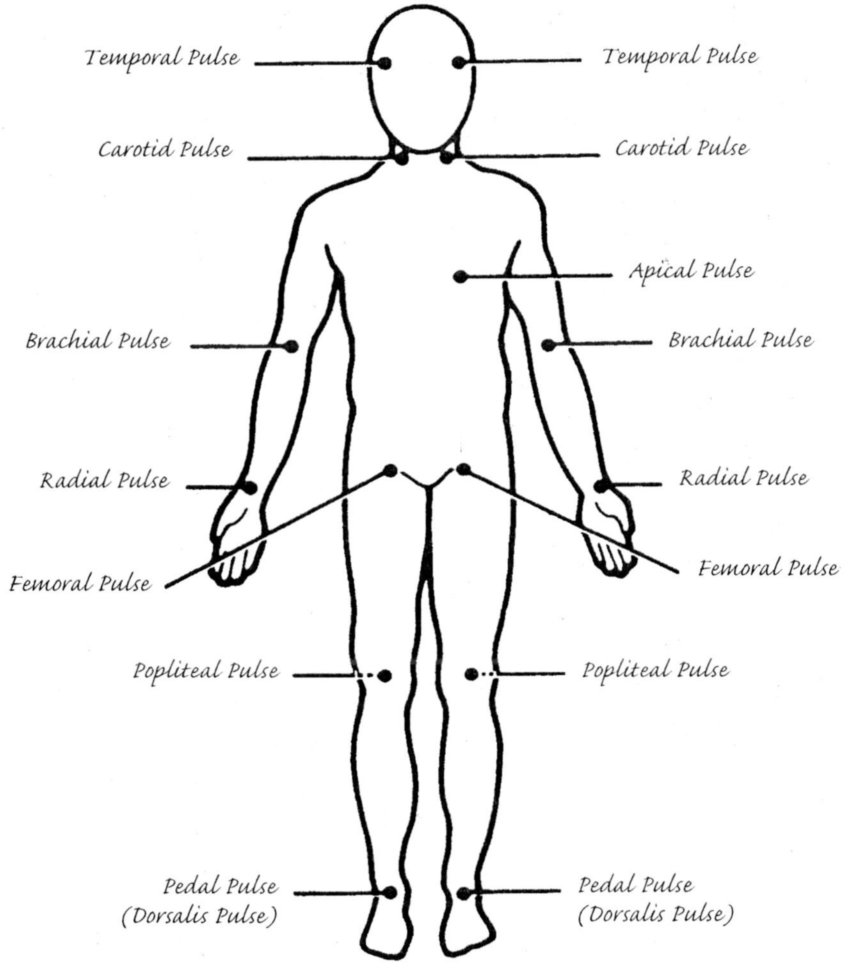

EXERCISE 19-4

Objective: To identify the correct technique for feeling the radial pulse.

Directions: Circle the letter next to the picture in Figure 19-3 that shows the correct technique for feeling the radial pulse.

FIGURE 19-3

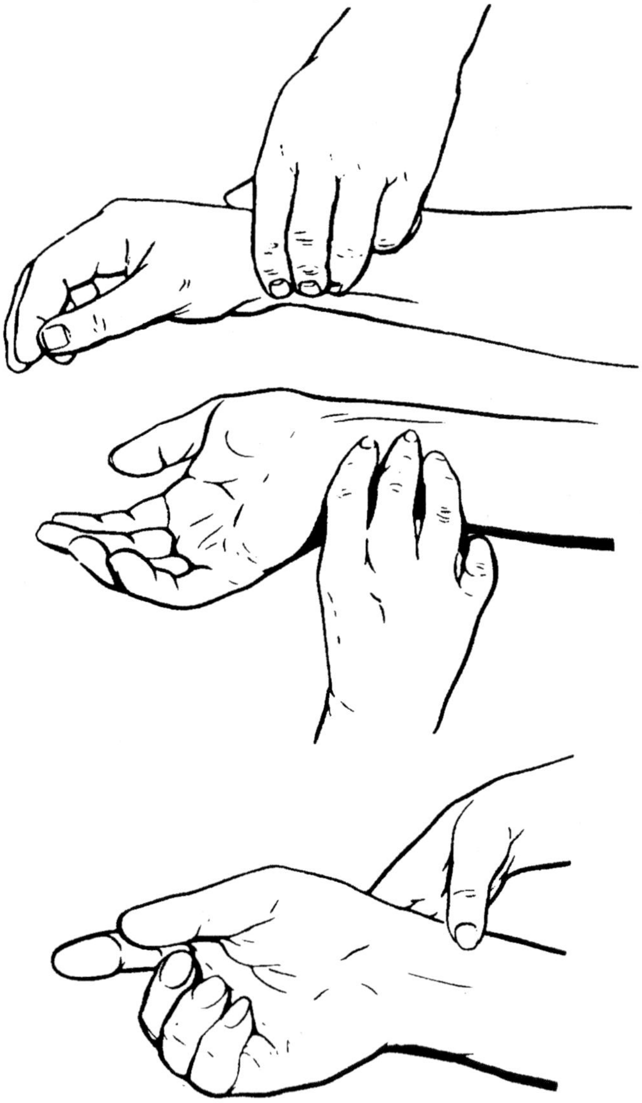

A.

B.

C.

EXERCISE 19-5

Objective: To recognize important aspects of procedures used to measure vital signs.

Directions: Select from the List of Procedures the letter of the procedure that best answers each question. Write the correct letter(s) on the blank line next to the question.

List of Procedures

A. Shaking down the glass thermometer
B. Reading a Fahrenheit thermometer
C. Reading a centigrade thermometer
D. Measuring an oral temperature
E. Measuring a rectal temperature
F. Measuring axillary temperature
G. Using a battery-operated electronic oral thermometer
H. Using a battery-operated electronic rectal thermometer
I. Using a battery-operated electronic oral thermometer to measure axillary temperature
J. Measuring the radial pulse
K. Measuring the apical pulse
L. Measuring the apical pulse deficit
M. Measuring respirations
N. Measuring blood pressure
O. Measuring pain in a child
P. Measuring pain in an adult

N **1.** Which procedure requires the use of a sphygmomanometer?

A, B, G D, E, F **2.** Which six procedures require the use of glass thermometers?

E, H **3.** Which two procedures could be used to get a measurement of R-100.4°F?

J, K, L **4.** In which three procedures would you observe the rate, rhythm, and force?

K, L, N **5.** Which three procedures involve the use of a stethoscope?

M **6.** For which procedure would the normal adult rate be from 16 to 20 times a minute?

L **7.** Which procedure could involve two nursing assistants working together?

B 8. Which procedure involves counting by twos like this: 2, 4, 6, 8?

J, M, N 9. Which three procedures would you follow if your immediate supervisor asked you to take vital signs?

E, H 10. Which two procedures could you use to measure temperature if the patient is receiving oxygen by cannula, catheter, face mask, or oxygen tent?

O 11. Which procedure involves a happy and sad face scale?

P 12. Which procedure involves using a 0–10 rating scale?

EXERCISE 19-6

Objective: To recognize important aspects of abnormal respirations.

Directions: Select the letters of the abnormal respiration from the Word List that match the definitions below. Write the letter next to the matching description.

Word List

A. stertorous respiration
B. abdominal respiration
C. shallow respiration
D. irregular respiration
E. Cheyne-Stokes respiration

C 1. Breathing with only the upper part of the lungs.

B 2. Using mostly abdominal muscles for breathing.

E 3. A pattern where the breathing is slow and shallow, then faster and deeper to peak, then slow and shallow again. The breathing may stop for 10 seconds before beginning the pattern again.

A 4. Abnormal sounds like snoring while breathing.

D 5. The depth and rate are not steady.

EXERCISE 19-7

Objective: To identify important techniques for measuring respirations.

Directions: Circle the letter of the phrase that best completes the sentence.

1. To be sure the patient will not know that you are watching his breathing, you should
   A. count respirations while taking his blood pressure.
   (B.) hold the patient's wrist just as if you were taking his pulse.
   C. distract him by talking about the weather.

2. What should you do if you cannot clearly see the chest rise and fall?
   (A.) Fold the patient's arm across his chest to feel his breathing as you hold his wrist.
   B. Place your hand on the patient's chin to feel his breathing.
   C. Use a disposable thermometer to distract the patient.
3. If you count the chest rising 15 times in 1 full minute, you would report
   A. 30 respirations per minute.
   (B.) 15 respirations per minute.
   C. 7 respirations per minute.
4. If you count 9 respirations in 30 seconds, you would report
   A. 27 respirations per minute.
   B. 9 respirations per minute.
   (C.) 18 respirations per minute.
5. If you count 19 respirations in 1 full minute, you would report
   (A.) 19 respirations per minute.
   B. 38 respirations per minute.
   C. 9 respirations per minute.

EXERCISE 19-8

Objective: To apply what you have learned about measuring the blood pressure.

Directions: Circle the letter of the word or phrase that best completes the sentence.

1. You are measuring the force of the blood flowing through the arteries when you
   A. measure a patient's temperature.
   B. count a patient's respirations.
   (C.) measure a patient's blood pressure.
   D. count a patient's pulse.
   E. measure a patient's vital signs.
2. "mm" is the abbreviation for
   A. mercury.
   B. centimeters.
   (C.) millimeters.
   D. cubic centimeters.
   E. systolic.
3. "Hg" is the abbreviation for
   (A.) mercury.
   B. centimeters.
   C. millimeters.
   D. oxygen.
   E. diastolic.

4. When a patient's blood pressure is higher than the normal range for his age and condition, it is referred to as
   A. hypotension.
   (B.) high blood pressure.
   C. diastolic pressure.
   D. millimeters mercury.
   E. low blood pressure.

5. When a patient's blood pressure is lower than the normal range for her age and condition, it is referred to as
   A. hypertension.
   B. high blood pressure.
   C. diastolic pressure.
   D. millimeters mercury.
   (E.) low blood pressure.

6. High blood pressure is also called
   A. hypotension.
   D. diastolic pressure.
   (B.) hypertension.
   E. Cheyne-Stokes pressure.
   C. systolic pressure.

7. Low blood pressure is also called
   A. systolic pressure.
   B. diastolic pressure.
   C. irregular pressure.
   (D.) hypotension.
   E. hypertension.

8. When you use a mercury sphygmomanometer, you will be
   (A.) watching the level of a column of mercury on a measuring scale.
   B. watching a pointer on a dial.
   C. counting respirations.
   D. watching a digital display.
   E. recharging the batteries.

9. When you use the aneroid sphygmomanometer, you will be
   A. watching the level of a column of mercury on a measuring scale.
   (B.) watching a pointer on a dial.
   C. counting respirations.
   D. watching a digital display.
   E. recharging the batteries.

10. When taking a patient's blood pressure you will be listening to how the brachial pulse sounds in the brachial artery in the patient's arm and at the same time
   A. pumping air into the cuff.
   (B.) watching an indicator (either a column of mercury or a dial) to take a reading.
   C. counting respirations.
   D. securing the cuff.
   E. watching the clock.

11. When recording blood pressure you should write it $\frac{120}{80}$ or 120/80. The top number stands for the
   (A.) systolic pressure.
   B. diastolic pressure.
   C. mercury pressure.
   D. blood pressure.
   E. millimeters mercury.

12. The bottom number of a recorded blood pressure stands for the
   A. systolic pressure.
   (B.) diastolic pressure.
   C. mercury pressure.
   D. blood pressure.
   E. millimeters mercury.

EXERCISE 19-9

Objective: To demonstrate your ability to correctly read an aneroid and a mercury sphygmomanometer.

Directions: Read the gauges in Figure 19-4 and write the correct answer on the blank line next to each gauge.

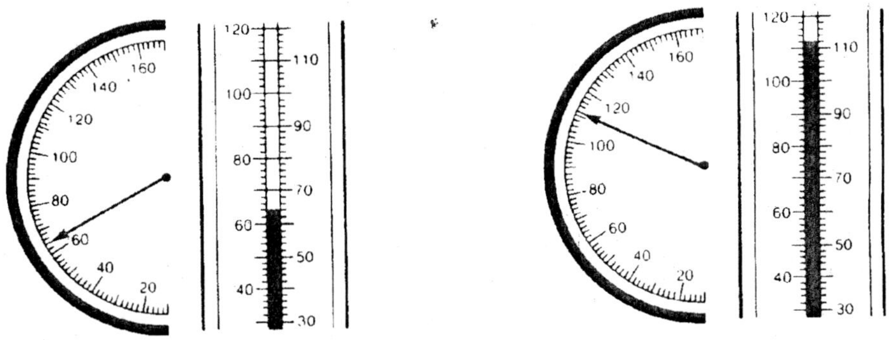

FIGURE 19-4

1. ___64___

2. ___112___

FIGURE 19-4 (cont.)

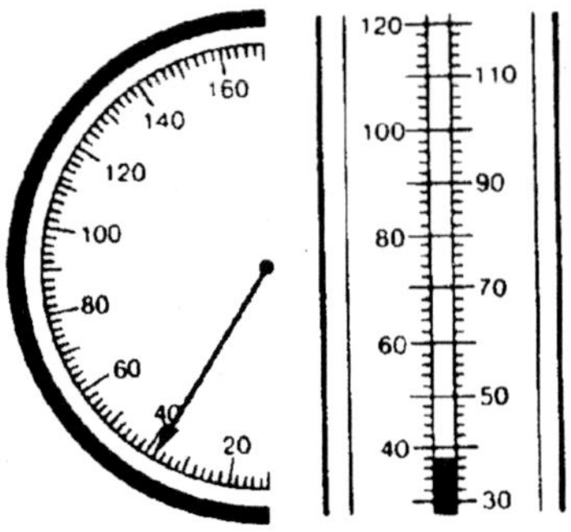

3. 38

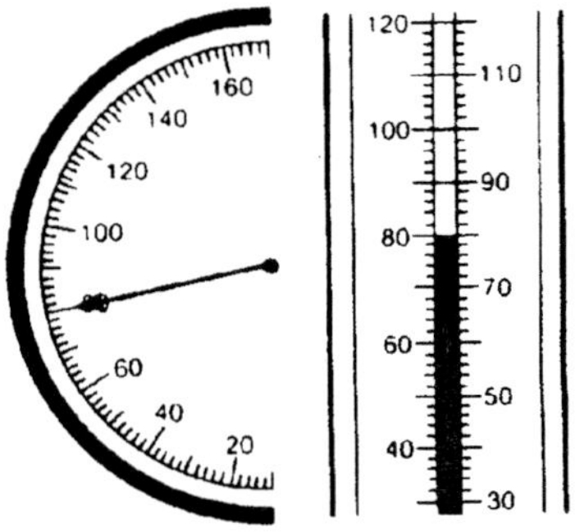

4. 80

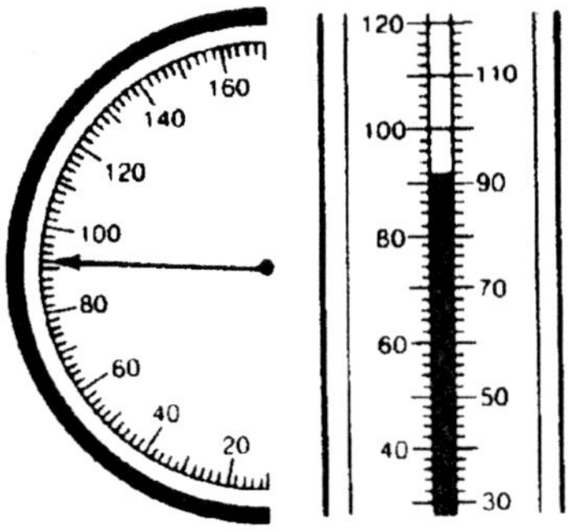

5. 92

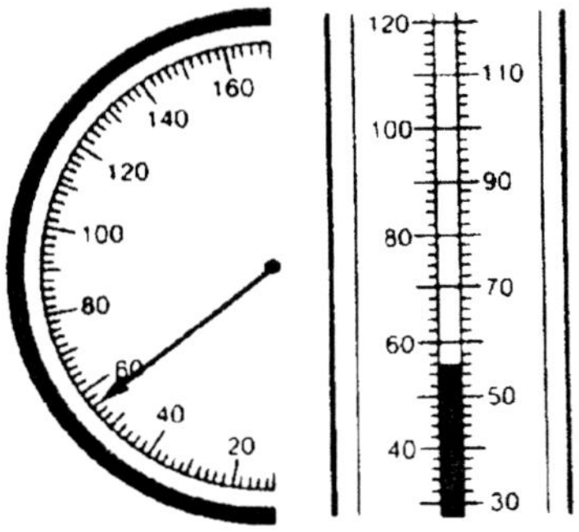

6. 56

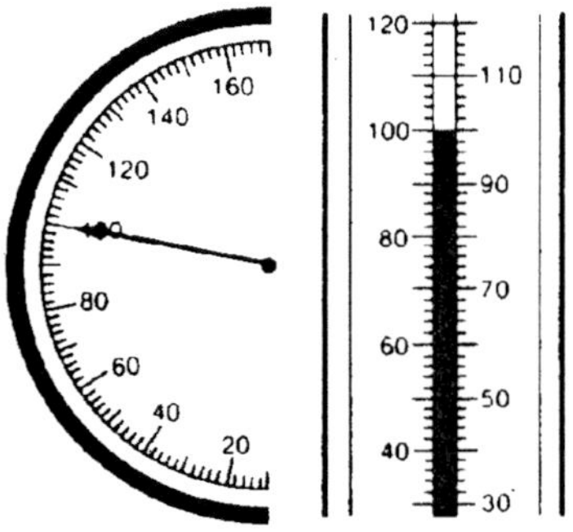

7. 100

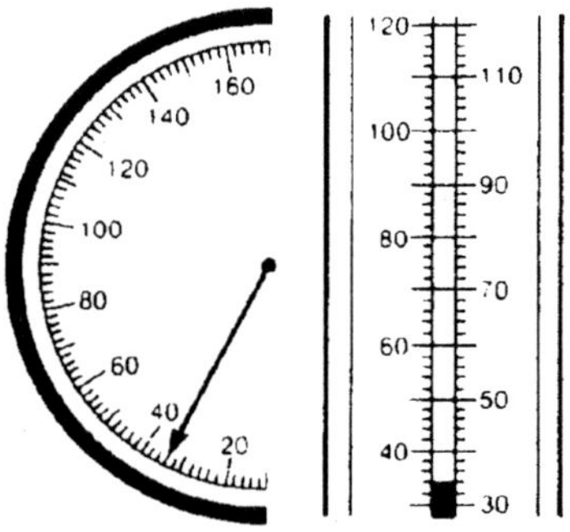

8. 34

FIGURE 19-4 (cont.)

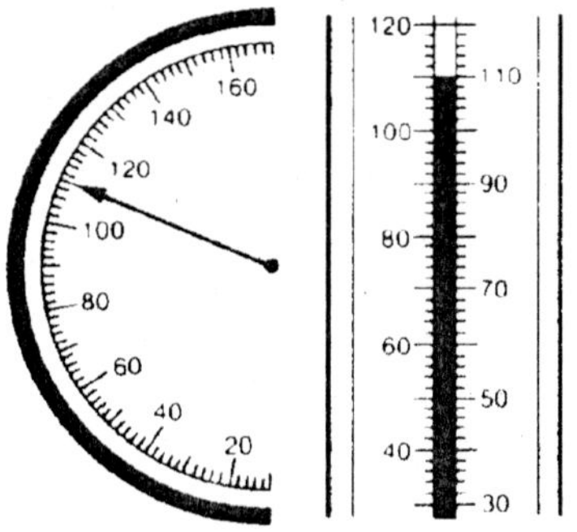

9. *110*

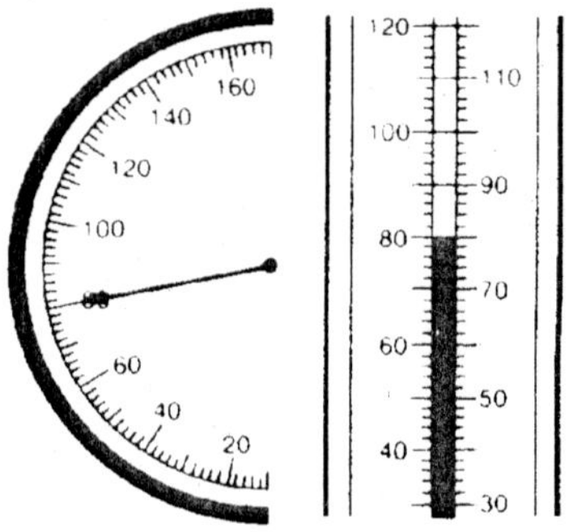

10. *80*

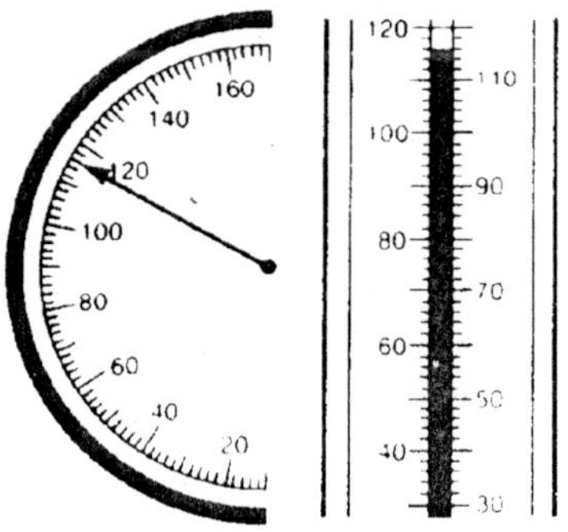

11. *116*

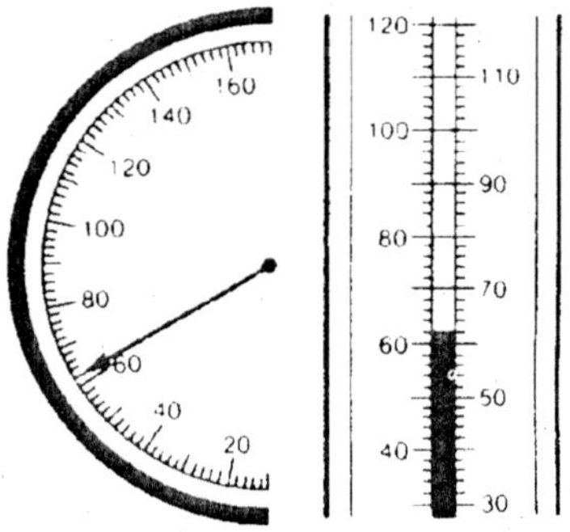

12. *62*

COMPETENCY CHECKLIST 19-1: VITAL SIGNS

ACTIVITY	S	U	COMMENTS
1. Student will correctly demonstrate the proper technique for:			
A. Shaking down a glass thermometer			
B. Reading a Fahrenheit thermometer			
C. Reading a centigrade thermometer			
D. Measuring an oral temperature			
E. Using a battery-operated electronic oral thermometer			
F. Measuring a rectal temperature using a glass thermometer			
G. Using a battery-operated electronic rectal thermometer			
H. Measuring an axillary temperature using a glass thermometer			
I. Using a battery-operated electronic oral thermometer to measure an axillary temperature			
J. Measuring a radial pulse			
K. Measuring an apical pulse			
L. Measuring an apical pulse deficit			
M. Measuring respiration			
N. Measuring blood pressure using a sphygmomanometer			

20

The Gastrointestinal System and Related Care

CHAPTER OVERVIEW

Instructor Notes

I. The Gastrointestinal System (Digestive System)
- A. Common Disorders and Diseases of the Gastrointestinal System

II. Tube Feedings
- A. Nasogastric Tubes
- B. Gastrostomy Tubes
- C. Enteral Feedings (Tube Feedings)

III. Diarrhea and Constipation
- A. Constipation
- B. Fecal Impaction

IV. Rectal Treatments
- A. Positioning the Patient for the Enema
- B. The Cleansing Enema
- C. The Prepackaged, Ready-to-Use Enema
- D. The Oil Retention Enema
- E. The Harris Flush (Return-Flow Enema)
- F. Disposable Rectal Tube with Connected Flatus Bag
- G. Rectal Suppositories

V. The Ostomy
- A. Psychological Aspects of Ostomies
- B. Caring for an Ostomy

Instructor Notes

OBJECTIVES

When the students have completed this chapter, they will be able to:

- Identify the major components of the gastrointestinal system and describe the digestive process.
- Describe the age-related changes in the gastrointestinal system.
- List the common disorders and diseases of the gastrointestinal system.
- Define and describe two different tubes used for tube feedings.
- Describe three ways that a nasogastric tube can be used.
- Describe how to recognize and manage diarrhea.
- Describe how to recognize and remove fecal impactions.
- List the steps for administering a cleansing enema.
- Describe what steps may be taken to help keep stool consistency soft and the bowels moving.
- Describe the procedures for the different types of rectal treatments.
- Describe the psychological aspects of caring for the ostomy patient.
- Give ostomy care.
- Define the key terms used in this chapter.

KEY TERMS

Absorption: Part of the digestive process in which digestive juices and enzymes break down food into usable parts

Anus: Muscular opening that controls elimination of stool from the rectum

Appendicitis: Inflammation (swelling and irritation) of the appendix, typically with pain in the right lower quadrant; surgery called an appendectomy is usually performed to remove the appendix

Bile: Substance manufactured by the liver that helps the food breakdown process

Constipation: Difficult, infrequent defecation, with passage of unduly hard and dry fecal material

Continuous: Uninterrupted, without a stop

Diarrhea: Abnormally frequent discharge of fluid fecal material from the bowel

Digestion: Breaking down the food that is eaten into a form that can be used by the body cells; this process is both mechanical and chemical

Duodenum: The first loop of the small intestine

Enema: Procedure of evacuation or washing out of waste materials (feces or stool) from a person's lower bowel

Evacuation: Discharge of the contents of the lower bowel through the rectum and anus

Fecal Impaction: Hard, puttylike fecal material resulting from prolonged retention of stool in the rectum

Instructor Notes

Flatus: Intestinal gas

Gastrointestinal (GI) System: The GI tract is about 30 feet long and consists primarily of the mouth, esophagus, stomach, small intestine, and large intestines

Gastrostomy: An opening made through the abdomen to the stomach for the purpose of feeding

Gastrostomy Tube (GT): Tube inserted into the abdomen for the introduction of fluids

Gavage: Feeding through a nasogastric tube

Intermittent: Alternating; stopping and beginning again

Large Intestine: Distal colon that absorbs water from stool

Lavage: The washing out of the stomach through a nasogastric tube, usually with normal saline

Liver: Responsible for manufacturing bile and is a storage area for glucose; the liver also is the place where toxins, or poisons, are removed from the blood

Nasogastric Tube: A tube placed through one of the patient's nostrils (naso-), down the back of the throat, and through the esophagus into the patient's stomach (-gastric)

Ostomy: A surgical procedure (operation) in which a new opening, called a stoma, is created in the abdomen, usually for the discharge of wastes (urine or feces) from the body

Ostomy Appliance: Collecting pouch usually attached to the skin around the stomach with adhesive

Pancreas: Produces digestive juices and enzymes responsible for food breakdown in the small intestines

Peristalsis: Rhythmic contractions of the muscle walls of the small and large intestines

Rectal Irrigation: Repeated washing out of the rectum; clean water runs into the rectum, gas (flatus) and water run out of the rectum, as in the Harris flush

Rectum: The lowest portion of the large intestine, which curves in an S-shape and stores fecal material

Retention: The patient keeps the enema fluid (oil) in the rectum for 20 minutes

Saliva: The secretion of the salivary glands into the mouth; saliva moistens the food and helps in swallowing; it contains an enzyme (protein) that helps digest starches

Sims's Position: Patient positioned on the left side with the right knee bent toward the chest; often called the enema position

Small Intestine: The first, smaller portion of the bowel, including the duodenum, where most of digestion and food breakdown occurs; also known as the small bowel

Sphincter: Ring-shaped muscle that surrounds and controls a natural opening in the body, such as the anus

Instructor Notes

Stoma: A surgically made opening connecting the urinary or intestinal tract with the outside, such as in a urostomy or colostomy

Suction: Using negative pressure to remove material, usually fluid

CORE STUDENT ASSIGNMENTS

Students should:

- Read this chapter in their textbook, *Being a Nursing Assistant*.
- Underline any words or sentences they do not understand. Write down any questions they have.
- Complete the Chapter Review in their textbook.
- Read the Time Management Tip for this chapter and think about how they might use this tip in their work.
- Complete the Nursing Assistant in Action exercise.

OPTIONAL STUDENT ASSIGNMENTS

Students should:

- Complete all workbook assignments for this chapter in their copy of *Workbook for Being a Nursing Assistant*.
- Use the CD/CD-Rom disk enclosed with their textbook to hear the pronunciation of the key terms in the chapter.
- Watch the "Handling of Infectious Waste" section of the "Infection Control" video from the Care Provider Skills series.
- Use the Website address **(www.prenhall.com/wolgin)** to access the free, interactive Companion Website created for this textbook. Get hints, instant feedback, and textbook references to chapter-related multiple-choice questions. Read and react to the Nursing Assistant in Action exercise. Link to other interesting sites.

METHODOLOGY AND SUGGESTED ACTIVITIES

I. Lecture/Discussion

- Answer any questions the students may have.
- Discuss the key terms and related abbreviations. Repeat them out loud and practice using them in sentences.
- Discuss the Time Management Tip for this chapter.
- Discuss the Nursing Assistant in Action exercise.
- Discuss the Critical Thinking points for this chapter.
- Discuss personal safety and protection. Emphasize the importance of following Standard Precautions.
- Review and discuss the anatomy of the GI system.
- Discuss the structure and function of the gastrointestinal system.
- Offer examples of case studies of common diseases and disorders of the gastrointestinal system.

Instructor Notes

- Review and discuss the different types of ostomies.
- Have an enterstomal therapy nurse talk with the group.
- Discuss the impact of an ostomy on patients of different age groups.
- Discuss the role of hydration and exercise with fecal impactions. Discuss ways nursing assistants can help avoid this condition with patients.
- Discuss the uses for the various kinds of enemas and when the nursing assistant may see them used. Review how to measure and report to the nurse the results of giving an enema.

II. Lab/Demonstration

- Show the video for this chapter. Discuss what kinds of precautions might be instituted with infections affecting the gastrointestinal tract. Have the students select the appropriate personal protective equipment to wear.
- Display and demonstrate feeding tubes.
- Display and explain use of equipment for rectal treatments. Have the students practice setting up the equipment and putting a patient at ease.
- Role play caring for patients with ostomies.
- Display and have the students practice using various samples of ostomy appliances.
- Demonstrate and have the students practice emptying and changing an ostomy bag.

III. Evaluation

- Review the answers to the Chapter Review with students.
- Review the answer to the workbook exercises with students.
- Review the students' understanding of the Time Management Tip.
- To evaluate student comprehension, give a quiz.
- To evaluate student skills, administer the competency checklist.
- Have the students visit the interactive Companion Website and take the quiz.

ANSWERS TO CHAPTER REVIEW

FILL IN THE BLANK

Read each sentence and fill in the blank line(s) with the word or words that complete the sentence. (Note: Hyphenated words get one line.)

1. The GI tract is about ___*thirty*___ feet long.
2. ___*Digestion*___ begins in the mouth, where food is chewed and mixed with saliva.
3. The rhythmic contractions of the muscle walls of the small and large intestine are called ___*peristalsis*___.

Instructor Notes

4. A feeding through a nasogastric tube is called a ___gavage___ feeding.

5. Intestinal gas is called ___flatus___.

MULTIPLE CHOICE

Choose the best answer for each question or statement.

1. All of the following are diseases and disorders of the gastrointestinal system *except*
   A. ulcers.
   B. jaundice.
   (C.) pericarditis.
   D. hemorrhoids.

2. When caring for a patient with a nasogastric tube, do all of the following *except*
   A. never pull on the tube when moving a patient.
   B. observe the patient's nostrils for signs of pressure.
   C. report any leakage to your supervisor immediately.
   (D.) remove the tube immediately if blood is noted.

3. When caring for a patient with a gastrostomy tube, do all of the following *except*
   A. cleanse around the gastrostomy site with mild soap and water, pat dry.
   B. twist the tube to ensure the tube is not adhered to the wall of the abdomen.
   C. watch for signs of irritation or leakage and report it to your supervisor immediately.
   (D.) All of the above.

4. Diarrhea is
   A. only unhealthy in children.
   B. not something you need to report to the supervisor.
   (C.) unhealthy and may result in severe illness or dehydration.
   D. always a sign of eating too much spicy food.

5. Which of the following guidelines for checking for a fecal impaction is incorrect?
   A. Be certain your state allows you to perform this procedure.
   B. Your supervisor should be available in case you have any questions or the patient experiences problems.
   (C.) Be aware that while performing this procedure the patient can experience an increased heart rate if you stimulate the vagus nerve in the rectum.
   D. Do not perform this procedure if you have not received the necessary training or met agency requirements to do so.

Instructor Notes

CRITICAL THINKING

CUSTOMER SERVICE

Encourage students to reflect and share their thoughts and experiences. Respect their privacy and confidentiality. Share your own viewpoints with the students.

CULTURAL CARE

Encourage students to reflect and share their thoughts and experiences. Respect their privacy and confidentiality. Share your own viewpoints with the students.

COOPERATION WITHIN THE TEAM

Encourage students to reflect and share their thoughts and experiences. Respect their privacy and confidentiality. Share your own viewpoints with the students.

NURSING ASSISTANT IN ACTION

Mr. Brammer has been receiving medications that cause his stools to become very hard. He tells you that he is constipated and has not had a bowel movement for several days. He is complaining of rectal pain and discomfort. He says in a frustrated voice, "I keep trying to go to the bathroom and nothing happens! Why didn't my doctor tell me about this sooner? I am afraid I will have hemorrhoids forever if this keeps up. I feel like there is a brick stuck in my rectum."

What Is Your Response/Action?

Report Mr. Brammer's condition to the nurse or your supervisor. A medication or treatment may be ordered for the patient after the professional nurse evaluates the situation. Do not suggest to Mr. Brammer that you know how to remove a fecal impaction. This procedure requires a physician's order.

Instructor Notes

20

Answers to Workbook Exercises

The following exercises will assist you to apply what you have read in Chapter 20, "The Gastrointestinal System and Related Care." For each exercise, read the objective and use information you have read in Chapter 20 to answer the questions, complete the sentences, or label the diagrams.

EXERCISE 20–1

Objective: To recognize and correctly spell words related to the gastrointestinal system and related care.

Directions: Label the diagram in Figure 20-1 with the correct words from the Word List below.

Word List

mouth	rectum	pharynx
appendix	tongue	gallbladder
large intestine	stomach	liver
teeth	small intestine	esophagus
pancreas	salivary glands	duodenum

FIGURE 20-1

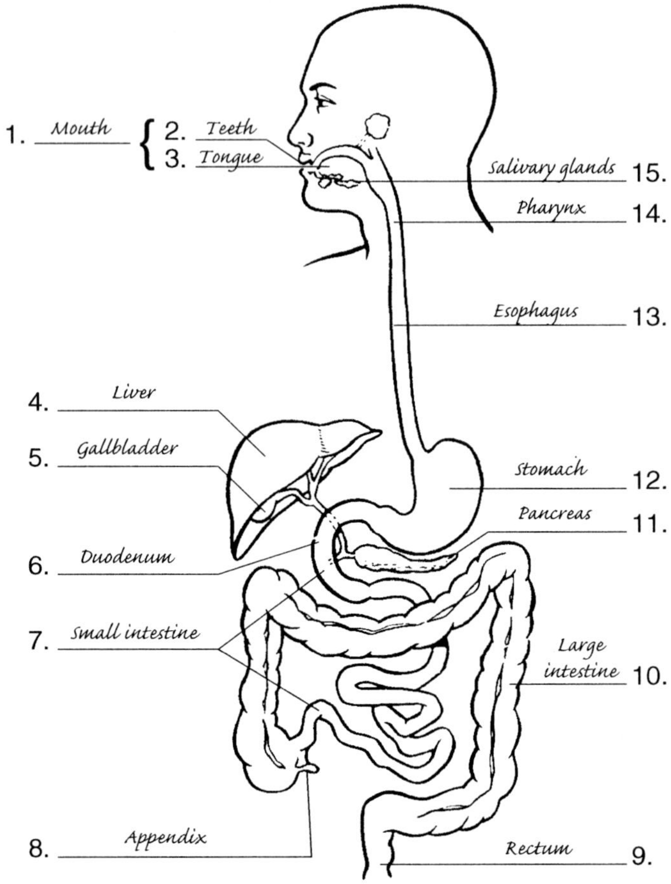

EXERCISE 20–2

Objective: To recognize and correctly spell words related to tube feedings and stomach lavage.

Directions: Label the diagram in Figure 20-2 with the correct words from the Word List below.

Word List

nostrils (naso)	gastric irrigation (lavage)
esophagus	nasogastric feeding (gavage)
stomach (gastric)	

FIGURE 20-2

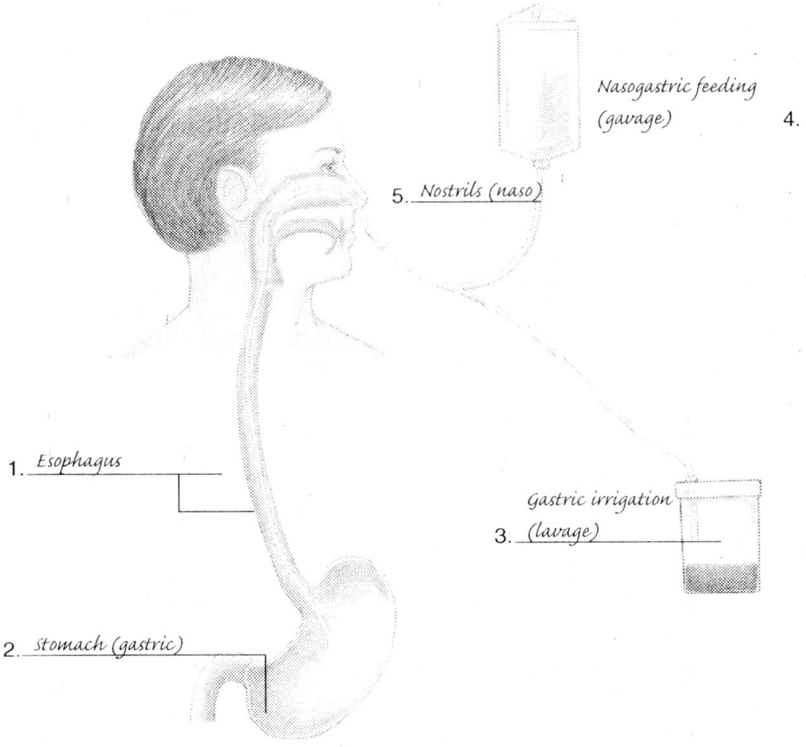

EXERCISE 20–3

Objective: To apply what you have learned about the gastrointestinal system and related care.

Directions: Read the following riddles carefully before writing the correct answer on the blank line.

1. These are 3 letters that stand for a certain kind of gastrostomy tube. What are the letters? *Hint:* An alternative meaning is something on which to hang your coat. ____PEG____

2. These are 4 letters that stand for a certain kind of diet that is a remedy for diarrhea. What is it? *Hint:* An alternative meaning is the name for an unruly child. ____BRAT____

3. This word means a discharge of the lower bowel through the rectum and anus. What is it? *Hint:* An alternative meaning is something we do to remove people before or after a disaster strikes. ____evacuation____

4. This lubricating substance is put onto a rectal tube before insertion. What is it? *Hint:* It has been said that Santa Claus's stomach shakes like a bowl full of this. ____jelly____

EXERCISE 20–4

Objective: To recognize the definitions of words related to the gastrointestinal system and related care.

Directions: Place the letter of the correct definition next to the matching word(s) from the Word List.

Word List

Q **1.** gastrointestinal (GI) system
P **2.** suction
E **3.** digestion
S **4.** anus
V **5.** absorption
Y **6.** small intestine
B **7.** enema
FF **8.** bile
O **9.** Sims's position
R **10.** lavage
DD **11.** gastrostomy tube (GT)
EE **12.** flatus
I **13.** retention
D **14.** diarrhea
G **15.** constipation
F **16.** continuous
W **17.** rectum
Z **18.** liver
J **19.** pancreas
T **20.** ostomy
AA **21.** nasogastric tube
CC **22.** intermittent
L **23.** gastrostomy
U **24.** ostomy appliance
M **25.** gavage
BB **26.** peristalsis
C **27.** duodenum
X **28.** rectal irrigation
A **29.** evacuation
H **30.** appendicitis
N **31.** large intestine
K **32.** saliva
GG **33.** fecal impaction

Definitions

A. Discharge of the contents of the lower bowel through the rectum and anus
B. Procedure of evacuation or washing out of waste materials (feces or stool) from a person's lower bowel
C. The first loop of the small intestine
D. Abnormally frequent discharge of fluid fecal material from the bowel
E. Breaking down the food that is eaten into a form that can be used by the body cells
F. Uninterrupted, without a stop
G. Difficult, infrequent defecation, with passage of unduly hard and dry fecal material

H. Inflammation (swelling and irritation) of the appendix, typically with pain in the right lower quadrant

I. The patient keeps the enema fluid (oil) in the rectum for 20 minutes

J. Produces digestive juices and enzymes responsible for food breakdown in the small and large intestines

K. The secretion of the salivary glands into the mouth; contains an enzyme (protein) that helps digest starches

L. An opening made through the abdomen to the stomach for the purpose of feeding

M. Feeding through a nasogastric tube

N. Distal colon that absorbs water from stool

O. Patient positioned on the left side with the right knee bent toward the chest, often called the enema position

P. Using negative pressure to remove material, usually fluid

Q. This tract is about 30 feet long and consists primarily of the mouth, esophagus, stomach, small intestine, and large intestine

R. The washing out of the stomach through a nasogastric tube, usually with normal saline

S. Muscular opening that controls elimination of stool from the rectum

T. A surgical procedure (operation) in which a new opening, called a stoma, is created in the abdomen, usually for the discharge of wastes (urine or feces) from the body

U. Collecting pouch usually attached to the skin around the stoma with adhesive

V. Part of the digestive process in which digestive juices and enzymes break down food into usable parts

W. The lowest portion of the large intestine, which curves in an S-shape and stores fecal material

X. Repeated washing out of the rectum; clean water runs into the rectum, gas (flatus) and water run out of the rectum, as in the Harris flush

Y. The first, smaller portion of the bowel, including the duodenum, where most of digestion and food breakdown occurs; also known as the small bowel.

Z. Responsible for manufacturing bile and is a storage area for glucose; also the place where toxins, or poisons, are removed

AA. A tube placed through one of the patient's nostrils (naso-), down the back of the throat, and through the esophagus into the patient's stomach (-gastric)

BB. Rhythmic contractions of the muscle walls of the small and large intestines

CC. Alternating; stopping and beginning again

DD. Tube inserted into the abdomen for the introduction of fluids

EE. Intestinal gas

FF. Substance manufactured by the liver that helps the food breakdown process

GG. Hard puttylike fecal material resulting from prolonged retention of stool in the rectum

EXERCISE 20–5

Objective: To apply what you have read about the gastrointestinal system and related care.

Directions: Circle the letter next to the word or statement that best completes the sentence or describes the sentence as true or false. If the sentence is false, draw a line through the incorrect part of the sentence and write the correction on the blank line.

1. Good nutrition and a functioning ________ are vital to a patient's health.
   A. nexus
   B. apex
   (C.) bowel
   D. tube

2. A large amount of ________ is necessary for the chemical breakdown of food.
   A. mercury
   B. lead
   (C.) water
   D. copper

3. The lining of the duodenum is composed of thousands of
   A. tilli.
   B. silli.
   C. billi.
   (D.) villi.

4. As a person ages, all of the following usually occur *except*
   (A.) the flow of saliva increases.
   B. the number of taste buds decreases.
   C. chewing and swallowing are more difficult.
   D. absorption of vitamins and minerals decreases.

5. All of the following are common disorders and diseases of the gastrointestinal system except
   (A.) myocardial infarction.
   B. hernias and ulcers.
   C. cholecystitis.
   D. constipation.

6. Varicose veins of the anal canal are called hemorrhoids.
   (A.) True
   B. False
   Correct Answer: ____________

7. ________ are growths on the lining of the intestines that can become cancerous if not treated.
   A. Jauntoids
   B. Rectoids
   (C.) Polyps
   D. All of the above

8. When fluids are removed with a gravity nasogastric tube, it is important that the collecting container is ~~higher~~ than the patient's body.
   A. True
   (B.) False
   Correct Answer: lower

9. For removing fluids from a patient's body, the degree of suction most commonly used is
   A. high.
   B. low.
   C. intermittent.
   (D.) B and C.

10. Before giving fluid through the NG tube, listen with a stethoscope over the stomach while inserting air into the tube. The sound of air in the stomach means
   A. the tube is not properly placed.
   B. the lungs are inflating.
   C. the tube is loose.
   (D.) the tube is properly placed in the stomach.

11. If you notice that the formerly greenish fluid in the drainage container connected to the nasogastric tube has suddenly become bright red, what would you do?
   A. Empty the container when it is full.
   B. Measure and record the amount and color of the drainage.
   (C.) Notify your immediate supervisor at once.
   D. Tell the patient at once.

12. The nursing assistant is responsible for watching the level of the feeding and making sure the formula is being fed ~~as fast as possible~~ into the patient's stomach.
   A. True
   (B.) False
   Correct Answer: slowly

13. In tube feeding, the formula is administered
A. when thoroughly shaken and chilled.
B. when it has reached boiling.
(C.) at room temperature.
D. at 98.6° F.

14. For adults, the NG tube must be flushed with ~~75 cc~~ of water before and after the feeding or every 8 hours.
A. True
(B.) False
Correct Answer: 40 cc

15. If the patient does not have a functioning GI tract, he may be able to receive a venous feeding called
(A.) total parenteral nutrition (TPN).
B. total food nutrition (TFN).
C. fast-food nutrition (FFN).
D. venous food nutrition (VFN).

16. If a patient has diarrhea, it is important to also note the amount of _________ output, because it may indicate dehydration.
A. blood
B. work
C. lavage
(D.) urine

17. The most common cause of constipation is lack of adequate fluid intake.
(A.) True
B. False
Correct Answer: ____________________

18. A device used to relieve flatus is
A. high bulk foods.
B. a rectal connector.
(C.) a rectal tube with connected bag.
D. a bowel bag.

19. Nursing assistants administer all of the following *except*
A. a rectal tube.
(B.) a medicated rectal suppository.
C. a nonmedicated rectal suppository.
D. a back rub.

20. A surgical procedure that may be done if the colon is diseased is
(A.) creation of a stoma.
B. a stapling of the stomach.
C. a hysterectomy.
D. all of the above.

21. A physician order is necessary to remove a fecal impaction.
(A.) True
B. False
Correct Answer: ____________________

22. Two diseases commonly treated with a stoma are
A. AIDS and pneumocystic disease.
B. diabetes and hypertension.
(C.) inflammatory bowel disease (IBD) and Crohn's disease.
D. diaphoresis and vertigo.

23. The nursing assistant should always report immediately if
A. there is slight bleeding around the stoma.
B. there is feces coming from the stoma.
C. there is an odor coming from the stoma.
(D.) there is bleeding from the stoma that doesn't stop.

24. Psychological changes that the ostomy patient may experience are all of the following *except*
A. being very anxious.
B. appearing to be depressed.
(C.) being cheerful and happy at the new changes.
D. being quiet and withdrawn.

25. Practicing with the patient to empty his ostomy bag will help him develop independence and confidence in his ability to care for it.
(A.) True
B. False
Correct Answer: ____________________

26. If the patient is able, the best time to empty an ostomy bag is
(A.) when the patient is on the toilet.
B. when the patient is in bed.
C. when the patient has visitors.
D. when the patient is sleeping.

COMPETENCY CHECKLIST 20-1: GASTROINTESTINAL CARE

ACTIVITY	S	U	COMMENTS
1. The student will demonstrate the correct method of giving			
A. A fecal impaction check			
B. A fecal impaction removal			
C. A cleansing enema			
D. The ready-to-use cleansing enema			
E. The ready-to-use oil retention enema			
F. The Harris Flush (return-flow enema)			
2. The student will demonstrate the correct method of using the disposable rectal tube with connected flatus bag.			
3. The student will demonstrate the correct method of administering a rectal suppository.			
4. The student will demonstrate the correct method for ostomy care:			
A. Emptying the ostomy pouch			
B. Changing the ostomy appliance			

21

Nutrition for the Patient

CHAPTER OVERVIEW

I. **A Well-Balanced Diet**

II. **What Are Nutrients?**

III. **Regular and Special Diets**
   A. Nutrition Status Assessment

IV. **Assisting Patients with Foods**
   A. Patients Requiring Assistance to Eat

V. **Between-Meal Nourishment**

VI. **Passing Drinking Water**

Instructor Notes

Instructor Notes

OBJECTIVES

When the students have completed this chapter, they will be able to:

- Define the components and importance of a well-balanced diet using the food group pyramid. Provide examples of foods included in each group.
- Describe the six classes of nutrients.
- List the three functions of essential nutrients.
- Identify examples of when a patient may be at nutrition risk.
- List conditions when a patient may need a special diet.
- Define examples of therapeutic diets and explain the purpose of each.
- Prepare the patient for mealtime and serve the food tray.
- Observe and record information concerning meals.
- Distribute between-meal nourishment and drinking water.

KEY TERMS

Calorie: Unit for measuring the energy produced when food is digested in the body

Calorie Count: Counting or adding up a total of all calories consumed in a 24-hour period

Enterally: Delivery of a nutrition formula through a tube for patients with a functional GI tract who are unable to take in adequate calories or food by mouth

Essential Nutrient: Nutrient needed for the human body to function; they must be consumed in the diet every day

Extra Nourishment: Snacks

Malnutrition: Poor nutrition status

Nutrient: Chemical substances found in foods

Nutrition Status Assessment: Assessment by an RN or RD as to what a patient eats and how the body uses it; determination of any special nutritional needs

Omit: Leave out

Parenteral Nutrition: Nutrition therapy delivered by an IV catheter for patients with a nonfunctioning GI tract

Registered Dietitian (RD): Person responsible for the preparation of well-balanced regular and therapeutic (special) diets to meet patients' nutritional needs

Regular Diet: A basic, or well-balanced, diet containing appropriate amounts of foods from each of the food groups

Therapeutic (Special) Diet: Any special diet

CORE STUDENT ASSIGNMENTS

Instructor Notes

Students should:

- Read this chapter in their textbook, *Being a Nursing Assistant*.
- Underline any words or sentences they do not understand. Write down any questions they have.
- Complete the Chapter Review in their textbook.
- Read the Time Management Tip for this chapter and think about how they might use this tip in their work.
- Complete the Nursing Assistant in Action exercise.

OPTIONAL STUDENT ASSIGNMENTS

Students should:

- Complete all workbook assignments for this chapter in their copy of *Workbook for Being a Nursing Assistant*.
- Use the CD/CD-Rom disk enclosed with their textbook to hear the pronunciation of the key terms in the chapter.
- Watch the "Transfer and Ambulation" video from the Care Provider Skills series.
- Use the Website address **(www.prenhall.com/wolgin)** to access the free, interactive Companion Website created for this textbook. Get hints, instant feedback, and textbook references to chapter-related multiple-choice questions. Read and react to the Nursing Assistant in Action exercise. Link to other interesting sites.

METHODOLOGY AND SUGGESTED ACTIVITIES

I. Lecture/Discussion

- Answer any questions the students may have.
- Discuss the key terms and related abbreviations. Repeat them out loud and practice using them in sentences.
- Discuss the Time Management Tip for this chapter.
- Discuss the Nursing Assistant in Action exercise.
- Discuss the Critical Thinking points for this chapter.
- Discuss personal safety and protection. Emphasize the importance of following Universal Precautions.
- Identify factors that enhance a meal, such as a pleasant environment, an attractive food tray with flavorful, well-prepared food, and an appetizing aroma.
- Stress the importance of checking special diets and nutritional snacks. Discuss how diet affects medications and various disease processes.
- Discuss multicultural differences in food selection.
- Stress the importance of hydration and the need for adequate water ingestion by patients.
- Discuss the role of socialization with meals.

Instructor Notes

II. Role Play/Lab

- Show the video for this chapter. Getting patients ready to eat often requires ambulating the patient to a chair or to a dining room. Review back safety tips and body mechanics prior to ambulating the patient.
- Assign students in groups to develop menus for 1 week to demonstrate daily intake as balanced according to the food group pyramid.
- Assign students in groups to develop a specific therapeutic diet.
- Invite a dietitian to speak to your class.
- Set up a tray of food to point out examples of dos and don'ts.
- Stress that hot food be served hot and cold food be served cold.
- Have students blindfold each other and practice feeding to better understand the feeding process.
- Stress feeding foods in variety.
- Demonstrate all procedures; have students return the demonstrations.
- Have the students demonstrate dysphasia precautions.
- Have the students practice counting the amount of foods eaten off a tray.

III. Evaluation

- Review the answers to the Chapter Review with students.
- Review the answer to the workbook exercises with students.
- Review the students' understanding of the Time Management Tip.
- To evaluate student comprehension, give a quiz.
- To evaluate student skills, administer the competency checklist.
- Have the students visit the interactive Companion Website and take the quiz.

ANSWERS TO CHAPTER REVIEW

FILL IN THE BLANK

Read each sentence and fill in the blank line(s) with the word or words that complete the sentence. (Note: Hyphenated words get one line.)

1. The process of counting or adding up all of the calories consumed in a 24-hour period is called a ___*calorie*___ ___*count*___.
2. The food group guide to a well-balanced diet that is divided into six categories is the ___*food*___ ___*pyramid*___.
3. Difficulty swallowing or chewing is called ___*dysphasia*___.
4. When feeding patients, it is important not to ___*rush*___ them while they eat.
5. A ___*nourishment*___ or snack is given to patients to provide energy or as part of their medical care.

MULTIPLE CHOICE

Choose the best answer for each question or statement.

Instructor Notes

1. How many servings of breads, cereals, and pastas are recommended on the food pyramid?
   A. 2–3
   B. 3–5
   C. 5–6
   (D.) 6–11
2. How many servings of vegetables are recommended on the food pyramid?
   A. 2–3
   (B.) 3–5
   C. 5–6
   D. 6–11
3. Which of the following is generally not allowed on a clear liquid diet?
   A. apple juice
   B. jello
   (C.) tomato juice
   D. tea
4. When feeding a patient who has dysphasia, do all of the following *except*
   A. position the patient with his head up 90 degrees.
   (B.) offer dry foods such as crackers.
   C. encourage the patient to swallow twice after each bite.
   D. be patient and offer verbal cues.
5. Obesity is an increasing problem because
   A. the fast-food industry encourages ordering the "Biggie Size."
   B. people are more physically active.
   C. parents cannot control their children's diets.
   (D.) many people are eating more food calories than they burn.

CRITICAL THINKING

CUSTOMER SERVICE

Encourage students to reflect and share their thoughts and experiences. Respect their privacy and confidentiality. Share your own viewpoints with the students.

CULTURAL CARE

Encourage students to reflect and share their thoughts and experiences. Respect their privacy and confidentiality. Share your own viewpoints with the students.

Instructor Notes

COOPERATION WITHIN THE TEAM

Encourage students to reflect and share their thoughts and experiences. Respect their privacy and confidentiality. Share your own viewpoints with the students.

NURSING ASSISTANT IN ACTION

Mrs. Smith has been hospitalized to control her diabetes and high blood pressure. She is ordered on a low-sodium, diabetic diet. After her family visits, you come to deliver her bedtime snack and find Mrs. Smith eating a hamburger, french fries and drinking a large soda. This meal contains a great deal of sodium and sugar. She says to you, "You know how I cannot eat the food you all serve me here. Let me just enjoy this one little meal and pretend you didn't see me eating just now."

What Is Your Response/Action?

Mrs. Smith is an adult so you should not ever scold her for eating the food from her family. Instead, you might say it was nice of her family to bring her a treat. Gently remind her of how the food will affect her blood sugar and blood pressure. Then inform the nurse that Mrs. Smith has eaten food off her diet.

21

Answers to Workbook Exercises

The following exercises will assist you to apply what you have read in Chapter 21, "Nutrition for the Patient." For each exercise, read the objective and use information you have read in Chapter 21 to answer the questions, complete the sentences, or label the diagrams.

EXERCISE 21-1

Objective: To recognize the definitions of words related to nutrition for the patient.

Directions: Place the letter of the correct definition next to the matching word(s) from the Word List.

Word List

_E_ **1.** therapeutic diet
_D_ **2.** extra nourishment
_G_ **3.** nutrient
_C_ **4.** enterally
_I_ **5.** omit
_K_ **6.** nutrition status assessment
_F_ **7.** essential nutrients
_B_ **8.** malnutrition
_H_ **9.** calorie
_M_ **10.** registered dietitian (RD)
_L_ **11.** regular diet
_A_ **12.** calorie count
_J_ **13.** parenteral nutrition

Definitions

A. Counting or adding up a total of all calories consumed in a 24-hour period
B. Poor nutrition status
C. Delivery of a nutrition formula through a tube for patients with a functional GI tract who are unable to take in adequate calories or food by mouth

D. Snacks
E. Any special diet
F. Nutrients needed for the human body to function; they must be consumed in the diet every day
G. Chemical substances found in foods
H. Unit for measuring the energy produced when food is digested in the body
I. Leave out
J. Nutrition therapy delivered by an IV catheter for patients with a nonfunctioning GI tract
K. Assessment by an RN or RD as to what a patient eats and how the body uses it; determination of any special nutritional needs
L. A basic, or well-balanced, diet containing appropriate amounts of foods from each of the food groups
M. Person responsible for the preparation of well-balanced regular and therapeutic (special) diets to meet patients' nutritional needs

EXERCISE 21-2

Objective: To apply what you have learned about serving food to the patient.

Directions: More than one action may apply. Select the action that most closely addresses the situation. Write the letter of the correct action next to the matching situation below.

Actions

A. Check the tray yourself.
B. Check the tray card against the ID band.
C. Help any patient who needs it.
D. Record this on appropriate form.
E. Correct anything that is wrong or missing.

Situations

_A_ **1.** Before you give a tray to a patient.
_B_ **2.** You find the tray for each patient.
_C_ **3.** A patient cannot cut his meat.
_E_ **4.** A patient tells you he didn't get a fork.
_D_ **5.** The patient ate only half his food.
_B_ **6.** A patient tells you he has the wrong tray.
_D_ **7.** The patient refuses to accept the tray and eats nothing.
_E_ **8.** Some food spills.
_C_ **9.** A patient seems too weak to pour his own coffee.
_E_ **10.** A patient on a regular diet didn't get any sugar on his tray, and he would like to have some.

__E__ **11.** You see a coffee pot on the patient's tray but no cup.

__A__ **12.** You look to be sure everything is on the tray.

__C__ **13.** A weak patient asks you to butter his bread.

__D__ **14.** The patient ate all the food served to him.

__E__ **15.** The patient tells you he didn't get any bread and butter, and you see none.

EXERCISE 21-3

Objective: To apply what you have learned about passing drinking water to patients.

Directions: Write Do or Don't next to each statement below as appropriate.

1. __Do__ pass fresh drinking water to patients at the assigned intervals each shift or day.

2. __Don't__ give ice to a patient whose pitcher is labeled "OMIT ICE."

3. __Do__ check to see which patients are NPO.

4. __Do__ check to see which patients are on restricted fluids.

5. __Do__ check to see which patients should get water without ice.

6. __Do__ return the same water pitcher to the patient from whom it was taken.

7. __Do__ remember to wash your hands before passing drinking water.

8. __Do__ wash your hands when done passing drinking water.

9. __Don't__ lower the head of bed to 10° for feeding patients.

10. __Don't__ feed patients one bite every 3 seconds.

EXERCISE 21-4

Objective: To apply what you have learned about food groups.

Directions: Beside each food write the letter of the food group to which it belongs.

Food Groups

A. milk, yogurt, and cheese
B. vegetables
C. fruits
D. meat, poultry, fish, dried beans, eggs, and nuts
E. breads, cereals, rice, and pasta
F. fats, oil, sweets

Foods

B **1.** peas	D **8.** dried beans	C **15.** apple
B **2.** onions	A **9.** yogurt	F **16.** butter
A **3.** milk	F **10.** cake	F **17.** candy bar
E **4.** macaroni	D **11.** nuts	C **18.** blueberries
B **5.** broccoli	B **12.** carrots	C **19.** banana
E **6.** rice	B **13.** potatoes	D **20.** chicken
E **7.** bread	A **14.** cheese	

EXERCISE 21-5

Objective: To apply what you have learned about essential nutrients.

Directions: For each food item listed below, find the nutrient that MOST CLOSELY matches that food item. Select each food item only once.

Nutrients

C = carbohydrates P = protein F = fat W = water
V = vitaminsM = minerals

Foods

F **1.** margarine	C **5.** cereal	M **9.** calcium
P **2.** beans	C **6.** fruits	V **10.** biotin
W **3.** beverages	P **7.** cheese	M **11.** iodine
M **4.** fluoride	P **8.** meat	F **12.** butter

EXERCISE 21-6

Objective: To apply what you have learned about the most common types of diets.

Directions: For each diet type listed, read the common purpose and then fill in the description column. You may describe the diet and/or give examples.

Examples of Different Types of Patient Diets

TYPE OF DIET	DESCRIPTION	COMMON PURPOSE
1. Regular	*Provides a well-balanced variety of complete nutrition. This diet must be tailored for age.*	To maintain or attain optimal nutritional status in patients who do not require a special diet
2. Clear liquid	*Clear broth and juices, ginger ale, gelatin, popsicles, clear coffee, and tea*	To provide calories and fluid in a form that requires minimal digestion. Commonly ordered after surgery.
3. Full liquid	*Strained soups/cereals, coffee, fruit and vegetable juices, ginger ale, gelatin, custard, ice cream, sherbet, pudding, tea*	For those unable to chew or swallow solid food. Used as a transitional diet between clear liquids and solid foods.
4. Soft	*Foods soft in consistency; no strongly flavored foods that could cause distress*	Used for patients who are unable to chew or swallow hard or coarse foods.
5. Mechanical soft	*Same food included in a soft diet except food is ground or strained.*	For patients with difficulty chewing or swallowing soft food.
6. Bland	*Foods mild in flavor, omits spicy food, caffeine, and alcohol*	Omits food that may cause excessive gastric acid secretion (ulcers).
7. Low residue	*Food low in fiber and bulk, also omits all foods that contain seeds*	Used for patients with acute colitis, enteritis, and diverticulitis.
8. High residue/fiber	*Food high in fiber such as whole grains, cereals, fruit, vegetables, and legumes*	Used for bowel regulation, high cholesterol, and high glucose; protects against colon cancer and diverticulosis.
9. Low calorie	*Low in calorically dense food such as fat*	For patients who need to lose weight.

TYPE OF DIET	DESCRIPTION	COMMON PURPOSE
10. Diabetic	Precise balance of carbohydrates, protein, and fats, devised according to the needs of the individual patient.	For diabetic patients; matches food intake with the insulin requirements.
11. High protein	Meals supplemented with high-protein foods, such as meat, fish, cheese, milk, and eggs, and oral supplements.	Assists in the repair of tissues wasted by disease. Used for increased protein needs (wound healing).
12. Low fat; low cholesterol	Limited amounts of butter, cream, oil, and margarine; limited fried food, high-fat meat, and dairy	For patients who have difficulty digesting fat. Examples include patients with pancreatitis, cholestasis, and heart and hepatic disease.
13. Lactose free/ low lactose	Excludes or limits food that contains lactose (milk products)	Used to prevent cramping and diarrhea in patients with a lactose deficiency.
14. Low sodium (low salt)	Limited amounts of foods containing sodium; no salt packet on tray. This diet may be restricted in protein, sodium, phosphorus, fluid, and potassium.	May be needed for patients with liver, cardiac, and renal disease. Used for patients with acute or chronic renal failure.
15. Gluten restricted	Restricts gluten-containing foods such as wheat, rye, barley, and oats	Used for patients with gluten-sensitive enteropathy.

EXERCISE 21-7

Objective: To apply what you have learned about nutrition for patients.

Directions: Circle the letter next to the word or statement that best completes the sentence or describes the sentence as true or false. If the sentence is false, draw a line through the incorrect part of the sentence and write the correction on the blank line.

1. If you eat the recommended number of portions of foods from each food group on the pyramid every day, your diet will be

A. adequate for body-builders.
B. adequate for fast growth.
(C.) adequate for good health.
D. inadequate for patients.

2. The number and size of portions of food will depend on
A. the age of the individual.
B. the size of the individual.
C. the activities of the individual.
(D.) all of the above.

3. Calories from fat should be less than ~~60%~~ of total calories.
A. True
(B.) False
Correct Answer: 30%

4. Fat has ________________ calories per gram of fat.
A. 100
(B.) 9
C. 4
D. 90

5. Water has ~~much~~ caloric value.
A. True
(B.) False
Correct Answer: no

6. Alterations to the patient's diet may be necessary for all the following reasons *except*
A. to increase or decrease the caloric content.
(B.) a desire for fad dieting.
C. to change the amounts of one or more nutrients.
D. cultural or religious requirements.

7. The nutrition status assessment may include chewing or swallowing problems.
(A.) True
B. False
Correct Answer: ________________

8. Most patients would prefer
A. to be fed.
(B.) to feed themselves.
C. to skip meals.
D. to eat when nauseated.

9. Providing a pleasant environment for the patient to eat may improve his appetite
(A.) True
B. False
Correct Answer: ________________

COMPETENCY CHECKLIST 21-1: NUTRITION

ACTIVITY	S	U	COMMENTS
1. Student will demonstrate how to assist patients with foods:			
A. Preparing the patient for a meal			
B. Serving the food			
C. Feeding the physically challenged patient			
D. Serving the between-meal snack			
2. Student will demonstrate the correct method of passing drinking water.			

The Urinary System and Related Care

22

CHAPTER OVERVIEW

Instructor Notes

I. **Anatomy and Physiology of the Urinary System**
   A. Kidneys
      1. Formation of Urine
   B. Ureters
   C. Bladder
   D. Urethra

II. **Diseases and Disorders of the Urinary System**

III. **Homeostasis**

IV. **Fluid Balance and Fluid Imbalance**
   A. Fluid Intake
   B. Fluid Output

V. **Unit of Measurement**
   A. Cubic Centimeters
   B. Graduate Containers

VI. **Measuring and Recording Fluid Intake**

VII. **Force Fluids, Restrict Fluids, and NPO**
   A. Force Fluids (FF)
   B. Restrict Fluids
   C. Nothing by Mouth

VIII. **Measuring and Recording Fluid Output**
   A. Urinary Catheters
   B. Daily Indwelling Catheter Care
   C. Fluid Output and the Incontinent Patient
   D. The Condom Catheter

IX. **Advanced Skills**
   A. Inserting an Indwelling Catheter

Instructor Notes

OBJECTIVES

When the students have completed this chapter, they will be able to:

- State the main function of the urinary system.
- Label the four components of the urinary system and explain the function of each.
- Describe three processes by which urine is formed.
- Differentiate normal and abnormal urine.
- List common diseases and disorders of the urinary system.
- Explain fluid balance and imbalance.
- List the reasons for recording accurate records of fluid intake and output.
- Accurately measure fluids using the metric system.
- Measure the capacity of serving containers.
- List ways to encourage a patient to increase fluid intake.
- Explain ways to restrict the patient's intake of fluid.
- List the ways in which the body loses fluid.
- Explain the function of urinary catheters and demonstrate their daily care.
- Apply a condom catheter.
- Discontinue an indwelling catheter.

KEY TERMS

Absorb: To take or soak in, up, or through

Anuria: Inability to urinate, no urine output

Balance of Fluids: See *fluid balance*

Bladder Distention: A stretching out of the bladder when urine produced is not excreted

Calibrated: Marked with lines and numbers for measuring

Catheter: A device for draining urine out of the body

Convert: Change

Cubic Centimeter: Having a volume equal to a cube whose edges are 1 centimeter long

Cystitis: In flammation of the urinary bladder

Dehydration: A decrease in the amount of water in the tissues occurring when fluid output exceeds input or intake

Discharge: Flowing out of material (secretion or excretion) from any part of the body such as pus, feces, urine, or drainage from a wound

Dysuria: Painful voiding

Edema: Abnormal swelling of a part of the body caused by fluid collecting in that area; usually the swelling is in the ankles, legs, hands, or abdomen

Eliminate: To rid the body of waste products, to excrete, expel, remove, put out

Instructor Notes

Evaporate: To pass off as vapor, as water evaporating into the air

Fluid: Applies to liquid substances

Fluid Balance: The same amount of fluid that is taken in by the body is given out by the body

Fluid Imbalance: When too much fluid is kept in the body or when too much fluid is lost

Fluid Intake: The fluid taken into the body, from whatever source

Fluid Output: The fluid passed or excreted out of the body, for example, urine, vomit, or diarrhea

Force Fluids: Extra fluids to be taken in by a patient according to the doctor's orders (FF)

Graduate: A measuring cup marked along its side to show various amounts so that the material placed in the cup can be measured accurately; the marks are called *calibrations*

Homeostasis: Stability of all body functions at normal levels

Incontinent: Unable to control urine or feces

Indwelling Urinary Catheter: A bladder drainage tube that is allowed to remain in place within the bladder

Insensible Fluid Loss: Fluid that is lost from the body without being noticed, such as in perspiration or air breathed out

Nothing by Mouth (NPO): Cannot eat or drink anything at all

Parenteral Intake: Fluids taken in intravenously

Peristaltic Waves: Waves of involuntary contraction

Perspiration: Sweat

Residual: Remaining or left over

Restrict Fluids: Fluids that are limited to certain amounts

Retain: To keep or hold in

Tissue Fluid: A watery environment around each cell that acts as a place of exchange for gases, food, and waste products between the cells and the blood

Urethra: A small tube that serves to empty urine from the bladder to the external environment

Urinary System (Excretory System): The group of body organs including the kidneys, ureters, bladder, and urethra that removes wastes from the blood and produces and eliminates urine

Urinate: To discharge urine from the body; other words for this function are void, micturate, and pass water

Urine: The fluid secreted by the kidneys, stored in the bladder, and excreted through the urethra

Void: To urinate, pass water

Instructor Notes

CORE STUDENT ASSIGNMENTS

Students should:

- Read this chapter in their textbook, *Being a Nursing Assistant*.
- Underline any words or sentences they do not understand. Write down any questions they have.
- Complete the Chapter Review in their textbook.
- Read the Time Management Tip for this chapter and think about how they might use this tip in their work.
- Complete the Nursing Assistant in Action exercise.

OPTIONAL STUDENT ASSIGNMENTS

Students should:

- Complete all workbook assignments for this chapter in their copy of *Workbook for Being a Nursing Assistant*.
- Use the CD/CD-Rom disk enclosed with their textbook to hear the pronunciation of the key terms in the chapter.
- Watch the "Infection Control" video from the Care Provider Skills series to learn about what kind of precautions you would take to protect yourself and your patient from infection.
- Use the Website address **(www.prenhall.com/wolgin)** to access the free, interactive Companion Website created for this textbook. Get hints, instant feedback, and textbook references to chapter-related multiple-choice questions. Read and react to the Nursing Assistant in Action exercise. Link to other interesting sites.

METHODOLOGY AND SUGGESTED ACTIVITIES

I. Lecture/Discussion

- Answer any questions the students may have.
- Discuss the key terms and related abbreviations. Repeat them out loud and practice using them in sentences.
- Discuss the Time Management Tip for this chapter.
- Discuss the Nursing Assistant in Action exercise.
- Discuss the Critical Thinking points for this chapter.
- Discuss personal safety and protection. Emphasize the importance of following Universal Precautions.
- Discuss the structure and function of the urinary system.
- Discuss the relationship of fluid intake and output to fluid balance.
- Discuss the human need for water (hydration).
- Offer examples of case studies of common diseases and disorders of the urinary system.
- Review the principles of sterile technique and asepsis.

Instructor Notes

II. Role Play/Lab

- Show the video for this chapter. Discuss precautions the students should take to prevent exposure to body fluids. Review what to do if body fluid exposure does occur in your institution.
- Demonstrate all procedures and have students return the demonstrations.
- Allow the students to measure and record container capacities.
- Assign the students to record their own fluid intake and output for a 24-hour period.
- Role play methods to maintain patient privacy and dignity in various cultures.

III. Evaluation

- Review the answers to the Chapter Review with students.
- Review the answer to the workbook exercises with students.
- Review the students' understanding of the Time Management Tip.
- To evaluate student comprehension, give a quiz.
- If applicable, practice sterile technique skills and drills with students.
- To evaluate student skills, administer the competency checklist.
- Have the students visit the interactive Companion Website and take the quiz.

ANSWERS TO CHAPTER REVIEW

FILL IN THE BLANK

Read each sentence and fill in the blank line(s) with the word or words that complete the sentence. (Note: Hyphenated words get one line.)

1. A patient may be *dehydrated* if there is a decrease in the amount of water in their tissues.
2. *fluid* *output* is the sum total of liquids that come out of the body.
3. Patients who need to increase their fluid intake may need to *force* *fluids*.
4. Patients are often NPO before and after *surgery*.
5. When a patient is incontinent, it means she is unable to control either her *urine* or *feces*.

Instructor Notes

MULTIPLE CHOICE

Choose the best answer for each question or statement.

1. Which of the following is not a structure of the urinary system?
- A. Ureters
- (B.) Valves
- C. Bladder
- D. Urethra

2. The following are all diseases and disorders of the urinary system *except*
- A. hematuria.
- B. acute renal failure.
- (C.) bursitis.
- D. renal colic.

3. All of the following may result in dehydration *except*
- A. vomiting.
- B. diarrhea.
- C. sweating.
- (D.) hypertension.

4. The unit of measurement health care providers use to measure intake and output is
- (A.) cc.
- B. oz.
- C. mm/hg.
- D. lbs.

5. When measuring the capacity of a container, you should do all of the following *except*
- A. place the container on a flat surface.
- B. view the container at eye level.
- (C.) swirl the fluid to get the best reading.
- D. carefully record your reading on paper.

CRITICAL THINKING

Instructor Notes

CUSTOMER SERVICE

Encourage students to reflect and share their thoughts and experiences. Respect their privacy and confidentiality. Share your own viewpoints with the students.

CULTURAL CARE

Encourage students to reflect and share their thoughts and experiences. Respect their privacy and confidentiality. Share your own viewpoints with the students.

COOPERATION WITHIN THE TEAM

Encourage students to reflect and share their thoughts and experiences. Respect their privacy and confidentiality. Share your own viewpoints with the students.

NURSING ASSISTANT IN ACTION

You are a student doing a clinical day working in a nursing care facility. Another student requests your help assisting Ms. Clark, a resident, to the bathroom. Before you get her positioned on the toilet, she has urinated and released some diarrhea on your uniform pant leg.

What Is Your Response/Reaction?

Mrs. Clark did not mean to do this so avoid expressing anger or acting frustrated. It is a good idea to keep an extra pair of scrubs in your work locker or in your car for just these kinds of accidents. If you do not have any other clothes to change into, wash out your pants in the staff bathroom and dry them with a hair dryer.

Instructor Notes

Answers to Workbook Exercises

22

The following exercises will assist you to apply what you have read in Chapter 22, "The Urinary System and Related Care." For each exercise, read the objective and use information you have read in Chapter 22 to answer the questions, complete the sentences, or label the diagrams.

EXERCISE 22-1

Objective: To recall the correct definitions of words used in reference to the urinary system and related care.

Directions: Choose the correct word(s) from the Word List and write it below the appropriate definition.

Word List

force fluids	fluid imbalance	incontinent
calibrated	urinary retention	edema
fluid intake	fluid output	eliminate
fluid balance	urinary system	dysuria
void	indwelling urinary catheter	NPO
anuria	catheter	homeostasis
	cystitis	urethra

Definitions

1. This word describes a measuring device marked with lines and numbers for measuring.
   calibrated

2. This term means to rid the body of waste products.
   eliminate

3. To voluntarily empty the bladder or urinate.

void

4. This term describes a patient who has a physician's order to not eat or drink, usually before surgery, a laboratory test, or a procedure or because his condition makes it necessary.

NPO

5. The group of body organs that includes the kidneys, ureters, bladder, and urethra.

urinary system

6. The state of having stability of all body functions at normal levels.

homeostasis

7. When a patient is unable to voluntarily urinate, this term refers to his condition.

urinary retention

8. This is a tubular device that stays in the bladder and is used to drain out the urine. It often has a collection bag for the urine attached to it.

indwelling urinary catheter

9. This term describes a patient who is unable to control the excretion of feces or urine.

incontinent

10. This situation can occur when either too much fluid stays in the body or too much fluid leaves the body.

fluid imbalance

11. The sum total of liquids that comes out of the body.

fluid output

12. This means that the amount of fluid eliminated is just about the same as the amount of fluid taken in.

Fluid balance

13. The sum total of liquids that goes into the body.

fluid intake

14. When the body retains excess fluid this condition can occur.

edema

15. This order means that a patient is encouraged to drink fluids.

fluids

16. This is the inability to urinate or no urine output.

Anuria

17. This device drains urine out of the body.

Catheter

18. This condition is an inflammation of the urinary bladder.

Cystitis

19. This condition results in painful voiding.

Dysuria

20. This part of the body is a small tube that empties urine from the bladder to the external environment.

Urethra

EXERCISE 22-2

Objective: To recognize and be able to correctly spell the parts of the urinary system.

Directions: Label the diagram in Figure 22-1 with the correct words from the Word List below.

Word List

ureters	nephron	left kidney
urethra	Bowman's capsule	right kidney
bladder	glomerulus	tubule

FIGURE 22-1

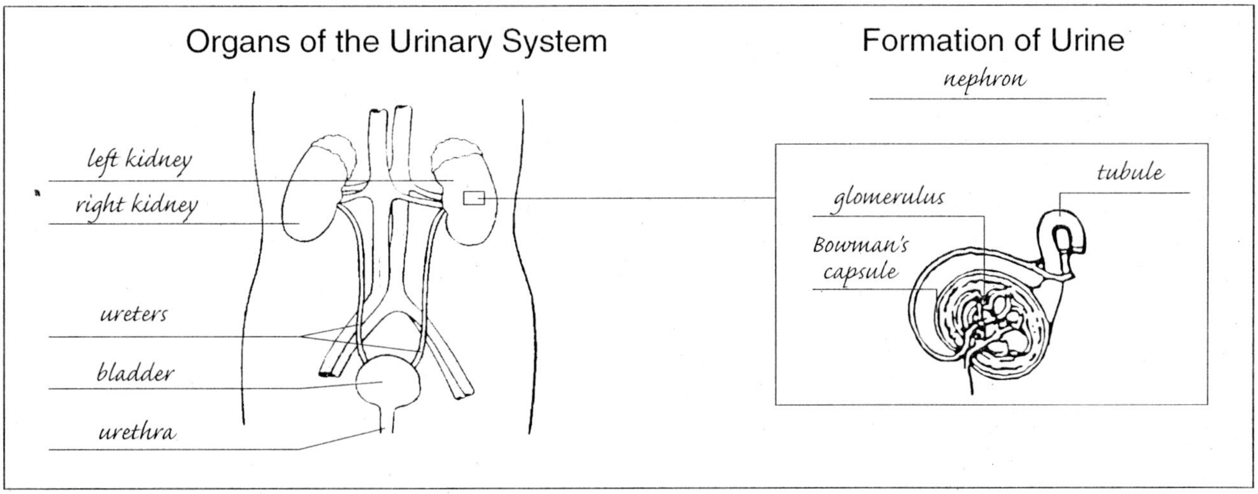

EXERCISE 22-3

Objective: To correctly define words that refer to diseases and disorders of the urinary system.

Directions: Label each disease or disorder with the letter of its correct definition.

Disease or Disorder

F 1. Acute renal failure
Q 2. Anuria
P 3. Cancer of the urinary bladder
T 4. Chronic renal failure
A 5. Cystitis
D 6. Dysuria
S 7. Hematuria
J 8. Hydronephrosis
V 9. Injury to the bladder
E 10. Nocturia
L 11. Oliguria
C 12. Polyuria
O 13. Pyelonephritis
N 14. Pyuria
H 15. Renal colic
M 16. Tuberculosis of the kidney
U 17. Tumors of the kidney
R 18. Urethral stricture
B 19. Urethritis
K 20. Urinary retention
G 21. Urinary tract infection (UTI)
I 22. Urolithiasis (renal calculi)
W 23. Dehydration

Definitions

A. Inflammation of the urinary bladder
B. Inflammation of the urethra often by sexually transmitted diseases such as chlamydia or gonorrhea.
C. Unusually large volume of urine in 24 hours
D. Painful voiding
E. Frequency of urination at night
F. Loss of kidney function
G. Presence of pathogenic microorganisms in the urinary tract
H. Sharp, severe pain in lower back over kidney, accompany forcible dilation of a ureter due to a stone or urinary calculus
I. Presence of stones in the urinary (excretory) system
J. Distention of the pelvis or one or both kidneys (urine being made but cannot be excreted due to urinary back up)
K. Inability to urinate
L. Very small amount of urine in 24 hours
M. Caused by Myeobacterium tuberculosis in the kidney
N. Pus in the urine infection

O. Infection of the kidney (acute or chronic)
P. Malignant tumor
Q. No urine
R. Narrowing of the urethra caused by infection or instrumentation; results in frequent voiding, dysuria, and hematuria (blood in the urine)
S. Blood in the urine
T. Progressive deterioration of kidney function
U. Considered malignant until proved otherwise
V. Due to trauma
W. Insufficient water in the tissues due to inadequate fluid intake or excessive fluid output

EXERCISE 22-4

Objective: To demonstrate the correct placement of intake and output information on the Intake and Output sheet.

Directions: Record the information in each statement in the correct place on the Intake and Output sheet in Figure 22-2. Total the amount for your shift. Refer to Figure 22-3 for the capacities of the serving containers.

PRACTICE STATEMENT: Mrs. Stavros is a patient who is dehydrated. She is on the Medicine Unit of the hospital where you are employed as a nursing assistant for the 7 A.M. to 3 P.M. shift. The doctor has ordered that she be put on a *liquid diet, force fluids,* and that her fluid intake and output be measured for the next 24 hours. The nurse communicates to you in the morning report meeting that Mrs. Stavros will be your patient and that she will be on Intake and Output (I&O). The patient has not been taking fluids well, and so the nurse would like you to encourage her to increase her fluid intake. If her fluid intake does not improve in the next 24 hours, the doctor stated that she will order that an IV be started. She would prefer that the patient try to take her fluids orally if possible. Mrs. Stavros has an indwelling catheter.

Statements

1. Your patient drank one 6-oz cup of juice, drank one-half of a 12-oz bowl of broth, and ate one 6-oz Jell-O cup for breakfast.
2. Between breakfast and lunch, with your encouragement, she drank one 12-oz. can of ginger ale.
3. Your patient drank one 8-oz cup of milk, drank one-half of a 12-oz bowl of broth, and ate one 6-oz Jell-O cup for lunch.
4. Between lunch and the time your shift was over, you convinced her to drink one 8-oz cup of water.
5. When you measured the amount of urine in the catheter bag, you determined that it filled the graduate container to the one-quart level.

FIGURE 22-2

INTAKE				OUTPUT			
ITEM	BY MOUTH	TUBE	PARENTERAL	URINE		GASTRIC	
				VOIDED	CATHETER	EMESIS	SUCTION
JUICE	180				1000		
BROTH	180						
JELL-O	180						
G. ALE	360						
MILK	240						
BROTH	180						
JELL-O	180						
WATER	240						
TOTAL							

FIGURE 22-3

Examples of Capacities of Serving Containers

4-oz juice cup	120 cc
6-oz cup	180 cc
8-oz cup	240 cc
12-oz cup	360 cc
1-cup milk carton	240 cc
4-oz ice cream cup	120 cc
6-oz Jell-O cup	180 cc
6-oz coffee cup	180 cc
1-qt water pitcher	1000 cc

EXERCISE 22-5

Objective: To apply what you have learned about the urinary system and related patient care.

Directions: Circle the letter next to the word or statement that best completes the sentence or describes the sentence as true or false. If the sentence is false, draw a line through the incorrect part of the sentence and write the correction on the blank line.

1. Homeostasis is the body's attempt
   (A.) to keep its internal environment stable or in balance.
   B. to increase its fluid intake.
   C. to gain weight through fluid intake.
   D. to stand very still.

2. Diagnostic studies of the urinary system are
   A. body fat analysis and QID urinalysis.
   B. difficult to interpret.
   C. key to predicting growth rates in children.
   (D.) able to indicate kidney function.

3. Some body fluid is lost through
   (A.) perspiration.
   B. delegation.
   C. undulation.
   D. constipation.

4. An abbreviation for cubic centimeter is
   A. cb.ctr.
   (B.) cc.
   C. cubo cento.
   D. cbcmtr.

5. The best time to record the patient's fluid intake is
   A. when you have time.
   B. when your immediate supervisor tells you to record ASAP.
   C. 20 minutes before the end of your shift.
   (D.) as soon as the patient consumes the fluids.

6. When measuring the capacity of serving containers, be sure to hold them at ~~waist level~~ while carefully observing the amount of fluid.
   A. True
   (B.) False
   Correct Answer: eye level

7. When measuring and recording intake and output, __________ __________ and __________ __________ are very important.
   A. good vision, good will
   B. exact observations, working fast
   C. disposable gloves, inline skates
   (D.) exact observations, accurate recordings

8. Fluids taken ____________ are recorded by the nurse.
   (A.) intravenously
   B. secretly
   C. copiously
   D. daily

9. NPO means "~~note patient order~~."
   A. True
   (B.) False
   Correct Answer: nothing by mouth

10. The indwelling catheter bag must always be kept
   A. above the head.
   B. above the waist.
   C. below the knee.
   (D.) below hip level.

COMPETENCY CHECKLIST 22-1: URINARY SYSTEM RELATED CARE

ACTIVITY	S	U	COMMENTS
1. Student correctly demonstrates the measuring of serving containers.			
2. Student correctly demonstrates determining amounts consumed.			
3. Student correctly demonstrates measuring urinary output.			
4. Student correctly demonstrates emptying urine from an indwelling catheter container.			
5. Student correctly demonstrates giving daily indwelling catheter care.			
6. Student correctly demonstrates applying a condom catheter.			
7. Student correctly demonstrates insertion of an indwelling urinary catheter in a woman.			
8. Student correctly demonstrates insertion of a straight urinary catheter in a man.			

Specimen Collection

23

CHAPTER OVERVIEW

Instructor Notes

I. **Specimen Collection**
   A. Asepsis in Specimen Collection

II. **Urine Specimens**
   A. Routine Urine Specimen
   B. Midstream, Clean-Catch Urine Specimen
   C. 24-Hour Urine Specimen
   D. Straining the Urine

III. **Sputum Specimen**

IV. **Stool Specimen**

Instructor Notes

OBJECTIVES

When the students have completed this chapter, they will be able to:

- List the types of specimens nursing assistants are expected to collect.
- Label specimens properly.
- Explain the need for accuracy in specimen collection.
- Explain the need for asepsis in specimen collection.
- Collect a routine urine specimen.
- Collect a routine urine specimen from an infant.
- Collect a midstream, clean-catch urine specimen.
- Collect a 24-hour urine specimen.
- Strain the urine.
- Collect a sputum specimen.
- Collect a stool specimen.

KEY TERMS

Asepsis: Free of disease-causing organisms

Clean Catch: Refers to the fact that urine for this specimen is not contaminated by anything outside the patient's body

Expectorate: To cough up matter from the lungs, trachea, or bronchial tubes and spit it out

Feces (Stool): Solid waste material discharged from the body through the rectum and anus; other names include excreta, excrement, bowel movement, and fecal matter

Genital: Refers to the external reproductive organs

Medical Asepsis: Special practices and procedures for preventing the conditions that allow disease-producing bacteria to live, multiply, and spread

Midstream: Catching the urine specimen between the time the patient begins to void and the time he stops

Saliva: The secretion of the salivary glands into the mouth; saliva moistens food and helps in swallowing

Specimen: A sample of material taken from the patient's body; examples are urine specimens, feces specimens, and sputum specimens

Sputum: Waste material coughed up from the lungs or trachea

CORE STUDENT ASSIGNMENTS

Students should:

- Read this chapter in their textbook, *Being a Nursing Assistant*.
- Underline any words or sentences they do not understand. Write down any questions they have.
- Complete the Chapter Review in their textbook.

Instructor Notes

- Read the Time Management Tip for this chapter and think about how they might use this tip in their work.
- Complete the Nursing Assistant in Action exercise.

OPTIONAL STUDENT ASSIGNMENTS

Students should:

- Complete all workbook assignments for this chapter in their copy of *Workbook for Being a Nursing Assistant.*
- Use the CD/CD-Rom disk enclosed with their textbook to hear the pronunciation of the key terms in the chapter.
- Watch the "Handling Infectious Waste" section of the "Infection Control" video from the Care Provider Skills series.
- Use the Website address **(www.prenhall.com/wolgin)** to access the free, interactive Companion Website created for this textbook. Get hints, instant feedback, and textbook references to chapter-related multiple-choice questions. Read and react to the Nursing Assistant in Action exercise. Link to other interesting sites.

METHODOLOGY AND SUGGESTED ACTIVITIES

I. Lecture/Discussion

- Answer any questions the students may have.
- Discuss the key terms and related abbreviations. Repeat them out loud and practice using them in sentences.
- Discuss the Time Management Tip for this chapter.
- Discuss the Nursing Assistant in Action exercise.
- Discuss the Critical Thinking points for this chapter.
- Discuss the importance of proper specimen collection for accurate medical diagnosis.
- Discuss personal safety and protection. Emphasize the importance of following Universal Precautions. Stress the need to wear protective equipment.
- Emphasize proper labeling technique for specimen collection. Also discuss accurate patient identification for safety.
- Arrange a field trip to a local lab.
- Discuss patient safety issues related to specimen collection and labeling. This is a frequent source of errors in health care.

II. Role Play/Lab

- Show the video for this chapter. Have the students practice emptying various types of urine collection devices while wearing the appropriate personal protective equipment.
- Demonstrate all the procedures and then have the students practice them.
- Have the students practice applying the infant collection devices on dolls.
- Review sample lab slips and containers.
- Have the students practice labeling the collection slips.
- Simulate 24-hour urine collection specimens for student practice.

Instructor Notes

III. Evaluation

- Review the answers to the Chapter Review with students.
- Review the answer to the workbook exercises with students.
- Review the students' understanding of the Time Management Tip.
- To evaluate student comprehension, give a quiz.
- To evaluate student skills, administer the competency checklist.
- Have the students visit the interactive Companion Website and take the quiz.

ANSWERS TO CHAPTER REVIEW

FILL IN THE BLANK

Read each sentence and fill in the blank line(s) with the word or words that complete the sentence. (Note: Hyphenated words get one line.)

1. When you ask a patient to cough up matter from the lungs, trachea, or bronchial tubes and spit it out, you are asking them to ___expectorate___.
2. By testing ___specimens___, physicians can get information to assist them in making a diagnosis and deciding on care for the patient.
3. When collecting specimens, you need to be very ___accurate___.
4. Always wear ___gloves___ when collecting a specimen.
5. After collecting the specimen, make sure you ___label___ it, to avoid mixups.

MULTIPLE CHOICE

Choose the best answer for each question or statement.

1. All of the following are important when collecting specimens *except*
   A. identifying the correct patient.
   B. accurately collecting the specimen.
   C. placing the correct label on the specimen.
   (D.) placing the specimens in alphabetical order.
2. Inaccurate or mislabeled specimens can lead to
   A. mistakes in diagnosis.
   B. delayed or unnecessary treatment.
   C. needing to repeat the procedure.
   (D.) all of the above.
3. Using medical asepsis to collect specimens includes all of the following *except*
   A. washing your hands before collecting the specimen.
   B. wearing gloves.
   (C.) sterilizing the specimen.
   D. washing your hands after collecting the specimen.

Instructor Notes

4. A clean-catch urine specimen means that the urine has
   (A.) not been contaminated by anything outside the patient's body.
   B. been obtained without dropping the sample.
   C. been collected while the patient was wearing gloves.
   D. been obtained with a catheter.

5. When collecting a 24-hour urine, do all of the following *except*
   A. throw out the first urine when collection begins.
   (B.) provide the patient with two times as much fluid to drink.
   C. post a sign indicating the patient is on a 24-hour urine collection.
   D. correctly label and date the container(s).

CRITICAL THINKING

CUSTOMER SERVICE

Encourage students to reflect and share their thoughts and experiences. Respect their privacy and confidentiality. Share your own viewpoints with the students.

CULTURAL CARE

Encourage students to reflect and share their thoughts and experiences. Respect their privacy and confidentiality. Share your own viewpoints with the students.

COOPERATION WITHIN THE TEAM

Encourage students to reflect and share their thoughts and experiences. Respect their privacy and confidentiality. Share your own viewpoints with the students.

NURSING ASSISTANT IN ACTION

You need to obtain a patient's urine sample to use in an analysis for illegal drug use. Your facility requires that you watch the patient while the specimen is voided. The patient offers you a bag with a bottle of urine in it. He tells you, "I brought you in a sample that you can test. Just use that one. How do you expect me to pee with you standing there watching me?"

What Is Your Response/Action?

Tell the patient that the sample brought in cannot be used. Tell the patient that you will be as unobtrusive as possible, but that you must watch the patient void the specimen per policy. Tell the patient that this policy is very strict and that you understand that it is a difficult test to take.

Instructor Notes

23

Answers to Workbook Exercises

The following exercises will assist you to apply what you have read in Chapter 23, "Specimen Collection." For each exercise, read the objective and use information you have read in Chapter 23 to answer the questions, complete the sentences, or label the diagrams.

EXERCISE 23-1

Objective: To recognize the definitions of words related to specimen collection.

Directions: Place the letter of the correct definition next to the matching word(s) from the Word List.

Word List

_F_ **1.** asepsis

_E_ **2.** medical asepsis

_G_ **3.** saliva

_I_ **4.** expectorate

_H_ **5.** clean catch

_J_ **6.** genital

_B_ **7.** specimen

_C_ **8.** feces (stool)

_D_ **9.** midstream

_A_ **10.** sputum

Definitions

A. Waste material coughed up from the lungs or trachea

B. A sample of material taken from the patient's body; examples are urine, feces, and sputum specimens

C. Solid waste material discharged from the body through the rectum and anus; other names include excreta, excrement, bowel movement, and fecal matter

D. Catching the urine specimen between the time the patient begins to void and the time he stops

E. Special practices and procedures for preventing the conditions that allow disease-producing bacteria to live, multiply, and spread

F. Free of disease-causing organisms
G. The secretion of the salivary glands into the mouth; it moistens food and helps in swallowing and also contains an enzyme (protein) that helps digest starches
H. Refers to the fact that the urine for this specimen is not contaminated by anything outside the patient's body
I. To cough up matter from the lungs, trachea, or bronchial tubes and spit it out
J. Refers to the external reproductive organs

EXERCISE 23-2

Objective: To apply what you have learned about specimen collection.

Directions: Read the following carefully before writing the correct answer on the blank line.

1. This process is done to urine samples to detect solids in the urine. What is it?
   straining
2. This word describes a clean-catch urine specimen. What is it?
   midstream
3. Feces is placed on this item when collected. What is it?
   slide
4. These can be found when the urine is strained. What are they?
   stones
5. When collecting a specimen, this item must be filled out with the proper information and sent to the laboratory with the specimen. What is it?
   laboratory slip

EXERCISE 23-3

Objective: To apply what you have learned about specimen collection.

Directions: Circle the letter next to the word or statement that best completes the sentence or describes the sentence as true or false. If the sentence is false, draw a line through the incorrect part of the sentence and write the correction on the blank line.

1. Most of the body's waste materials are discharged in the
   A. blood and sputum.
   B. sweat and mucus.
   (C.) urine and feces.
   D. stool and emesis.

2. If a person is sick, there will be noticeable changes in the body wastes when they are tested.
   (A.) True
   B. False
   Correct Answer: ______________________________

3. Specimens are to be collected
   A. within 2 hours of the ordered collection time.
   B. when the nursing assistant or nurse has time.
   (C.) at the time that is indicated by the medical order.
   D. "whenever."

4. The specimen collection procedure must be followed exactly
   A. or the specimen may not be useful.
   B. for the right patient.
   C. or the patient may be misdiagnosed.
   (D.) all of the above.

5. It is very important to identify the patient by name, ID number, and room number before obtaining the specimen.
   (A.) True
   B. False
   Correct Answer: ______________________________

6. The specimen must be completely ________ immediately to avoid mistakes.
   A. tested
   (B.) labeled
   C. stored
   D. shaken

7. If the specimen has the wrong name on it, all the following may occur *except*
   A. the wrong treatment may be ordered.
   B. the wrong medication may be ordered.
   C. the wrong problem may be identified.
   (D.) the patient will receive effective treatment.

8. It is important to wash your hands before and after collecting a specimen to avoid
   A. contamination of the specimen with your bacteria.
   B. spreading disease to the patient.
   C. contaminating yourself with disease-producing bacteria.
   (D.) all of the above.

9. The urine specimen that is the most common is the
   (A.) routine urine specimen.
   B. fecal specimen.
   C. common specimen.
   D. institutional specimen.

10. A clean-catch specimen must be free from
(A.) contamination.
B. harm.
C. cost.
D. high temperatures.

11. A clean-catch specimen procedure requires careful washing of the ~~abdominal~~ area.
A. True
(B.) False
Correct Answer: *genital*

12. Before a 24-hour urine specimen is started, the patient must
A. shower for 24 minutes.
B. be NPO for 24 hours.
(C.) empty her bladder.
D. measure her weight.

13. It is important to wear personal protective equipment while collecting patient specimens.
(A.) True
B. False
Correct Answer: ______

14. Sputum is a substance collected from the patient's
A. axilla.
B. navel.
C. sputola structures.
(D.) lungs.

15. The best time to obtain a sputum specimen is in the early morning after the patient has been sleeping all night.
(A.) True
B. False
Correct Answer: ______

16. The most common reason to test stool is to look for the presence of
(A.) blood or parasites.
B. stones or calculi.
C. *E. coli* bacteria.
D. bile.

17. Some stool specimens must be kept ~~cold~~ until tested.
A. True
(B.) False
Correct Answer: *warm*

18. It is important to explain to the patient
A. the reason for the test.
B. the results of the test.
(C.) what you are going to do before you do it.
D. all the steps to be followed in collecting specimens.

19. It may be necessary to remain with a small child to talk them through the process as a specimen is being collected.
(A.) True
B. False
Correct Answer: ______________________________

COMPETENCY CHECKLIST 23-1: SPECIMEN COLLECTION

ACTIVITY	S	U	COMMENTS
1. Student will demonstrate the correct method for collecting urine specimens:			
A. Routine urine			
B. Infant routine urine			
C. Midstream clean-catch urine			
D. 24-hour urine			
2. Student will demonstrate the correct method for straining urine.			
3. Student will demonstrate the correct method for collecting a sputum specimen.			
4. Student will demonstrate the correct method for collecting a stool specimen.			
5. Student will demonstrate the correct method for preparing a hemoccult slide for feces testing.			

24

The Endocrine System and Related Care of Diabetics

CHAPTER OVERVIEW

Instructor Notes

I. **Anatomy and Physiology of the Endocrine System**

II. **The Endocrine System and the Normal Aging Process**

III. **Common Diseases and Disorders of the Endocrine System**

IV. **Diabetes Mellitus**
   A. Terms Often Used with Diabetes Mellitus
   B. Signs and Symptoms of Diabetes Mellitus
   C. Signs and Symptoms of Insulin Shock
   D. Signs and Symptoms of Diabetic Coma
   E. Caring for the Diabetic Patient: Reducing Pressure Points
   F. Testing of Blood Glucose
   G. Urine Testing for Acetone

Instructor Notes

OBJECTIVES

When the students have completed this chapter, they will be able to:

- Label a diagram of the body showing the endocrine glands.
- Describe the function(s) of each gland.
- List the common diseases and disorders of the endocrine system.
- Recognize the signs and symptoms of diabetes mellitus, insulin shock, and diabetic coma.
- Teach the patient with diabetes how to avoid pressure points and skin problems.
- Test a patient's blood glucose level via a finger stick using a blood glucose meter.

KEY TERMS

Carbohydrate: Type of basic food element used by the body; composed of carbon, hydrogen, and oxygen; includes sugars and starches

Diabetes Mellitus: Disorder of carbohydrate metabolism caused by inability to convert sugar into energy because of inadequate production or utilization of insulin

Diabetic Coma: A coma (abnormal deep stupor) that can occur in a diabetic patient from lack of insulin

Endocrine Glands: Ductless glands that produce hormones and secrete them directly into the blood or lymph

Endocrine System: System composed of endocrine glands; regulates body function by secreting hormones

Exocrine Glands: Glands that produce hormones and secrete them either directly or through a duct to epithelial tissue, such as a body cavity or the skin surface

Gland: An organ that is able to manufacture and discharge a chemical that will be used elsewhere in the body

Glucose: A sugar formed during metabolism of carbohydrates; blood sugar

Hormones: Protein substances secreted by endocrine glands directly into the blood to stimulate increased activity

Hyperglycemia: Abnormally high blood sugar

Hypoglycemia: Abnormally low blood sugar

Insulin: Hormone that regulates the sugar content of the blood

Insulin Shock: Serious complication related to diabetes; occurs when the diabetic receives too much insulin, misses a meal, or has too much physical activity

Metabolism: The process through which food elements are converted energy for use in the human body

Secrete: Produce and release; glands secrete hormones

CORE STUDENT ASSIGNMENTS

Instructor Notes

Students should:

- Read this chapter in their textbook, *Being a Nursing Assistant*.
- Underline any words or sentences they do not understand. Write down any questions they have.
- Complete the Chapter Review in their textbook.
- Read the Time Management Tip for this chapter and think about how they might use this tip in their work.
- Complete the Nursing Assistant in Action exercise.

OPTIONAL STUDENT ASSIGNMENTS

Students should:

- Complete all workbook assignments for this chapter in their copy of *Workbook for Being a Nursing Assistant*.
- Use the CD/CD-Rom disk enclosed with their textbook to hear the pronunciation of the key terms in the chapter.
- Watch the portion related to care of the feet from the "Personal Care" video from the Care Provider Skills series.
- Use the Website address **(www.prenhall.com/wolgin)** to access the free, interactive Companion Website created for this textbook. Get hints, instant feedback, and textbook references to chapter-related multiple-choice questions. Read and react to the Nursing Assistant in Action exercise. Link to other interesting sites.

METHODOLOGY AND SUGGESTED ACTIVITIES

I. Lecture/Discussion

- Answer any questions the students may have.
- Discuss the key terms and related abbreviations. Repeat them out loud and practice using them in sentences.
- Discuss the Time Management Tip for this chapter.
- Discuss the Nursing Assistant in Action exercise.
- Discuss the Critical Thinking points for this chapter.
- Discuss personal safety and protection. Emphasize the importance of following Universal Precautions.
- Discuss the structure and function of the endocrine system. Use anatomy plates or play an anatomy matching game.
- Discuss the process of balancing carbohydrates with insulin production/use.
- Offer examples of case studies of common diseases and disorders of the endocrine system.
- Discuss the rapidly rising occurrence of diabetes in the American population and the factors causing it.

Instructor Notes

II. Lab/Demonstration

- Show the video for this chapter. Review the importance of careful foot care for diabetic patients and for patients with peripheral vascular disease. Reinforce that nursing assistants should never cut toenails.
- Demonstrate use of the One-Touch Profile meter.
- Review the signs and symptoms of hyperglycemia and hypoglycemia and steps the nursing assistant should take with patients who have these disorders.
- Assign the students practice time with the One-Touch meter.
- Explain use of equipment for urine acetone testing.
- Have the students practice reporting abnormal results and practice documenting them on your institution's flowsheet.
- Give the students case scenarios of hyperglycemia and hypoglycemia to respond to.

III. Evaluation

- Review the answers to the Chapter Review with students.
- Review the answer to the workbook exercises with students.
- Review the students' understanding of the Time Management Tip.
- To evaluate student comprehension, give a quiz.
- To evaluate student skills, administer the competency checklist.
- Have the students visit the interactive Companion Website and take the quiz.

ANSWERS TO CHAPTER REVIEW

FILL IN THE BLANK

Read each sentence and fill in the blank line(s) with the word or words that complete the sentence. (Note: Hyphenated words get one line.)

1. The hormone that regulates the sugar content of the blood is called *insulin*.
2. The process through which food elements are converted into energy for use in the body is called *metabolism*.
3. Abnormally low blood sugar is called *hypoglycemia*.
4. Abnormally high blood sugar is called *hyperglycemia*.
5. The most common way to test blood glucose is with a *blood* *glucose* *meter*.

MULTIPLE CHOICE

Instructor Notes

Choose the best answer for each question or statement.

1. The endocrine system consists of several glands that secrete liquids called
   (A.) hormones.
   B. urine.
   C. insulin.
   D. glucose.
2. The master gland of the endocrine system is the
   A. pancreas.
   (B.) pituitary.
   C. ovaries.
   D. thyroid.
3. Which of the following is not a disease or disorder of the endocrine system?
   A. Diabetes mellitus
   B. Hyperthyroidism
   (C.) Crohn's disease
   D. Addison's disease
4. The most common disorder of the endocrine system is
   A. cancer.
   B. hypoglycemia.
   C. impotence.
   (D.) diabetes mellitus.
5. Insulin shock occurs when the body has
   (A.) too much insulin.
   B. too little insulin.

CRITICAL THINKING

CUSTOMER SERVICE

Encourage students to reflect and share their thoughts and experiences. Respect their privacy and confidentiality. Share your own viewpoints with the students.

CULTURAL CARE

Encourage students to reflect and share their thoughts and experiences. Respect their privacy and confidentiality. Share your own viewpoints with the students.

COOPERATION WITHIN THE TEAM

Encourage students to reflect and share their thoughts and experiences. Respect their privacy and confidentiality. Share your own viewpoints with the students.

Instructor Notes

NURSING ASSISTANT IN ACTION

You are assigned to care for Mrs. Brauns, a 70-year-old diabetic. She is insulin dependent and supposed to be following a diabetic diet low in sugar. Her blood sugar is elevated after her grandchildren visit because they bring her favorite candy bars to eat. She says, "Please don't report anything about the candy. Sharing it with my grandchildren is one of the few joys I have since my husband died."

What Is Your Response/Action?

Assure Mrs. Brauns that you are not mad at her or going to get her in trouble, but that the nurse will need to know why her blood sugar is elevated today so that she can monitor it and give her the proper treatment.

24

Answers to Workbook Exercises

The following exercises will assist you to apply what you have read in Chapter 24, "The Endocrine System and Related Care of Diabetics." For each example, read the objective and use information you have read in Chapter 24 to answer the questions, complete the sentences, or label the diagrams.

EXERCISE 24-1

Objective: To recognize and correctly spell words related to the endocrine system and related care.

Directions: Label the diagram in Figure 24-1 with the correct words from the Word List below.

Word List

pineal	pituitary	parathyroids
thymus	thyroid	testes (in men)
pancreas	adrenals	ovaries (in women)

FIGURE 24-1

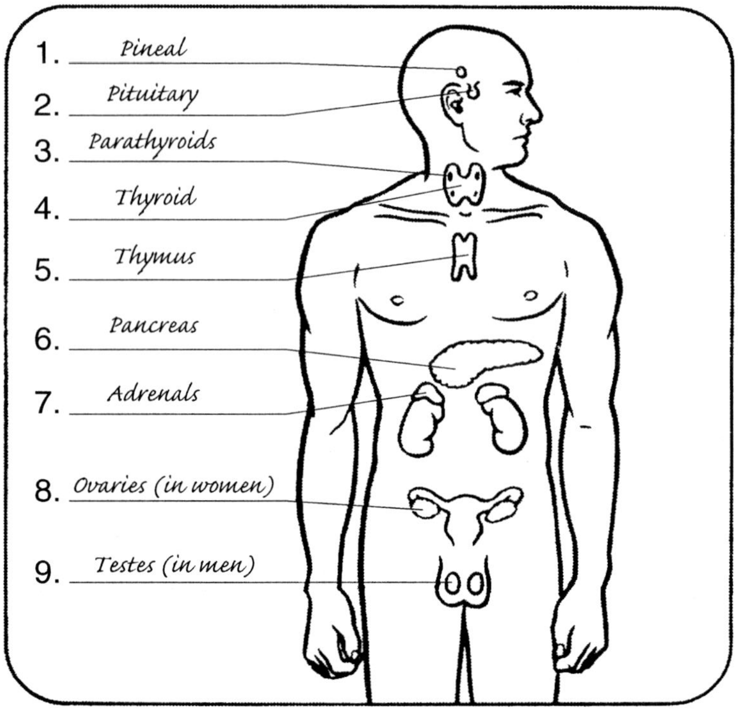

EXERCISE 24-2

Objective: To apply what you have learned about the endocrine system and related care of the diabetic.

Directions: Read the following riddles carefully before writing the correct answer on the blank line.

1. These are three classic symptoms of diabetes. What are they? *Hint:* The beginnings of all three words are the same and sound like a girl's name.
   polydipsia, polyphagia, polyuria
2. This item sounds like something you would write with, but it contains a point much sharper than a pen. What is it? *Hint:* It contains a lancet.
   penlet

EXERCISE 24-3

Objective: To recognize the definitions of words related to the endocrine system and related care of the diabetic.

Directions: Place the letter of the correct definition next to the matching word(s) from the Word List.

Word List

I 1. carbohydrate
K 2. exocrine glands
H 3. endocrine system
M 4. endocrine glands
N 5. hyperglycemia
D 6. insulin shock
J 7. diabetes mellitus
C 8. metabolism
L 9. gland
G 10. hypoglycemia
F 11. hormones
A 12. glucose
E 13. insulin
B 14. secrete
O 15. diabetic coma

Definitions

A. A sugar formed during metabolism of carbohydrates; blood sugar
B. To produce a special substance and release it
C. The process through which food elements are converted into energy for use in the human body
D. Serious complication related to diabetes; occurs when the diabetic patient receives too much insulin, misses a meal, or has too much physical activity
E. A hormone produced naturally by the pancreas that helps the body change sugar into energy
F. Protein substances secreted by endocrine glands directly into the blood to stimulate increased activity
G. Abnormally low blood sugar
H. System composed of endocrine glands; regulates body function by secreting hormones
I. Type of basic food element used by the body; composed of carbon, hydrogen, and oxygen; includes sugars and starches
J. Disorder of carbohydrate metabolism caused by inability to convert sugar into energy because of inadequate production or utilization of insulin
K. Glands that produce hormones and secrete them either directly or through a duct to epithelial tissue, such as a body cavity or the skin surface
L. An organ that is able to manufacture and discharge a chemical that will be used elsewhere in the body
M. Ductless glands that produce hormones and secrete them directly into the blood or lymph

N. Abnormally high blood sugar

O. A coma (abnormal deep stupor) that can occur in a patient from lack of insulin

EXERCISE 24-4

Objective: To apply what you have learned about the endocrine system and related care of the diabetic.

Directions: Circle the letter next to the word or statement that best completes the sentence or describes the sentence as true or false. If the sentence is false, draw a line through the incorrect part of the sentence and write the correction on the blank line.

1. The master gland of the body is the ________ gland.
   A. adrenal
   B. thyroid
   C. captain
   (D.) pituitary

2. The gland that is thought to be the link between our thinking, our emotions, and our body functions is the
   A. thinking link gland.
   (B.) hypothalamus gland.
   C. hippopotamus gland.
   D. emoto gland.

3. Insulin is produced in the
   A. hypoinsulin gland.
   B. sugar gland.
   C. parathyroids.
   (D.) pancreas.

4. The thymus gland gets ~~larger~~ with age.
   A. True
   (B.) False
   Correct Answer: smaller

5. In an emergency, the adrenal glands produce ________, which gives the body large amounts of energy.
   A. sugar
   B. insulin
   (C.) adrenalin
   D. progesterone

6. Two female hormones are ________ and ________
   A. insulin, protectin.
   B. estrogen, testosterone.
   C. testosterone, insulin.
   (D.) estrogen, progesterone.

7. The ________ produces a hormone that regulates growth.
A. pancreas
(B.) thyroid
C. heart
D. stomach

8. Insulin-dependent diabetes mellitus is
A. also known as Type I diabetes.
B. also known as juvenile-onset diabetes.
C. rapidly increasing in occurrence in the United States.
(D.) all of the above.

9. Male hormones are produced in the
A. ovaries.
(B.) testes.
C. pancreas.
D. liver.

10. Signs and symptoms of diabetes include all of the following *except*
A. excessive thirst.
B. poorly healing sores.
C. weight loss.
(D.) chest pain.

11. ________ is a male hormone.
A. Estrogen
B. Progesterone
(C.) Testosterone
D. Insulin

12. Cushing's syndrome occurs when the adrenal glands are
A. not active.
(B.) too active.
C. reactive.
D. absent.

13. The most common disorder caused by endocrine problems is
(A.) diabetes.
B. obesity.
C. pulmonary edema.
D. Cushing's syndrome.

14. Gangrene can occur when a body part does not get enough
A. insulin.
(B.) circulating blood.
C. gangrenite.
D. pituitrin.

15. Signs and symptoms of diabetes include all of the following *except*
A. polydipsia.
B. polyphasia.
C. polyuria.
(D.) polyinsulin.

16. Symptoms of insulin shock include all of the following *except*
A. faintness and dizziness.
(B.) hyperglycemia.
C. excessive sweating.
D. irritability.

17. Signs of diabetic coma include all of the following *except*
A. increased urination.
B. loss of appetite.
C. loss of consciousness.
(D.) blurred vision.

18. __________ care is very important for diabetic health.
(A.) Foot
B. Hair
C. Car
D. Home

19. Good awareness of blood sugar levels is dependent on use of
A. foot meters.
B. insulin meters.
C. carbohydrate meters.
(D.) blood glucose meters.

20. It is important that the patient learn to use a blood glucose meter and to administer his own insulin.
(A.) True
B. False
Correct Answer: ______________________________

21. For diabetics, shoes and stockings should fit correctly and not be
A. too tight.
B. too loose.
C. constrictive.
(D.) all of the above.

22. When using a blood glucose meter for several patients, the nursing assistant should
A. use a pipet to prevent contamination of the patient.
B. wash his or her hands between patients.
C. be sure to record the blood level after each test.
(D.) all of the above.

23. The nursing assistant must always wear disposable gloves when testing the patient's blood.

(A.) True

B. False

Correct Answer: ______________________________

24. Whenever testing the urine for glucose, use

(A.) a fresh sample.

B. a sample from the Foley bag.

C. a sample from the last test.

D. a sample from the toilet.

COMPETENCY CHECKLIST 24-1: GLUCOSE TESTING

ACTIVITY	S	U	COMMENTS
The student will demonstrate the correct method of testing for glucose using the One-Touch Profile diabetes tracking system.			

25

The Reproductive System and Related Care

CHAPTER OVERVIEW

Instructor Notes

I. **The Reproductive System**
   A. Female Reproductive System
   B. Male Reproductive System

II. **Sexuality**

III. **The Reproductive System and the Normal Aging Process**
   A. Aging of the Female Reproductive System
   B. Aging of the Male Reproductive System

IV. **Common Diseases and Disorders of the Reproductive System**
   A. Sexually Transmitted Diseases
   B. Caring for Patients with AIDS

V. **Care of the Gynecological Patient**
   A. Preparing the Patient for a Pelvic Exam
   B. Vaginal Douche or Nonsterile Irrigation

VI. **Postpartum Care**

Instructor Notes

OBJECTIVES

When the students have completed this chapter, they will be able to:

- Label a diagram with the female organs of the reproductive system and explain how each organ helps in the process of reproduction.
- Label a diagram with the male organs of the reproductive system and explain how each organ helps in the process of reproduction.
- Explain the meaning of sexuality and how the nursing assistant can appropriately respect the sexuality of patients.
- List the common disorders of the reproductive system.
- List the common sexually transmitted diseases (STDs).
- Explain HIV/AIDS precautions with all patients.
- Describe how to prepare a patient for a pelvic exam.
- Give a vaginal irrigation (douche).
- Identify important aspects of postpartum care.

KEY TERMS

AIDS: Viral infection characterized by decreased immunity to opportunistic infections

Estrogen: A female hormone that causes a buildup of the lining of the uterus to prepare it for possible pregnancy; also responsible for the development of secondary sexual characteristics

Fertile: Able to become pregnant; capable of reproduction

Fertilization: Joining of a sperm and ovum to form a new cell

Gynecological (GYN) Patient: Patient being treated for diseases or conditions of the female reproductive organs, including the breasts

HIV: Human immunodeficiency virus; the microorganism that causes AIDS

Menopause: Time during which menstruation stops, resulting in decreased hormone production and an end of fertility

Menstruation: Periodic (monthly) loss of some blood and a small part of the lining of the uterus when a woman is not pregnant

Ova/Ovum: The female reproductive cell(s) produced in the ovaries which is capable of uniting with a sperm cell and developing into a new organism

Ovulation: Process whereby an ovum is released from one ovary into the opening of the fallopian tube and moves to the uterus

Pelvic Inflammatory Disease (PID): Infection that spreads to all structures in the pelvic cavity.

Perineal Area: The area of the body between the thighs; includes the area of the anus and the external genital organs

Reproductive System: The group of body organs that makes possible the creation of a new human life

Instructor Notes

Sexually Transmitted Diseases (STDs): Diseases acquired as a result of sexual intercourse with an infected person

Sperm: The male reproductive cell produced in the testes that is released from the male during intercourse

Testosterone: The primary male sex hormone; manufactured in the testes

Vagina (Vaginal Canal): The canal leading from the cervix to the outside of the female body; serves as the organ for intercourse and the birth canal

Vaginal Irrigation (Douche): The introduction of a solution into the vagina with an immediate return of the solution by gravity; usually used for cleansing the vaginal canal or relieving inflammation of the vaginal tract

CORE STUDENT ASSIGNMENTS

Students should:

- Read this chapter in their textbook, *Being a Nursing Assistant*.
- Underline any words or sentences they do not understand. Write down any questions they have.
- Complete the Chapter Review in their textbook.
- Read the Time Management Tip for this chapter and think about how they might use this tip in their work.
- Complete the Nursing Assistant in Action exercise.

OPTIONAL STUDENT ASSIGNMENTS

Students should:

- Complete all workbook assignments for this chapter in their copy of *Workbook for Being a Nursing Assistant*.
- Use the CD/CD-Rom disk enclosed with their textbook to hear the pronunciation of the key terms in the chapter.
- Watch the "Age-Specific Competencies" video and the "Perineal Care" section of the "Bed Bath" video from the Care Provider Skills series.
- Use the Website address **(www.prenhall.com/wolgin)** to access the free, interactive Companion Website created for this textbook. Get hints, instant feedback, and textbook references to chapter-related multiple-choice questions. Read and react to the Nursing Assistant in Action exercise. Link to other interesting sites.

METHODOLOGY AND SUGGESTED ACTIVITIES

I. Lecture/Discussion

- Answer any questions the students may have.
- Discuss the key terms and related abbreviations. Repeat them out loud and practice using them in sentences.
- Discuss the Time Management Tip for this chapter.
- Discuss the Nursing Assistant in Action exercise.

Instructor Notes

- Discuss the Critical Thinking points for this chapter.
- Review Universal Precautions and infection control. Discuss personal safety and protection.
- Review and discuss the structure and function of the male and female reproductive systems.
- Offer case studies of the common diseases and disorders related to the reproductive system.
- Discuss the significance of HIV infection.
- Outline the special care of the gynecological patient.
- Discuss how cultural issues relate to a patient's view of sexuality.

II. Role Play/Lab

- Show the videos for this chapter. Discuss how the age of the patient will change the way the patient may react or feel during perineal care or during pelvic exams.
- Identify stages of growth and development of sexuality in the male and female based on age, disease process, social and cultural issues, and needs.
- Assign the students to teams to practice on a mannequin the procedure for preparing a patient for a pelvic exam.
- Role play scenarios to maintain the privacy and dignity of patients during reproductive related care.

III. Evaluation

- Review the answers to the Chapter Review with students.
- Review the answer to the workbook exercises with students.
- Review the students' understanding of the Time Management Tip.
- To evaluate student comprehension, give a quiz.
- To evaluate student skills, administer the competency checklist.
- Have the students visit the interactive Companion Website and take the quiz.

ANSWERS TO CHAPTER REVIEW

FILL IN THE BLANK

Read each sentence and fill in the blank line(s) with the word or words that complete the sentence. (Note: Hyphenated words get one line.)

1. The reproductive process begins with *ovulation*.
2. *Sexuality* is the group of characteristics that identify the differences between males and females.
3. Diseases that are acquired as a result of sexual intercourse are called *sexually* *transmitted* *diseases*.
4. HIV/AIDS is transmitted by *body* *fluids*.
5. Cleaning of the perineum after delivery is called *postpartum* care.

Instructor Notes

MULTIPLE CHOICE

Choose the best answer for each question or statement.

1. Which of the following is not a part of the female reproductive system?
   A. Cervix
   (B.) Prepuce
   C. Hymen
   D. Ovary
2. Which of the following is not a part of the male reproductive system?
   A. Prostate
   (B.) Hymen
   C. Epididymis
   D. Scrotum
3. Which of the following is not a disorder of the female reproductive system?
   A. Dysmenorrhea
   B. Pelvic inflammatory disease
   C. Fibroids
   (D.) Hydrocele
4. Which of the following is not a disorder of the male reproductive system?
   A. Prostatitis
   B. Varicocele
   (C.) Cystocele
   D. Benign prostate hyperplasia
5. HIV/AIDS cannot be transmitted by
   A. blood transfusions.
   B. direct contact with body fluids.
   (C.) touching the skin of a patient who has the infection.
   D. being stuck by an IV needle used with an AIDS patient.

CRITICAL THINKING

CUSTOMER SERVICE

Encourage students to reflect and share their thoughts and experiences. Respect their privacy and confidentiality. Share your own viewpoints with the students.

CULTURAL CARE

Encourage students to reflect and share their thoughts and experiences. Respect their privacy and confidentiality. Share your own viewpoints with the students.

Instructor Notes

COOPERATION WITHIN THE TEAM

Encourage students to reflect and share their thoughts and experiences. Respect their privacy and confidentiality. Share your own viewpoints with the students.

NURSING ASSISTANT IN ACTION

You are working in a community health center preparing Carrie Cooper, an 18-year-old woman, for a GYN exam. She is nervous about the pelvic exam and tells you her boyfriend is HIV positive, but refuses to use condoms when they have sex. Carrie says, "You know how men are, he will quit seeing me unless I do as he says. All my girlfriends keep telling me that he is so hot. I do not want to give him up!"

What Is Your Response/Action?

A good way to start to respond to Carrie would be to agree with her that it is important to use condoms. Reinforce that she is putting her own health at risk with this behavior. Ask Carrie how she feels about this boyfriend versus what her parents think. Suggest to Carrie to ask the physician more about HIV and how she can talk to her boyfriend about safe sex and HIV prevention for her.

25

Answers to Workbook Questions

The following exercises will assist you to apply what you have read in Chapter 25, "The Reproductive System and Related Care." For each exercise, read the objective and use information you have read in Chapter 25 to answer the questions, complete the sentences, or label the diagrams.

EXERCISE 25-1

Objective: To recognize and be able to correctly spell the parts of the female reproductive system.

Directions: Label in Figure 25-1 the parts of the female reproductive organs and specialized cells with the words from the Word List.

Word List

labia majora	urethral meatus	uterus
ovary tube	ovary	cervix
uterine neck	fallopian tube	vaginal orifice
clitoris	hymen	labia minora
ovum escaping	vagina or birth canal	

FIGURE 25-1

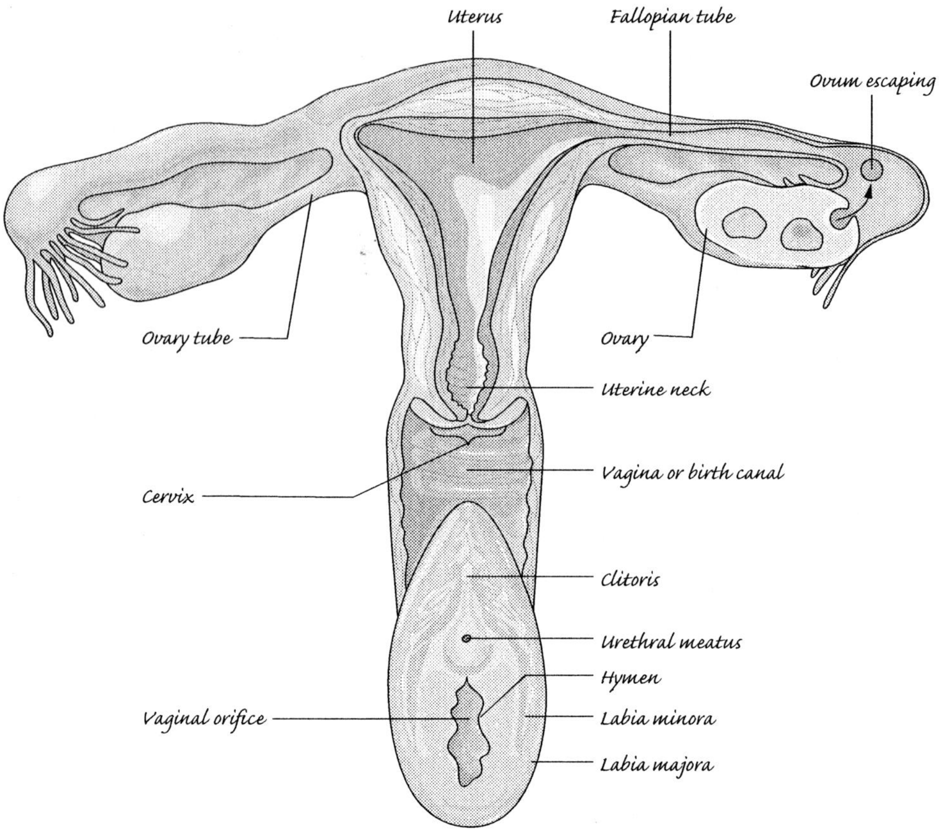

EXERCISE 25-2

Objective: To recognize and be able to correctly spell the parts of the male reproductive organs.

Directions: Label in Figure 25-2 the parts of the male reproductive organs and specialized cells with the words from the Word List.

Word List

bladder	testicle (testis)	glans penis
vas deferens	prostate	epididymis
ejaculatory duct	bulbo-urethral gland	seminal vesicle
rectum	urethral meatus	prepuce
scrotum		

FIGURE 25-2

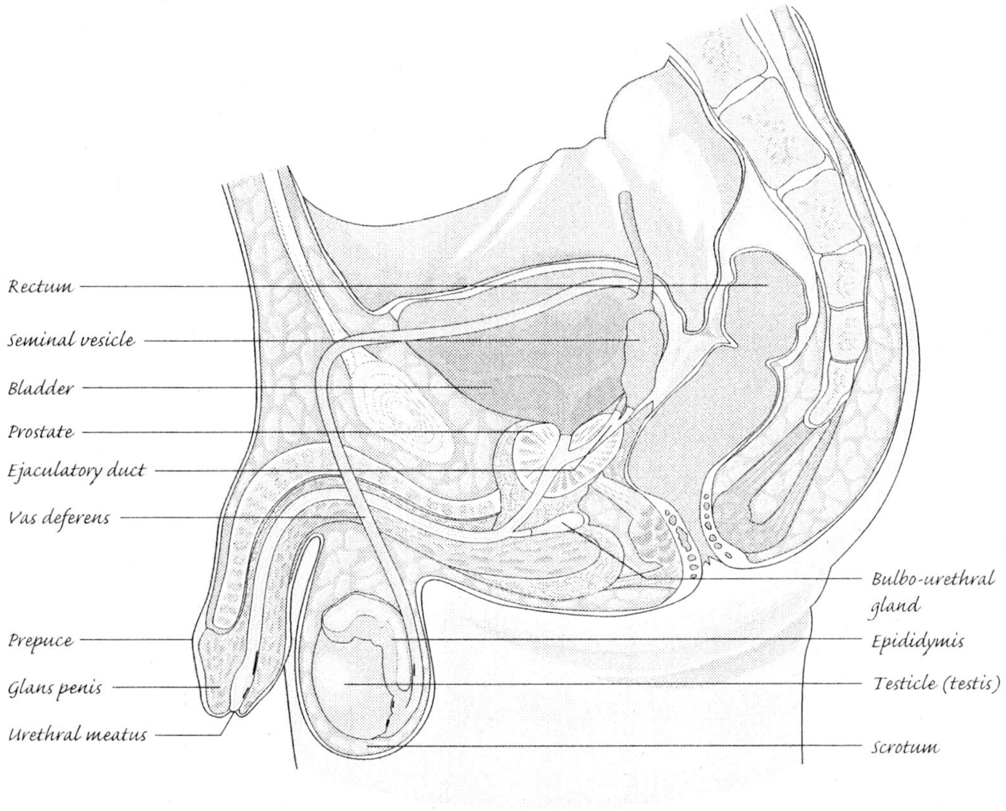

EXERCISE 25-3

Objective: To associate sexually transmitted diseases (STDs) with their responsible organisms.

Directions: Draw a line to connect the disease with the correct organism.

Disease	Organism
pelvic inflammatory disease	HPV virus
gonorrhea	herpes simplex virus
AIDS	Chlamydia
syphilis	gonococcus
genital warts	HIV virus
genital herpes simplex	*Treponema pallidum*

EXERCISE 25-4

Objective: To identify words that relate to postpartum care.

Directions: Unscramble the words in the Word List at the left. Then circle the same words in the Word Search grid at the right.

Word List

1. MUVO ____OVUM____
2. TRAPTUMPOS ____POSTPARTUM____
3. MERSP ____SPERM____
4. XVIRCE ____CERVIX____
5. TINMOLAUAB ____AMBULATION____
6. NEARCASE ECSTION ____CESAREAN SECTION____
7. IPRE TOLBET ____PERI BOTTLE____
8. CAVRIPY ____PRIVACY____

Word Search

O	Q	A	S	P	R	I	V	A	C	Y	X	W	U	P	X
V	Y	P	E	R	I	B	O	T	T	L	E	G	S	U	W
U	C	E	S	A	R	E	A	N	S	E	C	T	I	O	N
M	K	R	Q	A	M	B	U	L	A	T	I	O	N	Q	R
S	K	N	B	V	C	X	U	P	W	P	I	M	I	L	A
P	E	R	C	E	R	V	I	X	R	M	W	O	M	I	L
E	P	I	Q	P	O	S	T	P	A	R	T	U	M	K	F
R	C	V	E	T	Y	P	M	T	B	U	W	X	I	L	S
M	O	T	R	E	V	C	Q	R	T	X	W	E	E	N	C

EXERCISE 25-5

Objective: To recall important points to remember when preparing a female patient for a pelvic examination.

Directions: Complete the following sentences with the correct words from the Word List below. You are a nursing assistant who has been working for 6 months after completing your training. You work in a women's health clinic. The nurse asks you to prepare Ms. Smith for a pelvic exam.

Word List

call light	dorsal lithotomy	drape
examination	privacy	equipment
stirrup	wash	gloves
gown	comfort	hands
dress	condition	reproductive

1. This examination is very important for assessing the ____condition____ of the female ____reproduction____ organs.
2. This can be a difficult ____examination____ for a woman to receive.
3. It is important that ____privacy____ and ____comfort____ be maintained.
4. The typical position used in this exam is the ____dorsal____ ____lithotomy____ position.

5. ___Stirrups___ may be used to position the legs and the feet.

6. An additional ___drape___ may be used to cover the feet.

7. If you leave the patient alone in the room, make sure to leave the ___call___ ___light___ within her reach.

8. ___Wash___ your ___hands___ before and after handling equipment or specimens and use disposable ___gloves___.

9. Care for the ___equipment___ according to the clinic's policy.

10. After the examination, assist the patient to ___dress___ or put on a ___gown___. If she is able to dress herself, leave the room so that the patient can dress herself in private.

EXERCISE 25-6

Objective: To apply what you have learned about human reproduction and patient care.

Directions: Circle the letter next to the statement that best completes the sentence or describes the sentence as true or false. If the sentence is false, draw a line through the incorrect portion of the sentence.

1. There are several female organs of reproduction, but the primary reproductive organs are the
   A. uterus and the vagina.
   (B.) two ovaries.
   C. fallopian tubes.
   D. testes and the penis.

2. The primary reproductive organs of the male are the
   (A.) two testes.
   B. penis and the prostate gland.
   C. sperm cells.
   D. urethra and the penis.

3. Males may be unaware they have human papillomavirus and can spread it to their partners.
   (A.) True
   B. False
   Correct Answer: ______________________________

4. The process whereby an ovum is released from an ovary into the fallopian tubes and travels to the uterus is called
   A. conception.
   B. climax.
   C. menstruation.
   (D.) ovulation.

5. During intercourse, the sperm travel up the vas deferens to a point where they enter the urethra.
   (A.) True
   B. False
   Correct Answer: ____________________

6. Menstruation diminishes around age 45–52, leading to menopause.
   (A.) True
   B. False
   Correct Answer: ____________________

7. Females may have no symptoms of gonorrhea and still spread the diseases to sexual partners.
   (A.) True
   B. False
   Correct Answer: ____________________

8. There is only one duct in the penis that is used for the flow of urine and the flow of
   A. blood.
   B. milk.
   C. testosterone.
   (D.) semen.

9. Sexuality refers to the group of characteristics that identify the differences between
   A. sex and reproduction.
   B. good and bad.
   C. right and wrong.
   (D.) male and female.

10. Sexuality is a normal part of growth and development and ~~must always be associated with the sex organs~~.
   A. True
   (B.) False
   Correct Answer: *involves warm, caring feelings shared between people and must not always be associated with the sex organs.*

11. Sexually transmitted diseases (STDs) can be 100% prevented
   A. by luck and timing.
   (B.) through abstinence.
   C. by the use of male condoms.
   D. by the use of female condoms.

12. A person can carry the HIV virus for many years before developing AIDS.
   (A.) True
   B. False
   Correct Answer: ____________________

13. Three examples of STDs are
A. chlamydia, pneumonia, and gonorrhea.
B. chlamydia, gonorrhea, and amenorrhea.
(C.) HSV, HPV, and HIV.

14. Genital herpes simplex (HSV) can be contracted
A. only if sores are visible.
B. only if sores are open and draining.
(C.) from anyone having HSV.
D. only during menstruation.

15. Some forms of human papillomavirus (HPV) infection (genital warts) can be cancerous.
(A.) True
B. False
Correct Answer: ____________________

16. Examples of female reproductive disorders are
(A.) cystocele and rectocele.
B. tumors of the breast and hydrocele.
C. prostatitis and BPH.
D. varicocele and varicose veins.

17. Examples of male reproductive disorders are
(A.) prostatitis and benign prostatic hyperplasia (BPH).
B. tumors of the breast and cancer of the uterus.
C. vaginitis and pelvic inflammatory disease (PID).
D. menorrhagia and backaches.

18. Men being treated for impotence due to erectile dysfunction should see a ~~dermatologist~~ before taking topical or internal remedies.
A. True
(B.) False
Correct Answer: urologist

19. Another word for vaginal irrigation is
A. constipation.
B. enema.
(C.) douche.
D. perineal care.

20. An episiotomy is a small cut in the vagina made during childbirth to make the opening larger and to prevent tearing.
(A.) True
B. False
Correct Answer: ____________________

21. Postpartum perineal care is performed each time after the patient urinates and/or defecates.
(A.) True
B. False
Correct Answer: ____________________

22. Postpartum perineal care is important to prevent
(A.) infection.
B. herpes.
C. HIV.
D. chlamydia.

23. Excessive vaginal irrigation can wash away normal protective secretions.
(A.) True
B. False
Correct Answer: ____________________

24. Early ambulation is important to prevent circulation problems after childbirth, but before the patient gets up you must check with your immediate supervisor to see if the patient
A. has hardsole shoes to wear.
(B.) has numbness in her legs from the anesthesia.
C. has orders to walk more than a mile a day.
D. can request that her husband walk for her.

25. Some patients develop a severe ~~rash~~ if they ambulate when they have doctor's orders to lay flat or at a reduced angle for several hours after receiving spinal anesthesia.
A. True
(B.) False
Correct Answer: *headache*

26. The way a patient expects to be treated by a health care worker is influenced by
A. the time of day.
B. the nurse.
C. pain.
(D.) the cultural characteristics of that patient.

COMPETENCY CHECKLIST 25-1: CARE RELATED TO THE REPRODUCTIVE SYSTEM

ACTIVITY	S	U	COMMENTS
1. Student will demonstrate the proper procedure for preparing the female patient for a pelvic exam.			
2. Student will demonstrate the proper procedure for perforing postpartum perineal care.			

26

The Nervous System and Related Care

CHAPTER OVERVIEW

Instructor Notes

I. **Anatomy and Physiology of the Nervous System**
  A. Sensing and Responding to the Environment
  B. Protection of the Nervous System
  C. The Brain
  D. The Autonomic Nervous System
  E. The Sense Organs

II. **Care of the Artificial Eye**

III. **Care of Eyeglasses**

IV. **Hearing Aids**
  A. Parts of the Hearing Aid
  B. Placement of the Hearing Aid
  C. Checking the Batteries

V. **The Nervous System and the Normal Aging Process**
  A. Common Diseases and Disorders of the Nervous System

VI. **Care of the Seizure Patient**

VII. **The Cerebrovascular Accident (Stroke) Patient**
  A. Common Results of Cerebrovascular Accidents
  B. Psychological Aspects of Caring for a CVA Patient

VIII. **Patients with Aphasia**
  A. Transient Ischemic Attacks (TIAs)

Instructor Notes

OBJECTIVES

When the students have completed this chapter, they will be able to:

- Describe the functions of the nervous system, the brain, and the spinal cord.
- List two divisions of the autonomic nervous system.
- List the five sense organs.
- Describe the care of a patient's artificial eye, eyeglasses, and hearing aid.
- Describe common age-related changes in the nervous system.
- List common diseases and disorders of the nervous system.
- Describe four types of seizures.
- Discuss five safety measures for the patient having a seizure.
- List four causes and results of a cerebrovascular accident (stroke).
- Describe the nursing assistant's role in the care of a cerebrovascular accident patient.
- Describe the psychological aspects of caring for a patient who has had a cerebrovascular accident.
- Demonstrate how to communicate with an aphasic patient using correct technique.

KEY TERMS

Aphasia: Loss of language or speech

Autonomic Nervous System: The part of the nervous systems that carries messages without conscious thought

Canthus: The inner aspect of the eye closest to the nose

Cerebral Spinal Fluid: The fluid that circulates around and within the brain and spinal cord

Cerebrovascular Accident (CVA): Stroke; blockage or bleeding of blood vessels in the brain, interrupting the blood supply to that part of the brain and damaging the surrounding area of the brain

Complex Partial Seizure: A seizure with motor and possible sensory symptoms (such as muscle twitching and smelling a foul odor) and a change in the level of consciousness

Contracture: Drawing together, bunching up, or shortening of muscle tissue because of spasm or paralysis, either permanently or temporarily

Convulsive: Involving convulsions—rhythmic, involuntary contraction of muscles

Deficit: A temporary or permanent negative change in a patient's usual neurologic function

Embolus: Blood clot or mass of other undissolved matter that travels through the circulatory system from its place of formation to another site, lodges in a small blood vessel, and causes an obstruction

Environment: All the surrounding conditions and influences affecting the life and development of an organism

Instructor Notes

Hemiplegia: Paralysis of only one-half of the body

Hemisphere: Half of a sphere; in the nervous system, one-half of the brain

Hemorrhage: Excessive bleeding

Hypothalamus: An area of the brain responsible for control of the pituitary gland

Impulse: An electrical or chemical charge transmitted through certain tissues, especially nerve fibers and muscles

Intervertebral Discs: The material between the vertebral bodies that cushions the spinal column

Involuntary: Without conscious will, control, or decision

Meninges: The covering of the brain and spinal cord. There are three layers: the dura mater, the arachnoid, and the pia mater

Myelin Sheath: Protective covering around most nerves

Nervous System: The group of body organs consisting of the brain, spinal cord, and nerves that controls and regulates the activities of the body and the functions of the other body systems

Neuron: A type of nerve cell in the nervous system

Normal Pressure Hydrocephalus: A disorder caused by enlargement of the ventricles, fluid-filled spaces in the brain

Osteoporosis: Condition in which bones become brittle or thin and break easily

Plaque: Fatty deposits within blood vessels attached to vessel walls

Respond: React; begin, end, or change activity in reaction to stimulation

Rupture: Break open

Seizure: An episode, either partial or generalized, that may include altered consciousness, motor activity, or sensory phenomena or convulsions

Simple Partial Seizure: A seizure when the patient is aware of his surroundings but experiences either motor (muscle twitching or movement) or sensory changes (see or hear things not present)

Spasm: An involuntary sudden movement or convulsive muscular contraction

Stimuli: Changes in the external or internal environment strong enough to set up a nervous impulse or other responses in an organism

Thrombus: A blood clot that remains at its site of formation

Vascular: Pertaining to blood vessels

Vertebral Bodies: The bones around the spinal cord

Voluntary: Under control of the will; with conscious decision

Instructor Notes

CORE STUDENT ASSIGNMENTS

Students should:

- Read this chapter in their textbook, *Being a Nursing Assistant.*
- Underline any words or sentences they do not understand. Write down any questions they have.
- Complete the Chapter Review in their textbook.
- Read the Time Management Tip for this chapter and think about how they might use this tip in their work.
- Complete the Nursing Assistant in Action exercise.

OPTIONAL STUDENT ASSIGNMENTS

Students should:

- Complete all workbook assignments for this chapter in their copy of *Workbook for Being a Nursing Assistant.*
- Use the CD/CD-Rom disk enclosed with their textbook to hear the pronunciation of the key terms in the chapter.
- Watch the communication section of the "Dealing with Dementia" video from the Care Provider Skills series.
- Use the Website address **(www.prenhall.com/wolgin)** to access the free, interactive Companion Website created for this textbook. Get hints, instant feedback, and textbook references to chapter-related multiple-choice questions. Read and react to the Nursing Assistant in Action exercise. Link to other interesting sites.

METHODOLOGY AND SUGGESTED ACTIVITIES

I. Lecture/Discussion

- Answer any questions the students may have.
- Discuss the key terms and related abbreviations. Repeat them out loud and practice using them in sentences.
- Discuss the Time Management Tip for this chapter.
- Discuss the Nursing Assistant in Action exercise.
- Discuss the Critical Thinking points for this chapter.
- Discuss personal safety and protection. Emphasize the importance of following Universal Precautions. Stress the need to wear protective equipment.
- Discuss the structure and function of the nervous system.
- Discuss the impact of sensory losses in the geriatric population.
- Offer examples of case studies of common diseases and disorders of the nervous system.
- Clarify and explain any difficult terminology.
- Discuss care of patients with visual impairments and techniques for care that enhance independence.
- Invite an ophthalmologist to speak to the class and display an artificial eye.

Instructor Notes

- Invite a speaker from the local epilepsy foundation.
- Discuss the care of the patient who is hard of hearing. Discuss techniques for communication that preserve dignity and limit isolation and frustration.
- Arrange a field trip to a rehabilitation hospital.
- Invite a speech pathologist to speak to the class.

II. Role Play/Lab

- Show the video for this chapter. Role play scenarios where the student is working with a patient who has dementia and then one who is delirious. Emphasize techniques that work best with both kinds of patients.
- Demonstrate all the procedures and then have the students practice them.
- Have the students simulate having decreased visual and hearing senses by wearing earplugs or glasses smudged with petroleum jelly.
- Review and demonstrate correct procedures for seizure care. Dispel the myths.
- Review methods and techniques for stroke care. Review safe lifting and bending practices.

III. Evaluation

- Review the answers to the Chapter Review with students.
- Review the answer to the workbook exercises with students.
- Review the students' understanding of the Time Management Tip.
- To evaluate student comprehension, give a quiz.
- To evaluate student skills, administer the competency checklist.
- Have the students visit the interactive Companion Website and take the quiz.

ANSWERS TO CHAPTER REVIEW

FILL IN THE BLANK

Read each sentence and fill in the blank line(s) with the word or words that complete the sentence. (Note: Hyphenated words get one line.)

1. The nervous system controls and organizes all body movement including ___*voluntary*___ and ___*involuntary*___ types of movement.
2. The cerebrum is divided into two ___*hemispheres*___.
3. Changes in the external or internal environment strong enough to set up an impulse are called ___*stimuli*___.
4. When a patient can only move one-half of his body, he has ___*hemiplegia*___.
5. Loss of language or speech is called ___*aphasia*___.

Instructor Notes

MULTIPLE CHOICE

Choose the best answer for each question or statement.

1. The right hemisphere of the brain cerebrum controls
   (A.) the left side of the body.
   B. the right side of the body.
   C. a person's thought and reasoning ability.
   D. the hypothalamus.

2. The fight-or-flight response is activated
   A. in the parasympathetic division of the nervous system.
   (B.) in the sympathetic division of the nervous system.
   C. by the endocrine glands.
   D. None of the above.

3. When caring for a hearing aid,
   A. never wash it under water.
   B. check the batteries.
   C. do not expose it to heat.
   (D.) All of the above.

4. When caring for a patient who has had a seizure, do all of the following *except*
   (A.) note what kind of seizure the patient had.
   B. note what the seizure looked like.
   C. turn the patient's head to one side to prevent aspiration.
   D. protect the patient from injury.

5. You are working with a patient with aphasia. All of the following are helpful *except*
   A. communicating through writing.
   (B.) asking only yes/no questions.
   C. allowing enough time for a response.
   D. triggering the next sound for the patient.

CRITICAL THINKING

CUSTOMER SERVICE

Encourage students to reflect and share their thoughts and experiences. Respect their privacy and confidentiality. Share your own viewpoints with the students.

CULTURAL CARE

Encourage students to reflect and share their thoughts and experiences. Respect their privacy and confidentiality. Share your own viewpoints with the students.

Instructor Notes

COOPERATION WITHIN THE TEAM

Encourage students to reflect and share their thoughts and experiences. Respect their privacy and confidentiality. Share your own viewpoints with the students.

NURSING ASSISTANT IN ACTION

Mr. Joseph is an elderly patient who requires hearing aids. He has just returned from a whirlpool treatment where another staff member was assigned to supervise him. He tells you that no one removed his hearing aid prior to the treatment. Somehow the hearing aid fell into the water while he was in the whirlpool and now it is not working properly.

What Is Your Response/Action?

Apologize to Mr. Joseph for the damage to his hearing aid. Hearing aids are expensive pieces of equipment that are vital to Mr. Joseph. Tell him that you will report the damage to your supervisor. Follow through with this plan and fill out an incident report. Also consider changing the battery and working with others to create a communication plan for Mr. Joseph who now cannot hear as well.

Instructor Notes

26

Answers to Workbook Exercises

The following exercises will assist you to apply what you have read in Chapter 26, "The Nervous System and Related Care." For each exercise, read the objective and use information you have read in Chapter 26 to answer the questions, complete the sentences, or label the diagrams.

EXERCISE 26-1

Objective: To recognize and correctly spell words related to the nervous system and related care.

Directions: Unscramble the words in the Word List at the left. Then circle the same words in the Word Search at the right.

Word List

1. BEMOLSU _EMBOLUS_
2. ULESPMI _IMPULSE_
3. QAEULP _PLAQUE_
4. TRUPUER _RUPTURE_
5. UEZRESI _SEIZURE_
6. IHMPELGEAI _HEMIPLEGIA_
7. FDECITI _DEFICIT_
8. PASAHAI _APHASIA_
9. VAC _CVA_

Word Search

K	I	L	C	T	D	E	B	A	G	R	F	N	Q
D	R	T	K	F	O	S	F	O	I	U	U	D	S
H	W	E	M	B	O	L	U	S	L	P	I	E	A
E	O	U	K	Q	E	U	R	M	D	T	M	F	S
L	P	A	N	A	G	P	L	A	Q	U	E	I	H
P	Q	I	D	H	S	M	C	L	A	R	L	C	I
L	M	S	A	B	F	I	I	B	J	E	C	I	S
R	G	A	F	I	C	F	S	A	E	F	B	T	P
V	L	H	S	E	I	Z	U	R	E	D	G	G	M
A	R	P	E	R	D	G	J	B	Q	K	A	H	O
I	P	A	I	G	E	L	P	I	M	E	H	K	V
X	I	C	V	A	H	M	T	J	S	B	O	L	W
A	E	U	K	Z	L	O	S	W	N	N	I	D	T

EXERCISE 26-2

Objective: To apply what you have learned about the nervous system and related care.

Directions: Read the following riddles carefully before writing the correct answer on the blank line.

1. I often form on the inside of vessel walls. Who am I? *Hint:* My name sounds like an engraved award.

   plaque

2. When I occur, I can cause the patient to become unconscious. Who am I? *Hint:* Under different circumstances, I would take your possessions away.

   seizure

EXERCISE 26-3

Objective: To recognize the definitions of words used in patient rehabilitation activities.

Directions: Place the letter of the correct definition next to the matching word(s) from the Word List.

Word List

E **1.** cerebral spinal fluid
M **2.** intervertebral discs
G **3.** canthus
F **4.** aphasia
A **5.** hemorrhage
C **6.** autonomic nervous system
DD **7.** involuntary
P **8.** embolus
Q **9.** contracture
L **10.** myelin sheath
HH **11.** cerebrovascular accident (CVA)
R **12.** rupture
BB **13.** meninges
B **14.** hypothalamus
I **15.** environment
T **16.** convulsive
J **17.** deficit
H **18.** complex partial seizure
K **19.** plaque
X **20.** osteoporosis
GG **21.** stimuli
U **22.** seizure
EE **23.** spasm
II **24.** simple partial seizure
W **25.** voluntary
S **26.** nervous system
CC **27.** hemiplegia
FF **28.** vascular
D **29.** impulse
Y **30.** neuron
AA **31.** thrombus
V **32.** vertebral bodies
O **33.** respond
N **34.** hemisphere

Definitions

A. Excessive bleeding

B. An area of the brain responsible for control of the pituitary gland

C. The part of the nervous system that carries messages without conscious thought

D. An electrical or chemical charge transmitted through certain tissues, especially nerve fibers and muscles

E. The fluid that circulates around and within the brain and spinal cord

F. Loss of language or speech

G. The inner aspect of the eye closest to the nose

H. A seizure with motor and possible sensory symptoms (such as muscle twitching and smelling a foul odor) and a change in the level of consciousness

I. All the surrounding conditions and influences affecting the life and development of an organism

J. A temporary or permanent negative change in a patient's usual neurologic function

K. Fatty deposits within blood vessels attached to vessel walls

L. Protective covering around most nerves

M. The material between the vertebral bodies that cushions the spinal column

N. Half of a sphere; in the nervous system, one-half of the brain

O. React; begin, end, or change activity in reaction to stimulation

P. Blood clot or mass of other undissolved matter that travels through the circulatory system from its place of formation to another site, lodges in a small blood vessel, and causes an obstruction

Q. Drawing together, bunching up, or shortening of muscle tissue because of spasm or paralysis, either permanently or temporarily

R. Break open

S. The group of body organs consisting of the brain, spinal cord, and nerves that controls and regulates the activities of the body and the functions of the other body systems

T. Involving convulsions—rhythmic, involuntary contractions of muscles

U. An episode, either partial or generalized, that may include altered consciousness, motor activity, or sensory phenomena or convulsions

V. The bones of the spinal cord

W. Under control of the will

X. Condition in which bones become brittle or thin and break easily

Y. A type of nerve cell in the nervous system

AA. A blood clot that remains at its site of formation

BB. The covering of the brain and spinal cord; there are three layers: the dura mater, the arachnoid, and the pia mater

CC. Paralysis of only one-half of the body

DD. Without conscious will, control, or decision

EE. An involuntary sudden movement or convulsive muscular contraction

FF. Pertaining to blood vessels

GG. Changes in the external or internal environment strong enough to set up a nervous impulse or other responses in an organism

HH. Stroke; blockage or bleeding of blood vessels in the brain, interrupting the blood supply to that part of the brain and damaging the surrounding area of the brain

II. A seizure when the patient is aware of his surroundings but experiences either motor (muscle twitching or movement) or sensory changes (see or hear things not present)

EXERCISE 26-4

Objective: To recognize the structures and functions of the nervous system.

Directions: Label the drawings in Figure 26-1 utilizing the words from the Word List below. (Some answers may be used more than once.)

Word List

cerebrum	cerebellum	brain
spinal nerves	axon	muscle tissue
nucleus	dendrite	motor neuron
pons	neuron	spinal cord
myelin sheath	sensory message to the brain	
medulla	motor message from the brain	

FIGURE 26-1

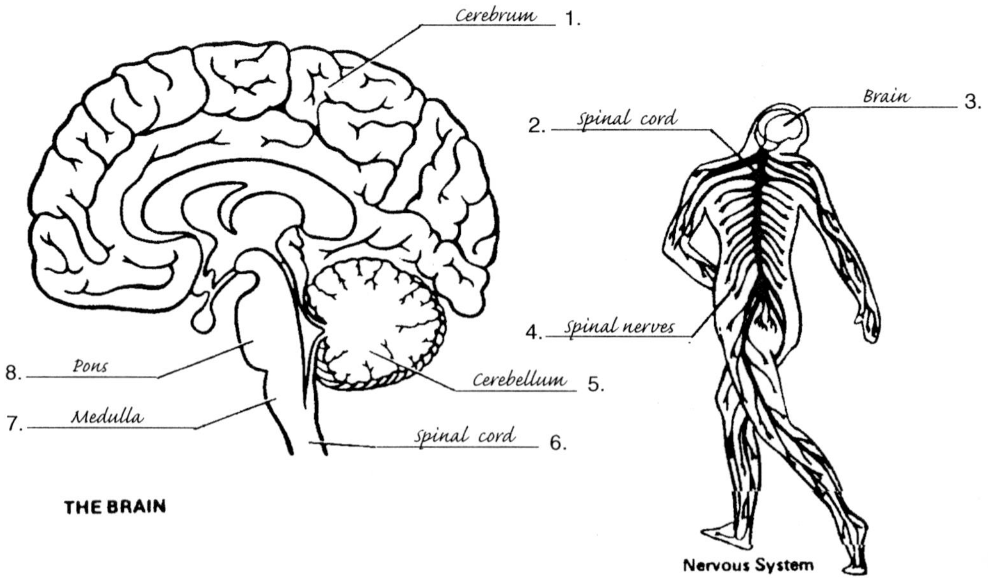

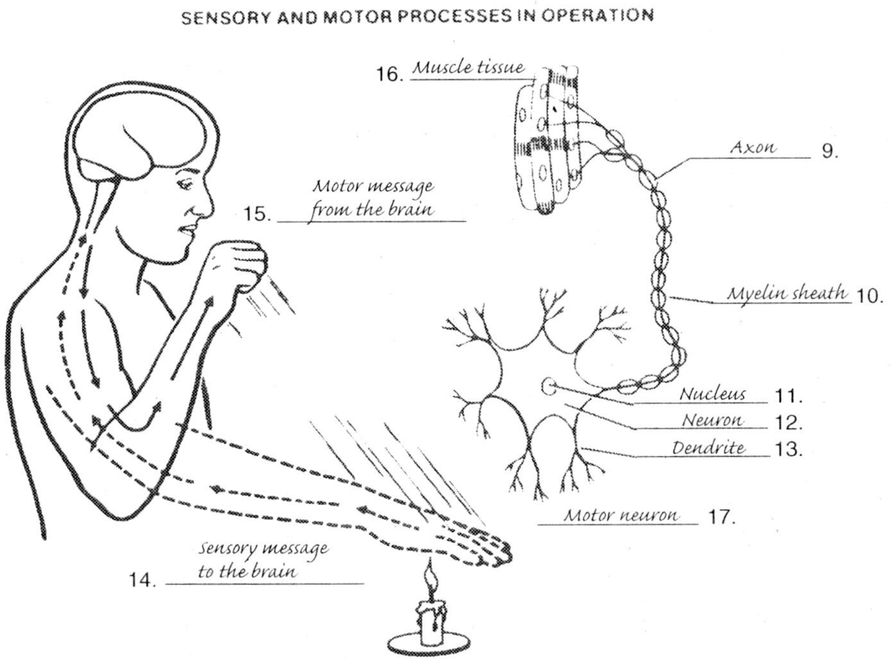

FIGURE 26-1 (cont.)

EXERCISE 26-5

Objective: To apply what you have learned about the nervous system and related care.

Directions: Circle the letter next to the statement that best completes the sentence or describes the sentence as true or false. If the sentence is false, draw a line through the incorrect part of the sentence and write the correction on the blank line.

1. CVAs may be caused by
   (A.) plaque.
   B. infection.
   C. cancer.
   D. All of the above.

2. For the patient who has a(n) ________, cleaning it is part of daily personal hygiene.
   (A.) artificial eye
   B. imagination
   C. missing canthus
   D. old injury

3. A hearing aid ~~will~~ restore full, normal hearing ability.
   A. True
   (B.) False
   Correct Answer: *will not*

4. Hemiplegia may result in which of the following?
A. Loss of sensation.
B. Loss of movement.
C. Loss of pain.
(D.) All of the above.

5. The weight and size of the brain decrease as a person ages.
(A.) True
B. False
Correct Answer: ______________________

6. ________ is a weakness or paralysis of one side of the face.
(A.) Bell's palsy
B. Bob's bell
C. Paul's bell
D. Belle's pal

7. ________ may be related to cerebral trauma.
A. Osteoporosis
B. Alopecia
C. Dermatitis
(D.) Epilepsy

8. A disease that is a type of dementia is
A. glaucoma.
B. vertigo.
(C.) Alzheimer's.
D. a detached retina.

9. Blisters along the path of certain nerves is known as
(A.) shingles *(Herpes zoster)*.
B. quadriplegia.
C. cataracts.
D. Meniere's disease.

10. Parkinson's disease is a progressive disorder, leading to loss of control of movement.
(A.) True
B. False
Correct Answer: ______________________

11. A TIA
A. is a permanent condition.
B. is a sign of cancer.
(C.) is a mini stroke.
D. is an endocrine condition.

12. To provide safe care for a patient having a seizure,
   A. put the patient in bed.
   (B.) move furniture or equipment the patient may bump.
   C. put a tongue depressor in the patient's mouth.
   D. put his head between his knees.

COMPETENCY SKILLS CHECKLIST 26-1: NERVOUS SYSTEM CARE

ACTIVITY	S	U	COMMENTS
1. Student will demonstrate the proper method of caring for the artificial eye.			
2. Student will demonstrate the proper method of caring for the patient's eyeglasses.			
3. Student will demonstrate the proper method of applying the hearing aid.			

27

Warm and Cold Applications

CHAPTER OVERVIEW

Instructor Notes

I. **Principles for Warm and Cold Applications**
   A. Moist and Dry Applications
   B. Keeping the Patient Safe and Comfortable
      1. Keeping the Patient Comfortable
   C. Heat Applications
   D. Cold Applications
      1. The Cooling (Tepid) Sponge Bath

Instructor Notes

OBJECTIVES

When the students have completed this chapter, they will be able to:

- Explain the principles of warm and cold applications.
- Explain the reasons warm and cold applications are used.
- Explain the difference between generalized and localized applications.
- Explain the difference between moist and dry applications.
- Demonstrate safe, correct, and comfortable applications.
- Demonstrate the application of the warm compress.
- Demonstrate the application of the warm soak.
- Demonstrate the application of the warm-water bottle.
- Demonstrate the application of the commercial unit heat pack.
- Demonstrate the application of the heat lamp.
- Demonstrate the application of the Aquamatic K-pad.
- Assist a patient with the disposable, portable, or built-in sitz bath.
- Demonstrate the application of the cold compress.
- Demonstrate the application of the cold soak.
- Demonstrate the application of the ice bag, ice cap, or ice collar.
- Demonstrate the application of the commercial unit cold pack.
- Perform the cooling bath.

KEY TERMS

Compress: Folded piece of cloth used to apply pressure, moisture, heat, cold, or medication to a specific part of the body

Continuous: Uninterrupted, without a stop

Constrict: Get smaller

Cyanosis: When the skin looks blue or gray, especially on the lips, nailbeds, and under the fingernails; in a black patient, it may appear as a darkening of color; occurs when there is not enough oxygen in the blood

Dilate: Get bigger; expand

Dry Application: A warm or dry application in which no water touches the skin

Generalized: Affecting, involving, or pertaining to the whole body

Generalized Application: A warm or cold application applied to the entire body

Hyperthermia: A higher than normal body temperature

Hypothermia: A very low body temperature

Inflammation: A reaction of the tissues to disease or injury; there is usually pain, heat, redness, and swelling of the body part

Intermittent: Alternating; stopping and beginning again

Instructor Notes

Localized: Limited to one place or part; affecting, involving, or pertaining to a definite area

Localized Application: A warm or cold application applied to a specific area or small part of the body

Moist Application: A warm or cold application in which water touches the body

Sitz Bath: A bath in which the patient sits in a specially designed chairtub or regular bathtub with the hips and buttocks in water

Soak: Immerse the body or body part completely in water

CORE STUDENT ASSIGNMENTS

Students should:

- Read this chapter in their textbook, *Being a Nursing Assistant*.
- Underline any words or sentences they do not understand. Write down any questions they have.
- Complete the Chapter Review in their textbook.
- Read the Time Management Tip for this chapter and think about how they might use this tip in their work.
- Complete the Nursing Assistant in Action exercise.

OPTIONAL STUDENT ASSIGNMENTS

Students should:

- Complete all workbook assignments for this chapter in their copy of *Workbook for Being a Nursing Assistant*.
- Use the CD/CD-Rom disk enclosed with their textbook to hear the pronunciation of the key terms in the chapter.
- Watch the "Bed Bath" video from the Care Provider Skills series.
- Use the Website address **(www.prenhall.com/wolgin)** to access the free, interactive Companion Website created for this textbook. Get hints, instant feedback, and textbook references to chapter-related multiple-choice questions. Read and react to the Nursing Assistant in Action exercise. Link to other interesting sites.

METHODOLOGY AND SUGGESTED ACTIVITIES

I. Lecture/Discussion

- Answer any questions the students may have.
- Discuss the key terms and related abbreviations. Repeat them out loud and practice using them in sentences.
- Discuss the Time Management Tip for this chapter.
- Discuss the Nursing Assistant in Action exercise.
- Discuss the Critical Thinking points for this chapter.

Instructor Notes

- Discuss personal safety and protection. Emphasize the importance of following Universal Precautions.
- Discuss the purpose, principle, and procedures involving warm or cold and moist or dry applications.
- Review the dangers of burns and how to prevent them through temperature control and frequent patient checks.
- Review cultural ideas about pain, pain relief, and comfort related to hot and cold applications.

II. Role Play/Lab

- Show the video for this chapter. Discuss how to determine if the temperature of the water is too hot or too cold for the patient. Have the students practice setting and checking the temperature of the applications.
- Demonstrate the procedure for warm and cold applications using the appropriate equipment. Emphasize patient safety during these applications.
- Allow adequate practical time for the students to use all equipment.
- Demonstrate ways to maintain privacy, comfort, and dignity for the patient during hot/cold treatments.

III. Evaluation

- Review the answers to the Chapter Review with students.
- Review the answer to the workbook exercises with students.
- Review the students' understanding of the Time Management Tip.
- To evaluate student comprehension, give a quiz.
- To evaluate student skills, administer the competency checklist.
- Have the students visit the interactive Companion Website and take the quiz.

ANSWERS TO CHAPTER REVIEW

FILL IN THE BLANK

Read each sentence and fill in the blank line(s) with the word or words that complete the sentence. (Note: Hyphenated words get one line.)

1. When a blood vessel expands in size, it ___*dilates*___.
2. When a blood vessel gets smaller in size, it ___*constricts*___.
3. ___*Inflammation*___ occurs when the tissue reacts to disease or injury. There is usually pain, heat, redness, and swelling of the body part.
4. When something is ___*localized*___, it means it is limited to one place or part, or affects a definite area of the body.
5. If a patient's lips, fingernails, eyelids, or skin look blue or a darker color, ___*cyanosis*___ is said to have occurred.

MULTIPLE CHOICE

Instructor Notes

Choose the best answer for each question or statement.

1. Heat may be used as treatment to
   A. decrease blood pressure.
   (B.) speed the healing process.
   C. improve the appearance of the skin.
   D. decrease age of the skin.
2. Cold applications may be used to
   (A.) prevent or reduce swelling.
   B. decrease blood pressure.
   C. improve the appearance of the skin.
   D. dilate the blood vessels.
3. Which of the following is not a moist heat or cold application?
   A. Sitz bath
   (B.) Heat lamp
   C. Cool compress
   D. Tub bath
4. In order to keep the patient safe during hot applications, you should do all of the following *except*
   A. be careful not to spill any water.
   B. watch for too much redness or darkened area.
   (C.) keep the patient covered.
   D. check the skin every 5 minutes.
5. When blood vessels become dilated,
   (A.) the increased blood supply carries away the fluids that cause inflammation.
   B. the increased blood supply increases inflammation.
   C. the decreased blood supply carries away the fluids that cause inflammation.
   D. the decreased blood supply increases inflammation.

CRITICAL THINKING

CUSTOMER SERVICE

Encourage students to reflect and share their thoughts and experiences. Respect their privacy and confidentiality. Share your own viewpoints with the students.

CULTURAL CARE

Encourage students to reflect and share their thoughts and experiences. Respect their privacy and confidentiality. Share your own viewpoints with the students.

Instructor Notes

COOPERATION WITHIN THE TEAM

Encourage students to reflect and share their thoughts and experiences. Respect their privacy and confidentiality. Share your own viewpoints with the students.

NURSING ASSISTANT IN ACTION

You are assigned to care for Curtis Brown, a 20-year-old man who has sprained his ankle. You are supposed to apply to cold pack to his ankle, but he does not want it on. He tells you, "Hey man, I am in serious pain and that is not helping. You can just get me some pain pills and take that thing out of here!"

What Is Your Response/Action?

Mr. Brown's telling you that he is in pain, so you should believe him. Tell him that you will report his pain to the nurse. Also tell him that the cold pack will help reduce swelling, which tends to cause more pain. If he responds to the cold pack, report that and his pain (have him rate it on a pain scale) to the nurse.

27

Answers to Workbook Exercises

The following exercises will assist you to apply what you have read in Chapter 27, "Warm and Cold Applications." For each exercise, read the objective and use information you have read in Chapter 27 to answer the questions, complete the sentences, or label the diagrams.

EXERCISE 27-1

Objective: To recognize and correctly spell words related to warm and cold applications.

Directions: Unscramble the words in the Word List at the left. Then circle the same words in the Word Search at the right.

Word List

1. NOITAMMALFNI ___*INFLAMMATION*___
2. CLAOLZIDE ___*LOCALIZED*___
3. OMSTI ___*MOIST*___
4. OASK ___*SOAK*___
5. MOCRSEPS ___*COMPRESS*___
6. ETHA ___*HEAT*___
7. CANYSOIS ___*CYANOSIS*___
8. DCLO ___*COLD*___

Word Search

C	G	B	L	S	O	A	S	E	F	C	N	K
B	H	E	A	T	V	I	L	D	F	O	C	L
V	D	I	K	J	S	C	F	G	I	M	B	X
F	R	P	A	O	Z	H	X	T	D	P	D	P
U	F	Q	N	R	D	G	A	Q	Y	R	H	O
L	X	A	K	O	A	M	L	A	B	E	C	H
H	Y	B	S	B	M	S	Y	M	C	S	O	Z
C	D	O	C	A	A	E	D	O	T	S	L	N
A	Z	J	L	O	C	A	L	I	Z	E	D	S
E	S	F	Y	I	D	V	L	S	F	A	L	Y
G	N	I	C	D	J	G	B	T	M	A	L	Z
I	A	F	B	S	O	A	K	H	K	B	C	J
K	H	N	L	P	V	O	W	S	T	X	O	W

EXERCISE 27-2

Objective: To apply what you have learned about warm and cold applications.

Directions: Read the following riddles carefully before writing the correct answer on the blank line.

1. I describe how something can get smaller or narrower. What am I? *Hint:* My alternate definition is legally binding.

   constricting

2. This is a treatment that patients report as warm and soothing. What is it? *Hint:* To walk, a person stands. To drive a car, he ________.

   sitz

3. This cold application can cool a warm head. What is it? *Hint:* There is also one of these at the North and South Poles.

   ice cap

EXERCISE 27-3

Objective: To recognize the definitions of words related to the use of warm and cold applications.

Directions: Place the letter of the correct definition next to the matching word(s) from the Word List.

Word List

I	1. continuous	N	9. generalized application
B	2. dilate	M	10. localized
F	3. localized application	A	11. sitz bath
H	4. cyanosis	C	12. moist application
J	5. compress	G	13. intermittent
K	6. dry application	O	14. inflammation
E	7. constrict	L	15. generalized
D	8. soak	P	16. hyperthermia

Definitions

A. A bath in which the patient sits in a specially designed chairtub or a regular bathtub with the hips and buttocks in water

B. Get bigger; expand

C. A warm or cold application in which water touches the body

D. Immerse the body or body part completely in water

E. Get smaller

F. A warm or cold application applied to a specific area or small part of the body
G. Alternating; stopping and beginning again
H. When the skin looks blue or gray, especially on the lips, nailbeds, and under the fingernails; in a black patient, it may appear as a darkening of color; occurs when there is not enough oxygen in the blood
I. Uninterrupted, without a stop
J. Folded piece of cloth used to apply pressure, moisture, heat, cold, or medication to a specific part of the body
K. A warm or dry application in which no water touches the skin
L. Affecting, involving, or pertaining to the whole body
M. Limited to one place or part; affecting, involving, or pertaining to a definite area
N. A warm or cold application applied to the entire body
O. A reaction of the tissues to disease or injury; there is usually pain, heat, redness, and swelling of the body part
P. A higher than normal body temperature

EXERCISE 27-4

Objective: To apply what you have learned about using warm and cold applications.

Directions: Circle the letter next to the statement that best completes the sentence or describes the sentence as true or false. If the sentence is false, draw a line through the incorrect part of the sentence and write the correction on the blank line.

1. Heat may be applied to an area of the body to
 A. improve the patient's appearance.
 B. improve the appearance of the skin.
 (C.) speed up the healing process by increasing the circulation.
 D. speed up the healing process by decreasing the circulation.

2. Heat may also be applied to the body to
 A. increase the pain to a joint.
 B. decrease the circulation.
 C. reduce the patient's weight.
 (D.) reduce the pain caused by inflammation and congestion.

3. Cold applications cause the blood vessels to constrict, which helps to
 (A.) prevent or reduce swelling.
 B. prevent or reduce weight.
 C. improve cyanosis.
 D. increase bleeding.

4. The blood flow to a part becomes slower when
   (A.) cold is applied.
   B. cold is reduced.
   C. heat is applied.
   D. heat is increased.

5. Cold ~~should never~~ be applied to the entire body.
   A. True
   (B.) False
   Correct Answer: may

6. All of the following are moist, warm applications *except*
   A. a sitz bath.
   B. a soak.
   C. a compress.
   (D.) a heat lamp.

7. An Aquamatic K-pad has water circulating inside and it is considered to be a
   A. moist application.
   (B.) dry application.
   C. steam application.
   D. dry-moist application.

8. You should be sure your hands are dry before you handle electrical equipment.
   (A.) True
   B. False
   Correct Answer: ____________

9. The part of the patient's skin that is receiving the heat or cold must be inspected often for excessive redness or grayness, indicating a burn or cyanosis, because
   (A.) the patient may not have feeling in the body area due to a disease process and may not realize there is a problem.
   B. this indicates the treatment is complete.
   C. your immediate supervisor wants you to do this.
   D. it makes the patient think you are doing a good job.

10. When applying the ice cap, be sure the metal or plastic stopper is positioned ~~close to~~ the patient's body.
   A. True
   (B.) False
   Correct Answer: away from

COMPETENCY CHECKLIST 27-1: WARM AND COLD APPLICATIONS

ACTIVITY	S	U	COMMENTS
1. The student will demonstrate the correct method of heat application:			
A. Moist applications			
1. The warm compress			
2. The warm soak			
3. The commercial unit heat pack			
4. The disposable sitz bath			
5. The portable chair or built-in sitz bath			
B. Dry applications			
1. The warm-water bottle			
2. The heat lamp (perineal)			
3. The Aquamatic Hydro-thermal (K-pad)			
2. The student will demonstrate the correct method of cold application:			
A. Moist applications			
1. The cold compress			
2. The cold soak			
3. The sponge bath			
B. Dry applications			
1. The ice bag, ice cap, or ice collar			
2. The commercial unit cold pack			

28

Care of the Surgical Patient

CHAPTER OVERVIEW

Instructor Notes

I. Surgery
- A. Surgery Types

II. Preoperative Care
- A. Preoperative Patient Education
- B. Psychological Aspects of Preoperative Care
  1. Preventing Chest Complications
- C. Preoperative Checklist

III. Skin Preparation
  1. Areas to be Shaved in Preparation for Surgery

IV. The Morning of Surgery
- A. Readying the Postoperative Patient's Unit

V. Postoperative Nursing Care
- A. When the Patient Comes Back from Surgery
- B. Anesthesia
- C. Turning the Postoperative Patient
- D. Coughing and Deep-Breathing Exercises

Instructor Notes

OBJECTIVES

When the students have completed this chapter, they will be able to:

- Describe the purpose of preoperative education and list the topics included.
- Identify the concerns and worries of preoperative patients.
- Complete a preoperative checklist accurately.
- Shave a patient in preparation for surgery.
- Name and describe the areas to be shaved in preparation for surgery.
- Describe the tasks they will perform the morning of surgery.
- Get the patient's unit ready for return from the operating or recovery room.
- Assist with the postoperative care when a patient returns to the unit.
- Observe the patient for signs of postoperative problems.
- Care for the patient who is vomiting.
- Carry out their responsibilities concerning the patient's first voiding after surgery.
- Explain four reasons chest complications may occur following anesthesia.
- Turn the postoperative patient.
- Assist the patient with deep-breathing exercises.

KEY TERMS

Abdominal Prep: The procedure for making the patient's abdomen ready for surgery; includes thorough cleansing of the skin and careful shaving of body hair in the abdominal area

Anesthesia: Loss of feeling or sensation in a part of or all of the body

Anesthesiologist: The medical doctor who administers the anesthetic to the patient in the operating room

Anesthetic: A drug used to produce loss of feeling that can be given orally, rectally, by injection, or by inhalation; a person who has been given an anesthetic is anesthetized

Anesthetist: The registered nurse who assists the anesthesiologist

Aspirate: Material (vomitus, food, or liquids) inhaled into the lungs

Complication: An unexpected condition, such as the development of another illness in a patient who is already sick

Elective Surgery: Chosen and not vital for health

Emergency Surgery: Surgery performed to save life or limb

General Anesthetics: Anesthetics that cause loss of sensation in the entire body

Local Anesthetics: Anesthetics that cause numbness or a loss of sensation in only a part of the body

NPO (nothing by mouth): Cannot eat or drink anything at all, usually past midnight the night before surgery or a procedure

Postoperative: After surgery

Instructor Notes

Preoperative: Before surgery

Scrotal Prep: The procedures for making the genital area of a male patient ready for surgery; the preparation includes thoroughly cleansing the skin and carefully shaving the hair in the area

Skin Prep: Shaving the area of the body where an operation is going to be performed in preparation for surgery

Spinal Anesthetics: Anesthetics that cause a loss of feeling in a large area of the body, usually from the umbilicus down to and including the legs and feet

Unconscious: Unaware of the environment; occurs during sleep and in temporary episodes ranging from fainting or stupor to coma

Vaginal Prep: The procedures for making the genital area of a female patient ready for surgery; the preparation includes thoroughly cleansing the skin and carefully shaving the pubic hair; it may also include a cleansing douche

Void: To urinate, pass water

CORE STUDENT ASSIGNMENTS

Students should:

- Read this chapter in their textbook, *Being a Nursing Assistant*.
- Underline any words or sentences they do not understand. Write down any questions they have.
- Complete the Chapter Review in their textbook.
- Read the Time Management Tip for this chapter and think about how they might use this tip in their work.
- Complete the Nursing Assistant in Action exercise.

OPTIONAL STUDENT ASSIGNMENTS

Students should:

- Complete all workbook assignments for this chapter in their copy of *Workbook for Being a Nursing Assistant*.
- Use the CD/CD-Rom disk enclosed with their textbook to hear the pronunciation of the key terms in the chapter.
- Watch the patient privacy portion of the "Bed Bath" video from the Care Provider Skills series.
- Use the Website address **(www.prenhall.com/wolgin)** to access the free, interactive Companion Website created for this textbook. Get hints, instant feedback, and textbook references to chapter-related multiple-choice questions. Read and react to the Nursing Assistant in Action exercise. Link to other interesting sites.

Instructor Notes

METHODOLOGY AND SUGGESTED ACTIVITIES

I. Lecture/Discussion

- Answer any questions the students may have.
- Discuss the key terms and related abbreviations. Repeat them out loud and practice using them in sentences.
- Discuss the Time Management Tip for this chapter.
- Discuss the Nursing Assistant in Action exercise.
- Discuss the Critical Thinking points for this chapter.
- Discuss personal safety and protection. Emphasize the importance of following Standard Precautions. Stress the need to wear protective equipment.
- Discuss all definitions and key terms.
- Emphasize the importance of accurate patient identification for patient safety.
- Stress safety rules for transporting the patient to the operating suite.
- Emphasize the responsibility for preparing the patient's unit to receive the patient after surgery.
- Stress safety for the patient who has been given preoperative medications by the skilled medication nurse.
- Discuss fears and concerns different age groups may have about having surgery.
- Review the concepts of pain and pain management and the role culture plays in relation to surgical care.

II. Role Play/Lab

- Show the video for this chapter. Discuss and role play what kind of things help to promote privacy, dignity, and comfort for the patient.
- Demonstrate the procedures. Have the students work in groups to practice the procedures.
- Write the names of the surgical preps on slips of paper. Give one to each student. Give each student a turn to explain his or her type of surgical prep and the area to be shaved.
- Assign students to teams of two to practice arranging the patient's unit to send a patient to surgery and to receive the patient postoperatively.
- Have the students practice identifying signs and symptoms of postoperative complications and what they would do to prevent them.

III. Evaluation

- Review the answers to the Chapter Review with students.
- Review the answer to the workbook exercises with students.
- Review the students' understanding of the Time Management Tip.
- To evaluate student comprehension, give a quiz.
- To evaluate student skills, administer the competency checklist.
- Have the students visit the interactive Companion Website and take the quiz.

ANSWERS TO CHAPTER REVIEW

Instructor Notes

FILL IN THE BLANK

Read each sentence and fill in the blank line(s) with the word or words that complete the sentence. (Note: Hyphenated words get one line.)

1. A complication is an unexpected condition, such as the development of an infection, in a patient who is already sick.
2. When a patient cannot eat or drink anything at all, it is called being NPO.
3. Shaving the area of the body where surgery is to be performed is called a skin prep.
4. Loss of feeling or sensation in a part of or all of the body is called anesthesia.
5. Exercises to expand the lungs after surgery are called deep-breathing exercises.

MULTIPLE CHOICE

Choose the best answer for each question or statement.

1. Things that might worry the patient going to surgery are
   - A. how his hair will look.
   - (B.) a possible disability or death because of the operation.
   - C. who his room mate might be.
   - D. None of the above.
2. Which type of surgery is usually not covered by health insurance?
   - A. Emergency
   - B. Urgent
   - C. Facial cosmetic surgical repair following a car accident
   - (D.) Elective
3. Which of the following is not a type of surgical skin prep?
   - A. Abdominal prep
   - B. Vaginal prep
   - (C.) Elbow prep
   - D. Scrotal prep
4. All of the following is included in postoperative care *except*
   - A. deep-breathing exercises.
   - B. measurement of intake and output.
   - (C.) skin prep.
   - D. measurement of vital signs.

Instructor Notes

5. Notify your supervisor immediately for all of the following *except*
   A. rise or fall of blood pressure.
   (B.) patient questions.
   C. bleeding.
   D. cyanosis.

CRITICAL THINKING

CUSTOMER SERVICE

Encourage students to reflect and share their thoughts and experiences. Respect their privacy and confidentiality. Share your own viewpoints with the students.

CULTURAL CARE

Encourage students to reflect and share their thoughts and experiences. Respect their privacy and confidentiality. Share your own viewpoints with the students.

COOPERATION WITHIN THE TEAM

Encourage students to reflect and share their thoughts and experiences. Respect their privacy and confidentiality. Share your own viewpoints with the students.

NURSING ASSISTANT IN ACTION

Mrs. Samson is a 44-year-old white female who had her gallbladder removed 12 hours ago. Her Foley catheter was removed earlier in your shift. She keeps telling you she feels the need to "go" but she has not been able to urinate when you put her on a bedpan.

What Is Your Response/Action?

You could try to run some water in the bathroom if it is nearby. Sometimes the sound of water stimulates people to be able to urinate. You could check with the nurse and find out if Mrs. Samson is allowed up out of bed yet. If so, with help from a coworker, assist Mrs. Samson to walk to the bathroom or commode chair. Be sure to ask for assistance because fainting is common in fresh postoperative patients. If she is still unable to void, notify the nurse who can check on an order to place a urinary catheter.

28

Answers to Workbook Exercises

The following exercises will assist you to apply what you have read in Chapter 28, "Care of the Surgical Patient." For each exercise, read the objective and use information you have read in Chapter 28 to answer the questions, complete the sentences, or label the diagrams.

EXERCISE 28-1

Objective: To recognize and correctly spell words related to the care of surgical patients.

Directions: Unscramble the words in the Word List at the left. Then circle these words in the Word Search grid at the right.

Word List

1. TCIHTSEEAN *ANESTHETIC*
2. RIPSATEA *ASPIRATE*
3. SRCTAOL PPER *SCROTAL PREP*
4. GAIVNLA EPRP *VAGINAL PREP*
5. GNREELA *GENERAL*
6. CAOLL *LOCAL*
7. PSNIAL *SPINAL*
8. OMCPILTIONAC *COMPLICATION*
9. PON *NPO*

Word Search

O	C	P	A	N	E	S	T	H	E	T	I	C	S	B
K	T	Q	S	C	R	O	T	A	L	P	R	E	P	D
V	B	H	P	S	H	E	A	G	L	L	M	F	I	H
E	J	Z	I	A	J	I	S	A	S	L	P	G	N	I
M	G	D	R	L	B	L	R	G	A	F	C	I	A	F
I	K	Q	A	F	O	E	D	C	I	P	N	J	L	B
U	E	Y	T	L	N	P	O	E	B	Q	A	P	K	O
D	N	S	E	E	I	L	N	K	C	D	I	D	O	G
X	V	A	G	I	N	A	L	P	R	E	P	Q	A	E
F	B	Z	J	H	O	M	H	O	L	J	M	I	H	N
L	U	C	O	M	P	L	I	C	A	T	I	O	N	K
I	J	T	D	E	C	I	K	Y	G	E	N	C	M	F
Q	P	M	R	X	P	U	T	Z	V	Q	R	S	O	A

EXERCISE 28-2

Objective: To apply what you have learned about care of the surgical patient.

Directions: Read the following riddles carefully before writing the correct answer on the blank line.

1. I carry the patient to surgery. What am I? *Hint:* After sitting for a long period of time, you may become this.

   stretcher

2. These must be measured before any surgery. What are they? *Hint:* This also describes a stop sign at a busy intersection.

   vital signs

3. This function must return to an adequate level after surgery. What is it? *Hint:* Another name for an empty space.

   voiding

EXERCISE 28-3

Objective: To recognize the definitions of words used in care of the surgical patient.

Directions: Place the letter of the correct definition next to the matching word(s) from the Word List.

Word List

L 1. local anesthetics
E 2. unconscious
D 3. nothing by mouth (NPO)
I 4. anesthetic
N 5. vaginal prep
O 6. scrotal prep
K 7. general anesthetics
A 8. skin prep
M 9. anesthesiologist
G 10. anesthesia
H 11. anesthetist
R 12. aspirate
Q 13. spinal anesthetics
C 14. complication
J 15. abdominal prep
F 16. postoperative
B 17. preoperative
P 18. void
S 19. elective surgery
T 20. emergency surgery

Definitions

A. Shaving the area of the body where an operation is going to be performed in preparation for surgery
B. Before surgery
C. An unexpected condition, such as the development of another illness in a patient who is already sick

D. Cannot eat or drink anything at all, usually past midnight the night before surgery or a procedure
E. Unaware of the environment; occurs during sleep and in temporary episodes ranging from fainting or stupor to coma
F. After surgery
G. Loss of feeling or sensation in a part of or all of the body
H. The registered nurse who assists the anesthesiologist
I. A drug used to produce loss of feeling
J. The procedure for making the patient's abdomen ready for surgery
K. Anesthetics that cause loss of sensation in the entire body
L. Anesthetics that cause numbness or the loss of sensation in a part of the body
M. The medical doctor who administers the anesthetic to the patient in the operating room
N. The procedures for making the genital area of a female patient ready for surgery
O. The procedures for making the genital area of a male patient ready for surgery
P. To urinate, pass water
Q. Anesthetics that cause a loss of feeling in a large area of the body, usually from the umbilicus down to and including the legs and feet
R. Material (vomitus, food, liquids) inhaled into the lungs
S. Surgery chosen and not vital for health
T. Surgery performed to save a life or limb

EXERCISE 28-4

Objective: To apply what you have learned about preoperative documentation.

Directions: Read the situation description below and then document the findings on the sample Preoperative Checklist.

It is 7 A.M. and you have just arrived at work. The nurse gives you the preoperative checklist for Tom Green. She tells you that he is scheduled to have surgery in two hours, explains the care you are to give him, and that she would like you to fill out the portion of the checklist labeled "Morning of Surgery."

After greeting Mr. Green and introducing yourself, you measure his vital signs, height, and weight. His temperature is 100.2°F. His pulse is 68 beats per minute. His respirations are 16 times per minute. His blood pressure is 120/80. His weight is 186 pounds, and his height is 5 feet 11 inches.

He is able to bathe himself and brush his own teeth. You obtain a urine sample and send it to the lab. After his bath, he dresses in a clean hospital gown. There is no urinary drainage bag. You ask him if he is allergic or sensitive to any drugs and he answers, "None." He has no false teeth, prosthesis, nail polish, sanitary belts, makeup, hairpieces, or hair pins. He removes his wedding ring and his contact lenses, which he gives to his wife to take home.

The nurse comes in at 8 A.M. to give him his preoperative medications; the side rails are up. At 8:30 A.M., the transportation attendant arrives and takes the patient to the operating room by stretcher.

Sample Preoperative Checklist Completed by Nursing Assistant

EVENING BEFORE SURGERY

Patient's Name: TOM GREEN

Identify the patient by checking his identification bracelet:	Yes ___	No ___	
Skin prep done by ______ at ___ P.M.			
Skin prep checked by ______ at ___ P.M.			
Food restrictions, if any, explained to the patient:	Yes ___	No ___	
"NPO AFTER MIDNIGHT" sign put on patient's bed and explained to the patient:	Yes ___	No ___	
Enema administered by ______ at ___ P.M.			

MORNING OF SURGERY:

Bath?	Yes ✓	No ___	N/A ___
Oral hygiene?	Yes ✓	No ___	N/A ___
False teeth (dentures) and removable bridges removed?	Yes ___	No ___	N/A ✓
(Jewelry) and pierced earrings removed? Ring	Yes ✓	No ___	N/A ___
Hairpiece, wig, hairpins removed?	Yes ___	No ___	N/A ✓
Lipstick, makeup, and false eyelashes removed?	Yes ___	No ___	N/A ✓
Sanitary belt removed?	Yes ___	No ___	N/A ✓
Nail polish removed?	Yes ___	No ___	N/A ✓
Eyeglasses and (contact lenses) removed?	Yes ✓	No ___	N/A ___
Prostheses (artificial hearing aid, eye, leg, arm, and so forth) removed?	Yes ___	No ___	N/A ✓
All clothing removed except clean hospital gown?	Yes ✓	No ___	N/A ___
Patient allergic or sensitive to drugs?	Yes ___	No ✓	N/A ___
Preop urine specimen obtained and sent to lab?	Yes ✓	No ___	N/A ___
Urinary drainage bag emptied?	Yes ___	No ___	N/A ✓
Side rails in up position?	Yes ✓	No ___	N/A ___

Temperature 100.2 F Pulse 68 Respiration 16

Blood pressure 120/80 Weight 186 lbs. Height 5 ft. 11 in.

Time patient leaves for the operating room: 8.30 A.M.

Observations: Ready for surgery

Signature: J. Smith, N.A. 4/2/96

EXERCISE 28-5

Objective: To recognize appropriate tasks in preparing the postoperative patient's unit.

Directions: Circle the letters of all the tasks you should do to prepare the patient's unit to receive the patient after surgery.

(A.) Bring the IV pole to the bedside.
B. Attach a urine drainage bag to the bed frame.
(C.) Strip the linen from the bed.
(D.) Make the operating room or surgical bed.
E. Mop the floor.
(F.) Place tissues and emesis basin only on the bedside table.
(G.) Remove the drinking water.
H. Place a clean gown at the foot of the bed.

EXERCISE 28-6

Objective: To recognize appropriate actions to take for the preoperative patient.

Directions: Decide which of the following Actions is the most appropriate for the Situation descriptions. Put the letter for that Action in the space next to the Situation. More than one letter may be appropriate for each situation.

Actions

A. Listen and show interest in what the patient says.
B. Report this to your immediate supervisor.
C. Check or record this information on the preoperative checklist.

Situations

B **1.** If you notice the patient is sneezing, sniffling, or coughing
A, C **2.** After you post the NPO sign and explain it to the patient
B, C **3.** After administering an enema the evening before surgery and noting the results
A **4.** The patient wants to talk a lot.
A **5.** The patient expresses concern for his family.
B **6.** The patient's temperature rises the evening before surgery.
A **7.** The patient begins to talk about the possibility of death or serious complications.
C **8.** You prepared the patient's skin as instructed at 7:30 P.M.

C 9. On the morning of surgery, you helped the patient remove false teeth, jewelry, hairpins, and nail polish.

B 10. The patient complains of chest pains.

C 11. After weighing and measuring the patient

C 12. After obtaining a urine specimen

EXERCISE 28-7

Objective: To recognize appropriate actions to take for the postoperative patient.

Directions: Decide which of the following Actions is the most appropriate for the Situation descriptions. Put the letter for that Action in the space next to the situation.

Actions

A. Signal for the nurse immediately.

B. Turn the patient.

C. Change the patient's gown and bed linens.

Situations

A 1. You notice that I am a patient who is bleeding and the blood is bright red. What should you do?

B 2. I am a patient who has been in the same position for two hours. What should you do for me?

C 3. I am a postoperative patient. My gown and linens have become wet. What should you do for me?

A 4. I am a postoperative patient. You just noticed a rise in my blood pressure. What should you do?

A 5. My lips and fingernails are turning very pale or blue. What should you do?

A 6. You have just measured my vital signs, and my pulse is below 60. What should you do?

B 7. I am a postoperative patient and I have got myself in an uncomfortable position.

EXERCISE 28-8

Objective: To recognize appropriate steps in assisting the patient with deep-breathing exercises.

Directions: Circle the letter of the correct response.

1. You are helping a patient with deep-breathing exercises. You have explained what you want the patient to do. You have pulled the curtain around the bed and offered the bedpan. What should you do next?
   A. Place the pillow on the patient's abdomen for support.
   (B.) Dangle the patient's legs over the side of the bed, if allowed.
   C. Identify the patient by checking the identification bracelet.
2. If the patient is not permitted to dangle his legs, what should you do?
   (A.) Place the patient in as much of a sitting position as possible.
   B. Do the exercises with the patient lying down.
   C. Prop the patient up with the pillows.
3. You placed a pillow on the patient's abdomen and asked him to breathe deeply ten times. What should you do while he breathes?
   A. Take care of another patient.
   B. Count his pulse.
   (C.) Count the respirations out loud to the patient.

EXERCISE 28-9

Objective: To apply what you have learned about care of the surgical patient.

Directions: Circle the letter next to the statement that best completes the sentence or describes the sentence as true or false. If the sentence is false, draw a line through the incorrect part of the sentence and write the correction on the blank line.

1. Preoperative patient education includes all of the following *except*
   A. deep-breathing and coughing exercises.
   B. leg and foot exercises.
   C. turning from side to side.
   (D.) self-surgical procedures.
2. Part of your job as nursing assistant is to make the patient who is going to have surgery feel
   A. lively and happy.
   B. sad and dejected.
   (C.) as calm and relaxed as possible.
   D. nervous and upset.

3. The preoperative patient may be worried about all of the following *except*
- (A.) fear of the known.
- B. financial concerns.
- C. family concerns.
- D. the possibility of death or serious complications.

4. One way to help reduce the patient's fears is to
- (A.) give him extra time and attention.
- B. ignore his childish behavior.
- C. report his fears to your team members while at lunch.
- D. tell him not to worry.

5. Preventing chest complications following surgery includes
- (A.) watching the patient for symptoms of respiratory infection before surgery.
- B. washing the chest with soap.
- C. shaving the chest regularly.
- D. wearing gloves at all times when doing the prep.

6. NPO means
- A. non promo otto.
- B. night procedures only.
- (C.) nothing by mouth.
- D. non-permanent only.

7. A sign should be posted at the ~~nurse's station~~ if the patient is NPO.
- A. True
- (B.) False

Correct Answer: *head or foot of the patient's bed*

8. Hair on the body is a breeding place for
- (A.) microorganisms.
- B. rumors.
- C. cattle.
- D. all of the above

9. It is important to measure the patient's ________ immediately after he returns to his unit after surgery.
- A. feet
- B. I.Q.
- C. height and weight
- (D.) vital signs

10. If the patient vomits, ________ if he is unconscious.
- A. rinse out his mouth
- B. raise the siderails immediately
- (C.) turn his head to one side and clear his mouth
- D. all of the above

11. If a patient appears to be unconscious, he ~~cannot~~ hear what you are saying.

A. True

(B.) False

Correct Answer: may be able to

12. It is very important that the patient void adequately within a certain period of time after surgery.

(A.) True

B. False

Correct Answer: ______

COMPETENCY CHECKLIST 28-1: POSTOPERATIVE CARE

ACTIVITY	S	U	COMMENTS
1. The student will demonstrate proper procedure for skin prep:			
A. Shaving the breast			
B. Shaving the chest			
C. Shaving the abdomen			
D. Shaving an extremity			
E. Shaving the back			
F. Shaving the vaginal area			
G. Shaving the scrotal area			
2. The student will demonstrate the proper procedure for assisting the patient with deep-breathing exercises.			

Special Procedures

29

CHAPTER OVERVIEW

I. **Intravenous Infusion (IV) Equipment**

II. **Caring for the Patient with an Intravenous Infusion**

III. **Binders**

IV. **Elastic Stockings and Elastic Bandages**
   A. Applying Antiembolism Elastic Stockings
   B. Applying Elastic Bandages

Instructor Notes

Instructor Notes

OBJECTIVES

When the students have completed this chapter, they will be able to:

- Label the parts of the intravenous infusion equipment on a diagram.
- Change the gown of the patient with an intravenous infusion.
- Check the intravenous bottle, drip chamber, tubing, and the patient's arm so that the student can promptly report anything unusual to the immediate supervisor.
- List three reasons for the use of binders.
- Apply the three types of binders.
- Explain the purpose of antiembolism elastic stockings and elastic bandages.
- Apply elastic bandages and antiembolism elastic stockings.

KEY TERMS

Antiembolism Stockings: Designed to stimulate blood flow and to prevent the formation of blood clots in the bloodstream

Binder: A type of bandage applied to a large body area (abdomen or chest) to secure a dressing in place or to put pressure on or support a body part

Infiltration: Occurs when an IV solution runs into nearby tissue instead of into a vein

Intravenous Infusion: The injection of fluids, nutrients, and medication into a vein

Phlebitis: Inflammation of a vein

Thrombophlebitis: Inflammation and blood clots in a vein

CORE STUDENT ASSIGNMENTS

Students should:

- Read this chapter in their textbook, *Being a Nursing Assistant.*
- Underline any words or sentences they do not understand. Write down any questions they have.
- Complete the Chapter Review in their textbook.
- Read the Time Management Tip for this chapter and think about how they might use this tip in their work.
- Complete the Nursing Assistant in Action exercise.

OPTIONAL STUDENT ASSIGNMENTS

Students should:

- Complete all workbook assignments for this chapter in their copy of *Workbook for Being a Nursing Assistant.*
- Use the CD/CD-Rom disk enclosed with their textbook to hear the pronunciation of the key terms in the chapter.

Instructor Notes

- Watch the "Dressing When an IV Catheter Is in Place" portion of the "Personal Care" video from the Care Provider Skills series.
- Use the Website address **(www.prenhall.com/wolgin)** to access the free, interactive Companion Website created for this textbook. Get hints, instant feedback, and textbook references to chapter-related multiple-choice questions. Read and react to the Nursing Assistant in Action exercise. Link to other interesting sites.

METHODOLOGY AND SUGGESTED ACTIVITIES

I. Lecture/Discussion

- Answer any questions the students may have.
- Discuss the key terms and related abbreviations. Repeat them out loud and practice using them in sentences.
- Discuss the Time Management Tip for this chapter.
- Discuss the Nursing Assistant in Action exercise.
- Discuss the Critical Thinking points for this chapter.
- Discuss personal safety and protection. Emphasize the importance of following Universal Precautions.
- Emphasize the importance of reporting immediately to the supervisor anything unusual or of concern when a patient is receiving an IV.
- Discuss and review the signs and symptoms of decreased or lack of circulation from a too tight binder.
- Review signs and symptoms of infection and need for care with IVs.

II. Lab/Demonstration

- Show the video for this chapter. Discuss the infection control reasons for being very careful about changing gowns on a patient with an IV in place. Have the students practice this procedure.
- Pass around IV equipment so that all students can observe how the tubing looks and feels.
- Demonstrate the procedure of applying antiembolism stockings. Students working in groups of two return the demonstration.
- Demonstrate how to change a patient's gown without disturbing the IV. Have pairs of students practice and then demonstrate the gown-changing procedure.
- Demonstrate application of types of binders. Have pairs of students practice application of binders.
- Have the students practice looking for signs of phlebitis and reporting them to their supervisor.
- Have the students practice monitoring the patient's comfort while applying binders and elastic stockings.

III. Evaluation

- Review the answers to the Chapter Review with students.
- Review the answer to the workbook exercises with students.
- Review the students' understanding of the Time Management Tip.
- To evaluate student comprehension, give a quiz.

Instructor Notes

- To evaluate student skills, administer the competency checklist.
- Have the students visit the interactive Companion Website and take the quiz.

ANSWERS TO CHAPTER REVIEW

FILL IN THE BLANK

Read each sentence and fill in the blank line(s) with the word or words that complete the sentence. (Note: Hyphenated words get one line.)

1. The injection of fluids, nutrients, or medications into a vein is called an ___*intravenous*___ ___*infusion*___.
2. Only a ___*nurse*___ or ___*doctor*___ may change or regulate the amount of flow from an IV solution.
3. An ___*infiltration*___ occurs when an IV solution runs into nearby tissue instead of into a vein.
4. ___*Phlebitis*___ is an inflammation of a vein.
5. Stockings that are designed to promote blood flow and prevent the formation of clots are called ___*antiembolism*___ stockings.

MULTIPLE CHOICE

Choose the best answer for each question or statement.

1. All of the following are tasks a nursing assistant should do when caring for a patient with an intravenous therapy *except* for which one?
   A. Check to make sure the IV fluid or blood is flowing through the tubing.
   B. Make sure the tubing is not kinked.
   (C.) Adjust the rate if it is not flowing.
   D. Notify your supervisor if the skin around the IV is swollen.
2. When changing the gown of a patient who has an IV,
   A. remove the gown from the arm with the IV.
   B. move the gown down the tubing and up to the bag.
   C. unhook the IV bag from the pole and slide the gown off.
   (D.) All of the above.
3. Binders are wide cloth bandages applied mainly to the abdomen, chest, and perineum to
   (A.) secure a dressing.
   B. reduce pressure on a body part.
   C. stop circulation.
   D. increase pain and discomfort.

Instructor Notes

4. A medical condition in which there is inflammation of the vein is
   A. thrombophlebitis.
   B. diabetes.
   (C.) phlebitis.
   D. hepatitis.

5. When caring for a patient with antiembolism hose, make sure the stockings are
   A. pulled up firmly and twisted.
   (B.) changed and replaced every 8 hours or as ordered.
   C. in place during the bath.
   D. applied after the patient is out of bed.

CRITICAL THINKING

CUSTOMER SERVICE

Encourage students to reflect and share their thoughts and experiences. Respect their privacy and confidentiality. Share your own viewpoints with the students.

CULTURAL CARE

Encourage students to reflect and share their thoughts and experiences. Respect their privacy and confidentiality. Share your own viewpoints with the students.

COOPERATION WITHIN THE TEAM

Encourage students to reflect and share their thoughts and experiences. Respect their privacy and confidentiality. Share your own viewpoints with the students.

NURSING ASSISTANT IN ACTION

You are assigned to Mr. Smith who has antiembolism stockings ordered. His stockings are supposed to be on for 8 hours. You enter his room and see he has removed the stockings. He says, "I do not like wearing these things. I feel like a woman wearing these support hose and do not want them on when my friends and family are visiting me."

What Is Your Response/Action?

You can remind Mr. Smith why the support stockings are important—to prevent blood clots in his legs. You could also suggest a pair of pajama bottoms to cover up the stockings or a lap blanket if he is in the chair. If he still does not want to wear them, report this to the nurse.

Instructor Notes

29

Answers to Workbook Exercises

The following exercises will assist you to apply what you have read in Chapter 29, "Special Procedures." For each exercise, read the objective and use information you have read in Chapter 29 to answer the questions, complete the sentences, or label the diagrams.

EXERCISE 29-1

Objective: To apply what you have learned about special procedures that nursing assistants may perform while caring for patients.

Directions: Look carefully at the items shown in Figure 29-1. Label each one of them with the number of the correct word(s) from the Word List.

Word List

1. T binder (female)
2. elastic bandage
3. breast binder
4. T binder (male)
5. straight abdominal binder
6. antiembolism elastic stocking
7. IV infusion
8. IV solution
9. IV drip chamber
10. IV tubing
11. IV insertion site
12. IV clamp
13. IV pump or controller
14. skin near IV site
15. IV pole

FIGURE 29-1

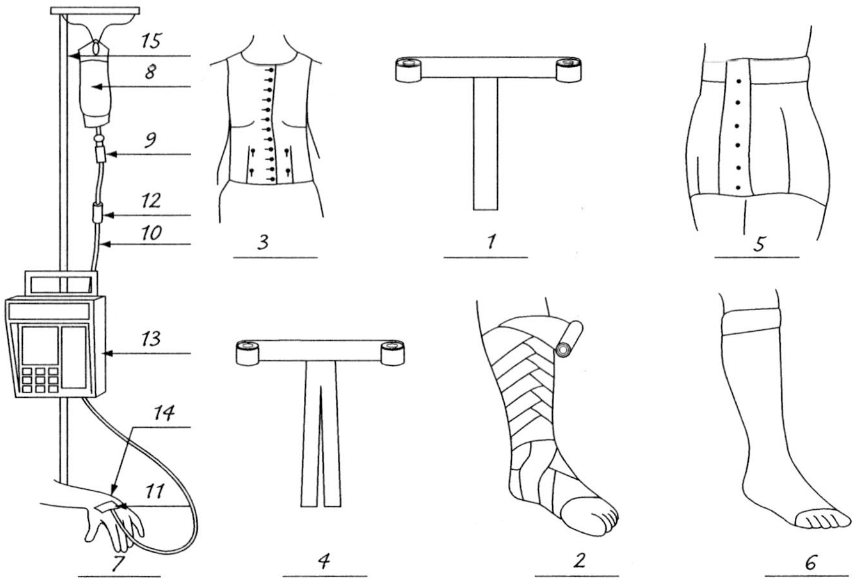

EXERCISE 29-2

Objective: To be able to recognize important safety measures related to performing special procedures.

Directions: Select the correct word(s) from the Word List to complete the sentences below.

Word List

overlap	circulation	Velcro	size	infiltration
kinked	one-half	hour	flow rate	interrupting

1. You must provide care for the patient or change his position without ___interrupting___ the flow of the IV solution.
2. Make sure the IV tubing is not ___kinked___ and that the patient is not lying on the tubing.
3. Nursing assistants do not independently adjust the ___flow___ ___rate___ using the IV clamp or electronic controller.
4. A(n) ___infiltration___ of the IV solution can cause the skin near the site to become painful or swollen. Report this condition immediately to the nurse.
5. If possible, choose a patient gown with ___Velcro___ to make changing the gown easier for the patient.

6. Binders, elastic bandages, and antiembolism stockings can be too tight and can reduce the patient's *circulation*.

7. The patient's legs must be measured to be sure the antiembolism stockings are the correct *size*.

8. The patient's fingers and toes should be checked each *hour* for pain, numbness, cyanosis, paleness, or lack of movement if he is wearing an elastic bandage on his arms or legs.

9. When applying an elastic bandage, it is important to apply pressure evenly and with each turn to overlap the bandage *one-half* the width of the one before it.

10. If more than one bandage is used, *overlap* them to prevent slipping or uneven pressure on the body part.

EXERCISE 29-3

Objective: To recognize and correctly spell words related to special procedures.

Directions: Unscramble the words in the Word List at the left. Then circle the same words in the Word Search grid at the right.

Word List

1. RAOUSVETNIN *INTRAVENOUS*
2. ISTPHBEIL *PHLEBITIS*
3. MSANMEIOBITL *ANTIEMBOLISM*
4. CITSALE *ELASTIC*
5. TIONARTLIFIN *INFILTRATION*
6. OODLB OSTCL *BLOOD CLOTS*
7. UBTGNI *TUBING*
8. DEELNE *NEEDLE*

Word Search

A	R	F	T	L	P	M	Z	N	E	E	D	L	E	T	L	S	B	C
J	H	A	R	Z	H	Q	A	X	C	A	O	R	H	F	W	Y	M	Z
B	I	E	V	E	L	D	O	Z	L	X	R	I	S	X	L	I	R	D
L	O	D	T	A	E	L	A	S	T	I	C	O	V	A	L	P	U	O
C	D	I	X	C	B	R	N	P	R	E	V	Q	B	K	G	I	G	H
K	U	N	Z	I	I	Y	T	O	I	A	L	H	P	N	O	J	B	J
D	K	T	K	N	T	Y	I	E	C	H	K	Y	I	K	Q	Z	L	E
E	B	R	I	Y	I	Z	E	I	V	Y	Z	B	E	X	A	F	O	W
E	U	A	F	X	S	C	M	L	Z	P	U	G	P	U	M	S	O	G
P	C	V	A	E	Z	O	B	L	F	T	N	Z	H	D	C	Y	D	C
L	L	E	O	Z	M	L	O	N	W	S	C	Y	A	J	P	Z	C	H
O	A	N	O	J	H	K	L	I	G	K	Z	O	W	G	K	E	L	Z
M	Y	O	T	Q	T	R	I	N	F	I	L	T	R	A	T	I	O	N
M	B	U	M	F	W	P	S	J	D	Z	F	D	X	A	V	E	T	K
O	L	S	V	D	Z	L	M	D	M	H	P	J	E	D	O	U	S	I
M	G	O	E	S	Q	R	F	V	Y	O	P	D	N	W	U	B	C	L
E	W	S	N	H	I	L	S	M	K	D	C	O	O	L	R	T	B	A

EXERCISE 29-4

Objective: To apply what you have learned about special procedures.

Directions: Circle the letter next to the statement that best completes the sentence or describes the sentence as true or false. If the sentence is false, draw a line through the incorrect part of the sentence and write the correction on the blank line.

1. Inflammation of a vein is called ~~infiltration~~.
   A. True
   (B.) False
   Correct Answer: *phlebitis*

2. Binders are used with patients to help
   A. relieve diarrhea.
   B. constrict body parts.
   C. secure blood clots to prevent movement.
   (D.) secure a dressing in place.

3. Bandages and stockings that provide support may contain ~~plastic~~.
   A. True
   (B.) False
   Correct Answer: *elastic*

4. The IV container should always be held ~~below~~ the IV site.
   A. True
   (B.) False
   Correct Answer: *above*

5. The amount of IV fluid that can flow into the patient's body is controlled and monitored by the ~~nursing assistant~~.
   A. True
   (B.) False
   Correct Answer: *professional nurse*

COMPETENCY CHECKLIST 29-1: APPLYING ELASTIC BANDAGES

ACTIVITY	S	U	COMMENTS
1. Student correctly demonstrates the steps involved in applying an elastic bandage:			
A. To a foot extending above the ankle			
B. To a foot and leg, extending above the knee			
C. To a foot and leg, extending over the entire thigh			
D. To a leg, extending from the ankle to over the knee			
E. To a knee			
F. To a hand, extending over the wrist			
G. To an arm, extending from the wrist over the elbow			
H. To an elbow			
I. To an entire arm from the wrist, extending over the entire upper arm			

30

Other Patients with Special Needs

CHAPTER OVERVIEW

I. **Cancer and Benign Tumors**
   A. Psychosocial Aspects of Cancer

II. **Immunosuppression**

III. **Mental Health and Mental Illness**

IV. **Substance Abuse**

Instructor Notes

Instructor Notes

OBJECTIVES

When the students have completed this chapter, they will be able to:

- Contrast benign and malignant tumors.
- Review risk factors and cancer prevention strategies.
- List the warning signs of cancer.
- Explain the psychosocial aspects of cancer.
- Give one example of a disease or treatment that results in immunosuppression.
- List three common misunderstandings about the transmission of AIDS.
- Name and describe a thought disorder and a mood disorder.
- Name the 3 spheres of orientation.
- List three signs or signals of substance abuse.

KEY TERMS

Acquired Immune Deficiency Syndrome (AIDS): Condition caused by a virus that destroys a key part of the body's immune response system

Benign Tumor: A tumor that stays at its site of origin and does not usually regrow once removed

Cancer: Refers to malignant neoplasms, or tumors

Chemotherapy: Refers to the use of drugs to treat cancer

Immunocompromised: Means that the immune system is not functioning normally; immunocompromised and immunosuppressed mean the same and are used interchangeably

Lumpectomy: Removal of a small part of the breast

Malignant (Neoplasms): New growths that spread, invade, and destroy organs

Mastectomy: Removal of the entire breast

Mental Health: Describes the best adjustment an individual can make at a given time, based on internal and external resources

Mental Illness: Describes a number of chemical imbalances in the brain or genetically based brain diseases that interfere significantly with people's abilities to live and work

Metastasis: Refers to the spreading of cancer cells through the systems of the body

Neoplasm (Tumor): New growth; the words *tumor* and *neoplasm* are interchangeable

Orientation: An individual's ability to identify who she is, where she is, and some information about time (month, year, time of day)

Radiation Therapy: The use of high doses of radiation, many times the dose used for x-ray exams, to treat cancer

Substance Abuse: The excessive use of mood-altering drugs, such as alcohol, cocaine, tobacco, or caffeine, that results in negative changes to a person's life

CORE STUDENT ASSIGNMENTS

Instructor Notes

Students should:

- Read this chapter in their textbook, *Being a Nursing Assistant.*
- Underline any words or sentences they do not understand. Write down any questions they have.
- Complete the Chapter Review in their textbook.
- Read the Time Management Tip for this chapter and think about how they might use this tip in their work.
- Complete the Nursing Assistant in Action exercise.

OPTIONAL STUDENT ASSIGNMENTS

Students should:

- Complete all workbook assignments for this chapter in their copy of *Workbook for Being a Nursing Assistant.*
- Use the CD/CD-Rom disk enclosed with their textbook to hear the pronunciation of the key terms in the chapter.
- Watch the "Communication"section of the "Age-Specific Competencies" video from the Care Provider Skills series.
- Use the Website address **(www.prenhall.com/wolgin)** to access the free, interactive Companion Website created for this textbook. Get hints, instant feedback, and textbook references to chapter-related multiple-choice questions. Read and react to the Nursing Assistant in Action exercise. Link to other interesting sites.

METHODOLOGY AND SUGGESTED ACTIVITIES

I. Lecture/Discussion

- Answer any questions the students may have.
- Discuss the key terms and related abbreviations. Repeat them out loud and practice using them in sentences.
- Discuss Time Management Tip for this chapter.
- Discuss the Nursing Assistant in Action exercise.
- Discuss the Critical Thinking points in this chapter.
- Discuss personal safety and protection. Emphasize the importance of following Universal Precautions. Stress the need to wear protective equipment.
- Review the differences between the terms *neoplasm, tumor, benign, malignant,* and *cancer.*
- Brainstorm with the students about common myths they have or have had about cancer.
- Discuss the treatment options of cancer (surgery, radiation therapy, chemotherapy, or combinations).
- Discuss common emotional and age-specific differences related to the impact of cancer on a patient.
- Review and discuss the transmission of AIDS.

Instructor Notes

- Review the different types of mental illness.
- Discuss the myths, stigmas, and confidentiality issues of mental illness.
- Review signs of substance abuse and the resources for assistance in your institution.
- Review and discuss how personal experiences with alcohol may influence caregiver behavior. Talk about ways to recognize and prevent caregiver beliefs from influencing care to patients.

II. Role Play/Lab

- Show the video for this chapter. Role play scenarios where the students practice talking to patients with depression problems.
- Role play caring for patients with cancer, mental illness, and substance abuse.
- Have the students answer/problem solve issues of confidentiality.
- Have the students explore their own feelings and attitudes about working with AIDS patients and mentally ill patients. Discuss and role play appropriate scenarios with good and bad communication styles.
- Have the students role play situations in which a coworker may be impaired.

III. Evaluation

- Review the answers to the Chapter Review with students.
- Review the answer to the workbook exercises with students.
- Review the students' understanding of the Time Management Tip.
- To evaluate student comprehension, give a quiz.
- Have the students visit the interactive Companion Website and take the quiz.

ANSWERS TO CHAPTER REVIEW

FILL IN THE BLANK

Read each sentence and fill in the blank line(s) with the word or words that complete the sentence. (Note: Hyphenated words get one line.)

1. The word neoplasm means ___new___ ___growth___.
2. ___Cancer___ is the leading cause of death in the United States.
3. When the immune system is not functioning normally and the body is unable to fight off infection as well, the patient is said to be ___immunocompromised___.
4. Mental illnesses are ___treatable___ illnesses.
5. Abuse of alcohol, cocaine, and other drugs can occur in people of ___all___ ages.

Instructor Notes

MULTIPLE CHOICE

Choose the best answer for each question or statement.

1. Treatment for cancer may include
   A. chemotherapy.
   B. radiation.
   C. surgery.
   (D.) All of the above.
2. Diseases that affect the immune system include
   A. cancer.
   B. HIV/AIDS.
   C. diabetes.
   (D.) All of the above.
3. HIV/AIDS is considered
   A. terminal.
   B. treatable with surgery.
   (C.) a chronic illness.
   D. an airborne infectious disease.
4. A person with depression has all of the following *except*
   A. persistent feelings of hopelessness.
   (B.) high blood pressure.
   C. tremendous feelings of sadness, worthlessness, or guilt.
   D. problems concentrating or making decisions.
5. Americans experience the highest rate of death and injury from
   A. anthrax.
   B. abuse of prescription drugs.
   C. abuse of illegal drugs.
   D. abuse of alcohol.

CRITICAL THINKING

CUSTOMER SERVICE

Encourage students to reflect and share their thoughts and experiences. Respect their privacy and confidentiality. Share your own viewpoints with the students.

CULTURAL CARE

Encourage students to reflect and share their thoughts and experiences. Respect their privacy and confidentiality. Share your own viewpoints with the students.

Instructor Notes

COOPERATION WITHIN THE TEAM

Encourage students to reflect and share their thoughts and experiences. Respect their privacy and confidentiality. Share your own viewpoints with the students.

NURSING ASSISTANT IN ACTION

You are assigned to care for Mr. Underwood, a 70-year-old man who has cancer and is clinically depressed. He takes antidepressant medication and was admitted to begin a course of chemotherapy. You find a bottle of vodka in his drawer when you are gathering equipment for his bath. He says, "Please don't tell anyone about the bottle. It is hard to get someone to bring me a drink. I really need a couple drinks to get through the day in this place. Give a dying man a break."

What Is Your Response/Action?

You tell Mr. Underwood that you must report the alcohol for his own safety. Alcohol may interact with his medications and the nurses and physicians will work to help him in other ways.

30

Answers to Workbook Exercises

The following exercises will assist you to apply what you have read in Chapter 30, "Other Patients with Special Needs." For each example, read the objective and use information you have read in Chapter 30 to answer the questions, complete the sentences, or label the diagrams.

EXERCISE 30-1

Objective: To recognize and correctly spell words related to the care of patients with special needs.

Directions: Unscramble the words in the Word List at the left. Then circle the same words in the Word Search grid at the right.

Word List

1. NCAREC _CANCER_
2. ASANEU _NAUSEA_
3. EBNGIN _BENIGN_
4. ASDI _AIDS_
5. BSUANCSTE BUAES _SUBSTANCE ABUSE_
6. TLAENM LILESNS _MENTAL ILLNESS_
7. SISATSATEM _METASTASIS_
8. PLOASNEM _NEOPLASM_

Word Search

M	A	N	T	I	R	P	I	C	M	L	H	N	J	B
E	Y	C	Z	V	G	Q	V	K	E	S	N	E	A	F
T	Z	S	A	X	S	B	Y	U	N	J	S	O	K	G
A	H	C	A	N	C	E	R	Z	T	W	N	P	D	P
S	K	J	I	O	N	N	Y	P	A	O	A	L	I	R
T	I	Q	D	I	W	I	E	L	L	X	U	A	M	G
A	X	G	S	Z	B	G	D	C	I	K	S	S	P	A
S	Y	R	U	O	L	N	U	O	L	H	E	M	O	M
I	E	S	F	R	D	M	P	A	L	B	A	A	K	P
S	V	L	J	H	J	X	M	G	N	J	Q	R	T	B
D	S	U	B	S	T	A	N	C	E	A	B	U	S	E
O	N	L	C	P	U	K	S	Y	S	X	S	O	H	C
A	E	T	Q	H	J	Y	B	W	S	D	N	K	I	F

EXERCISE 30-2

Objective: To demonstrate your ability to recognize the signs and symptoms of malignant tumors.

Directions: Circle the words in the Word List that are the signs and symptoms of malignant tumors.

Word List

1. A sore that does not heal
2. Weight loss
3. Unusual bleeding
4. All lumps in the breast
5. A rash that reappears
6. Change in bowel habits
7. Changes in the appearance of a mole
8. Nausea and vomiting
9. Diarrhea for 3 days
10. Unaccountable weight loss
11. A feeling of tiredness that lasts
12. Hoarseness, coughing, difficulty breathing or swallowing
13. Difficulty swallowing

EXERCISE 30-3

Objective: To recognize the definitions of words related to the special needs of patients.

Directions: Place the letter of the correct definition next to the matching word(s) from the Word List.

Word List

__D__ **1.** lumpectomy
__E__ **2.** Acquired immune deficiency syndrome (AIDS)
__K__ **3.** mental illness
__L__ **4.** substance abuse
__A__ **5.** neoplasm
__F__ **6.** benign (tumor)
__C__ **7.** mastectomy
__J__ **8.** orientation
__I__ **9.** immunocompromised
__G__ **10.** cancer
__M__ **11.** malignant (neoplasms)
__B__ **12.** metastasis
__H__ **13.** mental health

Definitions

A. New growth; or tumor
B. Refers to the spreading of cancer cells through the systems of the body
C. Removal of the entire breast
D. Removal of a small part of the breast
E. Condition caused by a virus that destroys a key part of the body's immune response system

F. Tumor that stays at its site of origin and does not usually regrow once removed

G. Refers to malignant neoplasms, or tumors

H. Describes the best adjustment an individual can make at a given time, based on internal and external resources

I. Means that the immune system is not functioning normally; immunosuppressed means the same and is used interchangeably

J. An individual's ability to identify who he is, where he is, and some information about time (month, year, time of day)

K. Describes a number of chemical imbalances in the brain or genetically based brain diseases that interfere significantly with people's abilities to live and work

L. The excessive use of mood-altering drugs, such as alcohol, cocaine, tobacco, or caffeine, that results in negative changes to one's life

M. New growths that spread, invade, and destroy organs

EXERCISE 30-4

Objective: To apply what you have learned about the special needs of patients.

Directions: Circle the letter next to the statement that best completes the sentence or describes the sentence as true or false. If the sentence is false, draw a line through the incorrect part of the sentence and write the correction on the blank line.

1. Breast cancer is one of the leading causes of death among women.
- (A.) True
- B. False

Correct Answer: ______________________________

2. The nursing assistant can help mastectomy patients by
- (A.) being calm and accepting of their responses.
- B. encouraging them to be happy.
- C. being absent from their unit as much as possible.
- D. all of the above.

3. __________ is a leading cause of death in the United States.
- A. Alopecia
- B. Dermatitis
- C. Gastritis
- (D.) Cancer

4. __________ is the use of drugs to treat cancer.
- A. Manipulation
- B. Psychotherapy
- C. Canceropathy
- (D.) Chemotherapy

5. Normal cells are also killed during radiation treatment.
(A.) True
B. False
Correct Answer: ____________________

6. Chemotherapy causes all of the following side effects *except*
A. nausea.
B. vomiting.
C. fatigue.
(D.) hair growth.

7. The cancer patient often undergoes surgical procedures that
A. may alter the bodily functions.
B. are not useful.
C. may alter the form of the body.
(D.) both A and C.

8. Special cells the body produces to fight bacteria and viruses are
A. osteoclasts.
B. immunocells.
(C.) antibodies.
D. super cells.

9. Examples of immunocompromising conditions are all of the following *except*
A. diabetes.
B. cancer.
C. AIDS.
(D.) influenza.

10. Substance abuse may affect up to what percent of hospitalized patients?
A. 10%
(B.) 25%
C. 40%
D. 50%

11. Substance abuse may be excessive use of all of the following *except*
(A.) chocolate.
B. alcohol.
C. prescription drugs.
D. controlled substances for pain relief.

12. A leading cause of automobile accidents in the United States is
A. drinking alcohol and driving.
B. taking illegal drugs and driving.
C. the use of a designated driver.
(D.) both A and B.

13. Drinking alcohol during pregnancy can cause a pattern of birth defects referred to as

A. drunk baby syndrome (DBS).
B. sad results syndrome (SRS).
(C.) fetal alcohol syndrome (FAS).
D. fetal death syndrome (FDS).

14. In situations of substance abuse, the

A. habit frees the user.
B. substance enhances the user.
C. user controls the substance.
(D.) habit controls the user.

15. The medical diagnosis of depression

A. is a mood disorder.
B. affects 10% to 12% of older adults.
C. has a negative social stigma attached to it.
(D.) all of the above.

31

Neonatal and Pediatric Care

CHAPTER OVERVIEW

Instructor Notes

I. Neonatal Care
   A. Feeding the Infant
      1. Feeding the Baby from a Bottle
   B. Helping a Mother Breast-feed
   C. Burping the Infant
   D. Observing the Infant's Stool
   E. Diarrhea in Infants
   F. Diapering
   G. Circumcision
   H. Umbilical Cord
   I. Bathing the Infant
      1. Sponge Bathing
      2. Tub Bathing
   J. Infant Safety

II. Pediatric Care
   A. Nursing Care of Pediatric Patients
   B. Safety
   C. Measuring Vital Signs
   D. Communicating with Pediatric Patients

Instructor Notes

OBJECTIVES

When the students have completed this chapter, they will be able to:

- Feed a baby using a bottle.
- Assist a mother to breast-feed.
- Feed and burp an infant.
- Describe a normal infant bowel movement.
- Diaper a baby.
- Demonstrate circumcision care.
- Demonstrate umbilical cord care.
- Demonstrate an infant bath.
- List five safety precautions when caring for infants.
- List eight safety precautions when caring for children.
- Measure vital signs in infants and children.
- List six things to remember when communicating with children.

KEY TERMS

Circumcise: Remove the foreskin of the penis by surgical procedure

Constipation: Difficult, infrequent defecation with passage of unduly hard and dry fecal material

Dehydrate: Loss of body fluids

Diaper: Washable or disposable covering applied to the perineal area for the purpose of containing stool or urine

Diarrhea: Abnormally frequent discharge of fluid fecal material from the bowel

Infant: A baby aged 1 month to 1 year

Pediatric Patient: Any patient under the age of 16 years

Stool: Solid waste material discharged from the body through the rectum and anus; other names include feces, excreta, excrement, bowel movement, and fecal matter

Umbilical Cord: A rather long, flexible, rough organ that carries nourishment from the mother to the baby; it connects the umbilicus of the unborn baby in the mother's uterus to the placenta

CORE STUDENT ASSIGNMENTS

Students should:

- Read this chapter in their textbook, *Being a Nursing Assistant*.
- Underline any words or sentences they do not understand. Write down any questions they have.
- Complete the Chapter Review in their textbook.

Instructor Notes

- Read the Time Management Tip for this chapter and think about how they might use this tip in their work.
- Complete the Nursing Assistant in Action exercise.

OPTIONAL STUDENT ASSIGNMENTS

Students should:

- Complete all workbook assignments for this chapter in their copy of *Workbook for Being a Nursing Assistant.*
- Use the CD/CD-Rom disk enclosed with their textbook to hear the pronunciation of the key terms in the chapter.
- Watch the infant and pediatric portions of the "Age-Specific Competencies" video from the Care Provider Skills series.
- Use the Website address **(www.prenhall.com/wolgin)** to access the free, interactive Companion Website created for this textbook. Get hints, instant feedback, and textbook references to chapter-related multiple-choice questions. Read and react to the Nursing Assistant in Action exercise. Link to other interesting sites.

METHODOLOGY AND SUGGESTED ACTIVITIES

I. Lecture/Discussion

- Answer any questions the students may have.
- Discuss the key terms and related abbreviations. Repeat them out loud and practice using them in sentences.
- Discuss the Time Management Tip for this chapter.
- Discuss the Nursing Assistant in Action exercise.
- Discuss the Critical Thinking points for this chapter.
- Discuss personal safety and protection. Emphasize the importance of following Universal Precautions.
- Discuss safety precautions when caring for infants and children and how they have changed over the years.
- Discuss guidelines for communicating with children of different ages.
- Discuss infant stools and signs to report immediately.
- Discuss burping methods.

II. Role Play/Lab

- Show the video for this chapter. (Note to the students safety measures during baby's bath.) Discuss other safety precautions to take when caring for small children.
- Display and demonstrate preparation and storage of different types of formula.
- Display and demonstrate use of various types of feeding bottles.
- Demonstrate a sponge and tub bath on a mannequin baby.
- Demonstrate umbilical cord care.
- Demonstrate how to diaper an infant.
- Demonstrate vital sign measurements in infants and children.

Instructor Notes

- Have students return demonstrations.
- Discuss when to report vital signs immediately to a supervisor.

III. Evaluation

- Review the answers to the Chapter Review with students.
- Review the answer to the workbook exercises with students.
- Review the students' understanding of the Time Management Tip.
- To evaluate student comprehension, give a quiz.
- To evaluate student skills, administer the competency checklist.
- Have the students visit the interactive Companion Website and take the quiz.

ANSWERS TO CHAPTER REVIEW

FILL IN THE BLANK

Read each sentence and fill in the blank line(s) with the word or words that complete the sentence. (Note: Hyphenated words get one line.)

1. Neonatal care refers to care given to newborn *infants*.
2. Diarrhea in the infant can result in *dehydration*.
3. Never *pull* on the umbilical cord. Let it fall off naturally.
4. Never *prop* a bottle and leave a baby unattended.
5. When taking a rectal temperature on a child, insert the thermometer *one-half* inch.

MULTIPLE CHOICE

Choose the best answer for each question or statement.

1. You can prevent a buildup of air in the baby's stomach by doing all of the following *except*
   A. feeding the infant slowly.
   (B.) feeding the infant with its head elevated.
   C. burping the baby every 1–2 ounces.
   D. None of the above.
2. The normal color of a breast-fed baby's stool is
   A. dark black.
   B. brown.
   (C.) mustard yellow.
   D. green.
3. The umbilical cord will generally dry and fall off in how many days?
   A. 1–2 days
   B. 3–5 days
   (C.) 5–10 days
   D. 14–20 days

Instructor Notes

4. When giving an infant a bath, you should do all of the following *except*
   A. assemble all of the equipment that you will need.
   B. line the sink or tub with a towel.
   (C.) fill the sink or tub with 3–4 inches of water.
   D. dry the infant well, including between skin folds.
5. When taking a rectal temperature in a baby, insert a well-lubricated thermometer
   (A.) ½ inch.
   B. 1 inch.
   C. 1½ inches.
   D. None of the above.

CRITICAL THINKING

CUSTOMER SERVICE

Encourage students to reflect and share their thoughts and experiences. Respect their privacy and confidentiality. Share your own viewpoints with the students.

CULTURAL CARE

Encourage students to reflect and share their thoughts and experiences. Respect their privacy and confidentiality. Share your own viewpoints with the students.

COOPERATION WITHIN THE TEAM

Encourage students to reflect and share their thoughts and experiences. Respect their privacy and confidentiality. Share your own viewpoints with the students.

NURSING ASSISTANT IN ACTION

You are assigned to care for Marta James, a new 20-year-old mother and her infant. Marta is to be discharged home tomorrow and she has not yet changed a diaper or fed her baby. Each time you try to encourage her to participate in the care of her newborn daughter, she says: "Leave me alone. I am too tired, and besides it is your job to care for my baby."

What Is Your Response/Action?

You could say that you are happy to take care of the baby, but it is also your job to take care of her. Part of getting ready to go home is to practice these skills. Say to Ms. James that you want to help prevent her from being overwhelmed at home. Mention Ms. James's behavior to the nurse as well so that she can also observe and talk with the patient.

Instructor Notes

31

Answers to Workbook Exercises

The following exercises will assist you to apply what you have read in Chapter 31, "Neonatal and Pediatric Care." For each exercise, read the objective and use information you have read in Chapter 31 to answer the questions, complete the sentences, or label the diagrams.

EXERCISE 31-1

Objective: To recognize definitions of words related to neonatal and pediatric care.

Directions: Place the letter of the correct definition next to the matching word(s) from the Word List below.

Word List

_D_ **1.** pediatric patient
_C_ **2.** infant
_H_ **3.** circumcise
_F_ **4.** diaper
_A_ **5.** dehydrate
_G_ **6.** stool
_B_ **7.** constipation
_E_ **8.** diarrhea

Definitions

A. Loss of body fluids
B. Difficult, infrequent defecation with passage of unduly hard and dry fecal material
C. A baby aged 1 month to 1 year
D. Any patient under the age of 16 years
E. Abnormally frequent discharge of fluid fecal material from the bowel
F. Washable or disposable covering applied to the perineal area for the purpose of containing stool or urine

G. Solid waste material discharged from the body through the rectum and anus; other names include feces, excreta, excrement, bowel movement, and fecal matter

H. Remove the foreskin of the penis by surgical procedure

EXERCISE 31-2

Objective: To apply what you have learned about neonatal and pediatric care.

Directions: Read the following riddles carefully before writing the correct answers.

1. When feeding the infant you look forward to this happening. What is it? *Hint:* If done in public by an adult it is rude.

   a burp

2. You feed this to an infant. What is it? *Hint:* Many mathematical calculations are solved with this.

   a formula

3. The appearance of this item can reveal much about the health of an infant. What is it? *Hint:* You can stand on this to reach items that are too high for you.

   stool

EXERCISE 31-3

Objective: To apply what you have learned about neonatal and pediatric care.

Directions: Circle the letter next to the statement that best completes the sentence or describes the sentence as true or false. If the sentence is false, draw a line through the incorrect part of the sentence and write the correction on the blank line.

1. An important part of any care given to infants and children is being careful of
   A. speed.
   B. fecal tolerance.
   (C.) safety measures.
   D. bowel and bladder training.

2. When feeding formula, the bottle ~~may~~ be propped, ~~if~~ the caregiver is too busy to hold the infant.
   A. True
   (B.) False
   Correct Answer: may never, even if

3. Most infants eat every ________ hours on average.
   A. 12
   (B.) 4
   C. 2
   D. 8

4. The nursing assistant helps the mother breast-feed when he provides
   A. food and nourishment.
   B. fun and laughter.
   C. formula preparation.
   (D.) privacy and comfort.

5. When breast-feeding, the arm holding the baby should be
   (A.) supported by a pillow or folded blanket.
   B. wrapped in an ace bandage.
   C. chilled in ice water.
   D. washed thoroughly before use.

6. If the mother is sleepy, do not
   A. disturb her while holding the infant.
   (B.) leave her alone while she is holding the baby.
   C. worry because she can sleep and breast-feed at the same time.
   D. give her the baby until she has slept 8 hours.

7. The ________ should be notified if the mother appears to be having difficulty breast-feeding.
   A. father
   B. doctor
   (C.) nurse
   D. family

8. When performing infant care, it is important to prevent the spread of microorganisms by doing which of the following?
   A. Apply infection control measures
   B. Wash hand frequently
   C. Avoid coughing and sneezing
   (D.) All of the above

9. If the breast tissue blocks the infant's nose when breast-feeding, the baby will stop feeding and let go of the breast; therefore,
   (A.) the mother should keep the breast tissue away from the infant's nose by pressing down on the breast in that area with her finger or thumb.
   B. the mother should be prepared for the infant to cry often during the time he is nursing.
   C. women with large breasts should bottle-feed.
   D. extend the feeding time by 15 minutes.

10. An important infant feeding skill for the nursing assistant to develop is
    A. changing the diaper.
    (B.) burping the baby.
    C. fast-food delivery.
    D. a taste for formula.

11. When burping the baby, gently rub and pat
    A. the infant's feet.
    B. the infant's stomach.
    C. the mother's back.
    (D.) the infant's back.

12. When changing the diaper, the nursing assistant should observe the stool for
    A. at least 5 minutes after changing the diaper.
    (B.) color, consistency, amount, and frequency.
    C. seeds and pits.
    D. microorganisms.
13. Diarrhea can be a serious, life-threatening condition for infants.
    (A.) True
    B. False
    Correct Answer: ______________________
14. Microorganisms from spoiled formula or the contaminated hands of those who handle the infant can cause diarrhea.
    (A.) True
    B. False
    Correct Answer: ______________________
15. Cloth diapers are held in place with
    A. tabs.
    B. tape.
    (C.) safety pins.
    D. waterproof pants.
16. An infant with watery stools can become dehydrated
    (A.) in 2 days or less.
    B. in 2 hours.
    C. within 2 weeks.
    D. within 1 week.
17. When the baby has had a circumcision, the nursing assistant
    A. should check with his immediate supervisor for care instructions.
    B. should be gentle when changing diapers.
    C. should be gentle when cleaning the area.
    (D.) all of the above.
18. Within 5 to 10 days the umbilical cord will
    A. turn green and develop an odor.
    B. turn red and bleed.
    C. grow 1 inch and turn black.
    (D.) dry, turn black, and eventually fall off.
19. While the umbilical cord is still attached, the baby should only be given sponge baths and not immersed in water.
    (A.) True
    B. False
    Correct Answer: ______________________

20. In the home, it is important to
(A.) never use heating pads on infants or children.
B. never use blankets on babies.
C. never use incubators.
D. take the infant's temperature every day.

21. An infant who has not yet learned to roll over ~~can~~ be left lying on the couch.
A. True
(B.) False
Correct Answer: *cannot*

22. Keep all medications and cleaning solutions out of reach of
A. the nurse.
(B.) the child.
C. the nursing assistant.
D. the mother.

23. Before measuring the vital signs of children it is important that the nursing assistant
A. check the identification band first.
B. use the right size cuff for the blood pressure.
C. inform the child what is going to be done.
(D.) all of the above.

24. Good communication with the ________ as well as the child is an important skill for the nursing assistant to develop.
A. family pet
(B.) parents
C. child's playmates
D. neighbors

25. Providing good care for the child is ~~worrisome~~ to the family members.
A. True
(B.) False
Correct Answer: *reassuring*

26. The nursing assistant should allow the family to help in the care of the child if possible.
(A.) True
B. False
Correct Answer: ________

27. It is important that you report to your immediate supervisor if the family seems to be worried about
A. a problem with the child's illness.
B. the child's response to care received.
C. the care the child is receiving in the hospital.
(D.) all of the above.

28. Safety must always be a concern of the nursing assistant because
(A.) children are unpredictable and can be easily injured.
B. it's a nice thing to be aware of.
C. he or she will be blamed if a child is injured.
D. the nursing assistant is unpredictable and could be easily injured.

COMPETENCY CHECKLIST 31-1: NEONATAL AND PEDIATRIC CARE

ACTIVITY	S	U	COMMENTS
1. The student will demonstrate the correct method of:			
A. Bottle-feeding the infant			
B. Burping the infant			
1. Method A			
2. Method B			
C. Diapering the infant			
1. Disposable diaper			
2. Cloth diaper			
D. Tub bathing the infant			
2. The student will demonstrate the correct method of:			
A. Measuring the child's pulse rate			
B. Measuring the child's respiratory rate			
C. Measuring the child's blood pressure			

32

The Older Adult Patient and Long-Term Care

CHAPTER OVERVIEW

Instructor Notes

I. Physical Changes of the Geriatric Person

II. Psychosocial and Psychological Aspects of Aging
- A. Common Disease Conditions
- B. Meeting the Older Adult Person's Psychosocial Needs
- C. Restorative Care

III. Reality Orientation for the Confused Patient

IV. Validation Therapy
- A. Stages of Confusion—Helping Measures
  1. Stage One—Malorientation Description
  2. Stage Two—Time Confusion Description
  3. Stage Three—Repetitive Motion Description
  4. Stage Four—Vegetative Description

V. Safety for the Older Adult Patient
- A. Ambulation Safety With and Without the Walker
- B. Assisting the Older Adult Resident with Nutrition

VI. Nursing Care for the Older Adult Patient
- A. Skin Care
- B. The Bed-bound Older Adult Patient

VII. Maintaining Dignity and Quality of Life

Instructor Notes

OBJECTIVES

When the students have completed this chapter, they will be able to:

- Describe the older adult patient in terms of physical and emotional changes.
- Define common chronic conditions of the older adult patient.
- Describe validation therapy.
- Provide opportunities to foster health and well-being in the older adult patient.
- Provide functional or restorative care.
- Assist with reality orientation.
- Create a safe environment for the older adult patient.
- Assist with ambulation.
- Understand nutrition for the older adult patient.
- Provide skin care appropriate for hygiene as well as prevention of pressure ulcers.
- Describe patient rights.

KEY TERMS

Dangling Position: Sitting up on the edge of the bed with the feet hanging down loosely

Dementia: An irreversible mental condition in which intellectual abilities are continuously reduced

Deteriorate: To make or grow worse; degenerate

Disoriented: Unaware of or unable to remember, recognize, or describe people, places, or times; confused perception of reality

Dysphagia: Difficulty in swallowing usually requiring evaluation by speech therapist to prescribe a certain diet and method of feeding

Flammable: Something that can be easily set on fire and burns quickly

Geriatric Person: An aged person; elderly; over 65 years of age

Pathologic: Involved with or caused by a disease

Pouching: Also known as pocketing of food; the retaining or holding of food in the mouth between the cheek and teeth

Restorative Care: Care given to help a patient attain or maintain their highest level of function and independence

Sundowning Syndrome: A term used to describe a state of increased confusion and disorientation that usually occurs in persons with cognitive dysfunction as evening approaches

Validation Therapy: A way of communicating with confused people

Vertigo: Dizziness

CORE STUDENT ASSIGNMENTS

Instructor Notes

Students should:

- Read this chapter in their textbook, *Being a Nursing Assistant.*
- Underline any words or sentences they do not understand. Write down any questions they have.
- Complete the Chapter Review in their textbook.
- Read the Time Management Tip for this chapter and think about how they might use this tip in their work.
- Complete the Nursing Assistant in Action exercise.

OPTIONAL STUDENT ASSIGNMENTS

Students should:

- Complete all workbook assignments for this chapter in their copy of *Workbook for Being a Nursing Assistant.*
- Use the CD/CD-Rom disk enclosed with their textbook to hear the pronunciation of the key terms in the chapter.
- Watch the "Dealing with Dementia" and the "Transfer and Ambulation" videos from the Care Provider Skills series.
- Use the Website address **(www.prenhall.com/wolgin)** to access the free, interactive Companion Website created for this textbook. Get hints, instant feedback, and textbook references to chapter-related multiple-choice questions. Read and react to the Nursing Assistant in Action exercise. Link to other interesting sites.

METHODOLOGY AND SUGGESTED ACTIVITIES

I. Lecture/Discussion

- Answer any questions the students may have.
- Discuss the key terms and related abbreviations. Repeat them out loud and practice using them in sentences.
- Discuss the Time Management Tip for this chapter.
- Discuss the Nursing Assistant in Action exercise.
- Discuss the Critical Thinking points for this chapter.
- Discuss personal safety and protection. Emphasize the importance of following Standard Precautions.
- Emphasize common physical changes in the older adult person.
- Discuss the differences and similarities of dementia and delirium.
- Emphasize the responsibility for meeting the psychosocial needs of the patient.
- Stress creating a safe environment for the older adult patient.
- Emphasize ambulation safety.
- Discuss the age-specific issues often encountered by the elderly.

Instructor Notes

II. Role Play/Lab

- Show the videos for this chapter. Have the students role play ambulating a confused older patient. Emphasize communication techniques that promote understanding between caregiver and patient.
- Offer case studies or scenarios that include theory appropriate to the older adult, and have students role play the situations.
- Invite a geriatric specialist to speak to the class about adult daycare centers in your community.
- Practice responding to patients showing signs of confusion in role-playing situations.
- Invite a dermatologist to speak to the class.
- Invite a physical therapist to speak to the class.
- Arrange a field trip to a local long-term facility.
- Have the students practice validation therapy.

III. Evaluation

- Review the answers to the Chapter Review with students.
- Review the answer to the workbook exercises with students.
- Review the students' understanding of the Time Management Tip.
- To evaluate student comprehension, give a quiz.
- Have the students visit the interactive Companion Website and take the quiz.

ANSWERS TO CHAPTER REVIEW

FILL IN THE BLANK

Read each sentence and fill in the blank line(s) with the word or words that complete the sentence. (Note: Hyphenated words get one line.)

1. As patients age, there are many ___*physical*___ changes that occur in the body.
2. ___*Dementia*___ is an irreversible mental condition in which intellectual abilities are continuously reduced.
3. ___*Disorientation*___ is when a person is unable to remember, recognize, or describe people, places, or times.
4. The specialty within health care that cares for the older adult is known as ___*geriatrics*___.
5. A patient's ___*Bill of Rights*___ is a document that outlines ways the institution will protect the dignity and privacy of the older adult.

Instructor Notes

MULTIPLE CHOICE

Choose the best answer for each question or statement.

1. Which of the following is not generally a major life change for a geriatric patient?
   A. Isolation from friends and family
   B. Change in income
   C. Fear of illness
   (D.) Child care pressures
2. Which of the following is not a common disease of the elderly?
   A. Dementia
   (B.) Head injuries
   C. Emphysema
   D. Cataracts
3. Alzheimer's disease is a degenerative disorder that produces
   (A.) dementia.
   B. diabetes mellitus.
   C. delirium.
   D. double vision.
4. To meet the needs of the older adult, you should
   A. provide a variety of activities that are mentally stimulating.
   B. provide purposeful activities.
   C. encourage the patient to participate and interact with others.
   (D.) All of the above.
5. Reorienting the disoriented person includes all of the following *except*
   A. telling the patient what day it is.
   B. telling the patient who you are.
   (C.) requiring the patient to verify the correct day, time, etc.
   D. making sure they have an accurate name band on.

CRITICAL THINKING

CUSTOMER SERVICE

Encourage students to reflect and share their thoughts and experiences. Respect their privacy and confidentiality. Share your own viewpoints with the students.

CULTURAL CARE

Encourage students to reflect and share their thoughts and experiences. Respect their privacy and confidentiality. Share your own viewpoints with the students.

Instructor Notes

COOPERATION WITHIN THE TEAM

Encourage students to reflect and share their thoughts and experiences. Respect their privacy and confidentiality. Share your own viewpoints with the students.

NURSING ASSISTANT IN ACTION

An 85-year-old, Hispanic woman, Maria De Rosa, is admitted to your Long-Term Care unit. While in the hospital, she had been in bed for several days and became quite weak. Her English is very poor. Her family expresses concern that she has not been eating or drinking very much and, since her admission, appears confused at times.

What Is Your Response/Action?

You can take care to approach Mrs. De Rosa calmly and with a gentle tone of voice. Use interpretors if you can or communication boards to help describe what you want her to do. Be alert for signs of fear or anger she may be expressing. Work with the nurse and other nursing assistants to provide a comforting environment of care.

32

Answers to Workbook Exercises

The following exercises will assist you to apply what you have read in Chapter 32, "The Older Adult Patient and Long-Term Care." For each example, read the objective and use information you have read in Chapter 32 to answer the questions, complete the sentences, or label the diagrams.

EXERCISE 32-1

Objective: To recognize the definitions of important diseases and conditions of the older adult.

Directions: Place the letter of the correct definition next to the matching word(s) from the Word List.

Word List

D **1.** cataracts
F **2.** emphysema
G **3.** fractures
H **4.** gallstones
E **5.** dementia
I **6.** hypertension
A **7.** arthritis
C **8.** diabetes
B **9.** hemorrhoids
M **10.** congestive heart disease
L **11.** varicose veins
J **12.** pneumonia
K **13.** Parkinson's disease
O **14.** gastritis
N **15.** cerebrovascular accident (CVA)
Q **16.** myocardial infarction (heart attack)
P **17.** arteriosclerosis
S **18.** Alzheimer's disease
R **19.** incontinence
T **20.** pathologic
U **21.** dysphagia

Definitions

A. Inflammation of the body joints, causing pain, swelling, loss of movement, and changes in structure
B. Engorged, blood-filled vessels around the anus or rectum
C. A disturbance of the carbohydrate metabolism
D. Clouding of the lens of the eye, causing decreased vision
E. Irreversible deteriorative mental state
F. Tiny bronchioles of the lungs become plugged with mucus
G. Breaks in the bones due to loss of mineralization or injury
H. Crystals that settle out of the bile stored in the gallbladder
I. High blood pressure
J. Acute inflammation or infection in the lungs
K. A chronic disease of the central nervous system, causing tremors in the body
L. Type of vascular disease in which the veins are distended, especially in the legs
M. The inability of the heart to pump out all of the blood returned to it from the veins
N. Blood supply to the brain is reduced; also called a stroke
O. Inflammation of the stomach caused by bacteria, viruses, vitamin deficiency, excessive eating, or overindulgence in alcoholic beverages
P. A pathological condition in which there is a thickening, hardening, and loss of elasticity of the walls of the arteries
Q. Arteries that supply the heart muscle become blocked; the heart muscle does not receive an adequate blood supply and parts of the heart muscle die
R. Inability to control urination
S. A degenerative disorder that produces progressive dementia
T. Involved with or caused by a disease
U. Difficulty in swallowing usually requiring evaluation by a speech therapist to prescribe a certain diet and method of feeding

EXERCISE 32-2

Objective: To recognize common physical changes in older adults as they age.

Directions: Place the correct letters representing a system change next to the matching physical change.

System Change

SKS = skeletal system
US = urinary system
ES = endocrine system
GS = gastrointestinal system
MS = muscular system
CVS = cardiovascular system
RS = respiratory system
NS = nervous system
IS = integumentary system
MH = mental health

Physical Change

ES 1. Decreased ability to heal
US 2. Decreased bladder tone (incontinence)
NS 3. Shorter memory, forgetfulness
SKS 4. Decreasing strength
MS 5. Decreased muscle mass and tone
RS 6. Decreased lung capacity
IS 7. Increased pigmentation (aging spots)
MH 8. Increased incidence of depression
MH 9. Changes in sleeping patterns
GS 10. Decreased appetite
ES 11. Increased incidence of diabetes
CVS 12. Decreased cardiac output
US 13. Decreased kidney function
SKS 14. Bones become brittle
NS 15. Decreased elasticity of ear drum

EXERCISE 32-3

Objective: To apply what you have learned about the older adult and long-term care.

Directions: Circle the letter next to the statement that best completes the sentence or describes the sentence as true or false. If the sentence is false, draw a line through the incorrect part of the sentence and write the correction on the blank line.

1. Examples of meeting the older adult patient's psychosocial needs are all of the following *except*
   A. providing meaningful activities in which he can participate.
   B. encouraging him to do as much as he is able.
   C. showing respect for him as an individual.
   (D.) leaving him isolated from others for long periods of time.
2. The nursing assistant can help to keep the patient oriented by
   A. displaying a clock and calendar where the patient can see them easily.
   B. referencing daily events such as, "It will be lunchtime soon."
   C. telling the patient where he is.
   (D.) all of the above.

3. The spiritual needs of the patient can be met by involving the minister, priest, rabbi, or other spiritual leader in the plan of care.
   (A.) True
   B. False
   Correct Answer: ______________________

4. Patients who are disoriented
   A. have clear recall of events that recently happened.
   B. may be quite lucid.
   (C.) may have difficulty remembering people, places, and times.
   D. should always be physically restrained.

5. ________ is a state of confusion and disorientation that may occur in persons with cognitive dysfunction as evening approaches.
   A. Moonbeaming
   B. Stargazing
   C. Sunstroke
   (D.) Sundowning

6. Keeping the room well lighted can reduce disorientation.
   (A.) True
   B. False
   Correct Answer: ______________________

7. An important responsibility of the health care team members is to provide safety for the older adult by all of the following *except*
   A. protecting from overexposure to sunlight.
   B. making sure the patient is in a full sitting (dangling) position for a few minutes before standing up after lying in bed.
   C. keeping the patient closest to the nurses station for observation.
   (D.) rushing the patient to complete simple tasks.

8. An unsteady patient may be permitted to ambulate ~~by himself~~ if he is provided a walker or cane.
   A. True
   (B.) False
   Correct Answer: *only with assistance*

9. The walker and the patient's feet ~~should~~ be moving at the same time to ensure safety for the older adult when ambulating.
   A. True
   (B.) False
   Correct Answer: *should not*

10. To make mealtime a positive experience, the nursing assistant should do all of the following *except*
   (A.) remove patient's dentures.
   B. set up the tray for the patient.
   C. do not rush if feeding the patient.
   D. identify the foods and tell patients with visual impairments where to find them on the tray.

11. ~~It is not~~ the responsibility of the nursing assistant to be aware of what kind of special diet the patient may be required to follow.

A. True

(B.) False

Correct Answer: *It is*

12. Because you will have to reposition and turn the nonambulatory patient many times each day,

A. you should not worry about good body mechanics.

B. you should not ask your team members to help you.

(C.) you should use a pull (turn) sheet properly to prevent damage to the patient's fragile skin.

D. reddened areas on the patient's skin should be expected.

13. The patient should be repositioned

A. only every 2 hours.

(B.) whenever necessary to keep her in good body alignment and promote good circulation.

C. only when awake.

D. only when she asks to be moved.

14. Pillows ~~should~~ be placed behind the knees if the patient is going to be sitting for an extended period of time.

A. True

(B.) False

Correct Answer: *should not*

15. A serious problem that can develop in bed-bound patients who do not move around is

(A.) constipation.

B. muscle growth and increased strength.

C. an increased interest in food.

D. a dangerous increase in time spent watching television.

16. As you care for the older adult, remember to treat her

A. with dignity and respect.

B. as you would want to be treated.

C. with kindness and gentleness.

(D.) all of the above.

17. A specialty within health care that relates to the care of older adults is

A. pediatrics.

B. energetics.

C. orthopedics.

(D.) geriatrics.

18. Included in patients' rights are all of the following *except*

A. a choice of doctors.

B. prompt response to reasonable requests.

C. privacy.

(D.) unreasonable treatment of caregivers.

19. According to the Omnibus Budget Reconciliation Act (OBRA), long-term care facilities must

A. provide free care.
(B.) inform the patient of his or her rights.
C. discharge the patient within 7 days.
D. all of the above.

20. Providing daily hygiene to the bed-bound patient will help the patient feel better and more relaxed.

(A.) True
B. False

Correct Answer: ______________________

33

Rehabilitation and Return to Self-Care

CHAPTER OVERVIEW

Instructor Notes

I. **The Holistic Approach to Rehabilitation**
   A. Cultural Care
   B. The Rehabilitation Program

II. **OBRA Requirements**

III. **The Professional Rehabilitation Team**
   A. The Role of the Rehabilitation Nurse
   B. The Role of the Physical Therapist
   C. The Role of the Occupational Therapist
   D. The Nursing Assistant's Role in Rehabilitation

IV. **Psychological Aspects of Rehabilitative Care**
   A. The Role of the Nursing Assistant

V. **Psychosocial Aspects of Rehabilitative Care**

VI. **Personal Care of the Patient Who Has a Disability**
   A. Assisting the Patient with Bathing and Grooming
   B. Feeding the Patient Who Has a Disability
   C. Bowel and Bladder Rehabilitation for the Incontinent Patient
      1. Rectal Suppositories
   D. Range of Motion

VII. **Pediatric Rehabilitation**

VIII. **Subacute Care**

Instructor Notes

OBJECTIVES

When the students have completed this chapter, they will be able to:

- Explain the goals of a holistic rehabilitation program.
- List key members of the rehabilitation team.
- Describe the roles of the rehabilitation nurse, physical therapist, and occupational therapist, as well as their role in helping these team members.
- Define their role in the rehabilitation and restorative care process.
- Describe psychological aspects of rehabilitative care.
- Discuss how they can help address psychosocial concerns related to rehabilitation.
- Help the patient with a disability to bathe, dress, and groom.
- Assist the patient with a disability to eat and drink.
- Assist with bowel and bladder rehabilitation and retraining for the incontinent patient.
- Insert nonmedicated rectal suppositories.
- Explain the principles and rules of range-of-motion exercises.
- Perform active or passive range-of-motion exercises with a patient.
- Explain the difference between subacute and acute care settings and the reasons for growth in subacute care.
- Follow guidelines when caring for a patient on a ventilator.

KEY TERMS

Active Motion: Producing, involving, or participating in activity or movement

Apathy: A lack of feeling or interest in things

Depression: Low spirits that may or may not cause a change in activity

Fatigue: A feeling of tiredness or weariness

Holistic: Intended to meet the needs of the whole patient; based on the belief that human beings function as complete units and cannot be effectively treated part by part

Incontinence: Inability to control the bowels or bladder; inability to control urination or defecation

Mobility: Ability to move

Mobilization: Making movable; putting into action

Motivation: Reason, desire, need, or purpose that causes a person to do something

Occupational Therapist: Person trained to assist the patient with performing activities of daily living

Orthotics: The science concerned with making and fitting prosthetic devices

Passive Motion: Not active, but acted upon; enduring without effort or resistance

Instructor Notes

Physical Therapist: Person trained to assist the patient with activities related to motion

Prosthetics: Artificial limbs or substitutes for missing body parts

Psychological: Involving aspects of the mind, such as feelings and thoughts

Psychosocial: Involving aspects of living together in a group of people

Range-of-Motion (ROM) Exercises: Exercises that move each muscle and joint through its full range of motion and help a confined patient exercise the muscles and joints

Rehabilitation: The process by which people who have been disabled by injury or sickness are helped to recover as much as possible of their original abilities for the activities of daily living

Rehabilitation Nurse: A nurse with special training in the causes and treatment of disabilities; may be certified in this specialty with the title certified rehabilitation registered nurse (CRRN)

Restorative Care: Care given to help a patient attain and maintain the highest level of function and independence

Subacute Care: Ongoing medical, nursing, rehabilitative, or dietary care provided to patients who need a lower level of care than an acute care (i.e., hospital) setting provides; categories of subacute care are based on the patient's health status and the type and length of care needed

Suppository: A semisolid preparation, sometimes medicated, that is inserted into the vagina or rectum

Unilateral Neglect: Failure of a patient disabled on one side of the body to dress, bathe, or otherwise care for that side because the patient forgets that side exists

Ventilator: Machine that mechanically breathes for and provides oxygen to sustain a patient unable to inhale and exhale on his own

CORE STUDENT ASSIGNMENTS

Students should:

- Read this chapter in their textbook, *Being a Nursing Assistant*.
- Underline any words or sentences they do not understand. Write down any questions they have.
- Complete the Chapter Review in their textbook.
- Read the Time Management Tip for this chapter and think about how they might use this tip in their work.
- Complete the Nursing Assistant in Action exercise.

Instructor Notes

OPTIONAL STUDENT ASSIGNMENTS

Students should:

- Complete all workbook assignments for this chapter in their copy of *Workbook for Being a Nursing Assistant*.
- Use the CD/CD-Rom disk enclosed with their textbook to hear the pronunciation of the key terms in the chapter.
- Watch the "Assisting with Dressing" portion of the "Personal Care" video from the Care Provider Skills series.
- Use the Website address **(www.prenhall.com/wolgin)** to access the free, interactive Companion Website created for this textbook. Get hints, instant feedback, and textbook references to chapter-related multiple-choice questions. Read and react to the Nursing Assistant in Action exercise. Link to other interesting sites.

METHODOLOGY AND SUGGESTED ACTIVITIES

I. Lecture/Discussion

- Answer any questions the students may have.
- Discuss the key terms and related abbreviations. Repeat them out loud and practice using them in sentences.
- Discuss the Time Management Tip for this chapter.
- Discuss the Nursing Assistant in Action exercise.
- Discuss the Critical Thinking points for this chapter.
- Discuss personal safety and protection. Emphasize the importance of following Universal Precautions.
- Present case studies and discuss them.
- Invite a rehabilitation psychologist to speak to the class.
- Invite an occupational therapist to speak to the class.
- Invite a physical therapist to speak to the class.
- Invite a respiratory therapist to speak to the class.
- Discuss patient motivation and how important it is in rehabilitation.
- Explain how a ventilator works and review care of a patient on one.
- Discuss the importance of bowel and bladder rehabilitation and ways to help the patient's rehabilitation be successful.

II. Role Play/Lab

- Show the video for this chapter. Have the students practice putting scrubs or other clothes on each other (over current clothes). Have the students "coach" each other to get dressed with one side "paralyzed."
- Write titles of professional rehabilitation team members on cards. Have the students choose cards and role play the interaction among the members as they provide services to a patient.
- Demonstrate range-of-motion exercises and have students return the demonstration.
- Assign students to groups of three to practice range-of-motion exercises.

Instructor Notes

- Display and demonstrate adaptive devices. Have students return demonstration and practice using adaptive devices.
- Have the students practice encouraging each other as they perform ADLs as rehabilitation patients.

III. Evaluation

- Review the answers to the Chapter Review with students.
- Review the answer to the workbook exercises with students.
- Review the student's understanding of the Time Management Tip.
- To evaluate student comprehension, give a quiz.
- To evaluate student skills, administer the competency checklist.
- Have the students visit the interactive Companion Website and take the quiz.

ANSWERS TO CHAPTER REVIEW

FILL IN THE BLANK

Read each sentence and fill in the blank line(s) with the word or words that complete the sentence. (Note: Hyphenated words get one line.)

1. The process of helping a person regain a state of health is called *rehabilitation*.
2. The *physical* *therapist* is trained to assist patients with activities related to motion.
3. The *occupational* *therapist* is trained to increase the functional ability of patients to do their activities of daily living.
4. Low spirits that may or may not cause a change in activity are called *depression*.
5. *Fatigue* is a feeling of tiredness or weariness.

MULTIPLE CHOICE

Choose the best answer for each question or statement.

1. Rehabilitation
   A. usually is a waste of time.
   B. is a process done to the patient.
   (C.) can help the patient recover as much as possible.
   D. is not influenced by cultural and religious beliefs.
2. Activities of daily living include all of the following *except*
   A. toileting.
   B. bathing.
   (C.) computer skills.
   D. homemaking.

Instructor Notes

3. In a rehabilitation program, the nursing assistant should
   A. do as much as possible for the patient.
   B. instruct the patient in exactly what to do.
   (C.) watch for signs that the patient is tired.
   D. All of the above.

4. A condition that occurs when the patient who is disabled on one side of the body forgets that side of the body even exists is called
   A. exercise neglect.
   B. exhaustion.
   C. exercise fatigue.
   (D.) unilateral neglect.

5. Subacute care is appropriate in all of the following cases *except*
   A. long-term transitional care (ventilator-dependent patients).
   (B.) Critical Care unit (newly admitted trauma patient).
   C. chronic subacute (long-term comatose patients).
   D. transitional subacute (stroke patients with > 6 days of hospitalization).

CRITICAL THINKING

CUSTOMER SERVICE

Encourage students to reflect and share their thoughts and experiences. Respect their privacy and confidentiality. Share your own viewpoints with the students.

CULTURAL CARE

Encourage students to reflect and share their thoughts and experiences. Respect their privacy and confidentiality. Share your own viewpoints with the students.

COOPERATION WITHIN THE TEAM

Encourage students to reflect and share their thoughts and experiences. Respect their privacy and confidentiality. Share your own viewpoints with the students.

NURSING ASSISTANT IN ACTION

Mrs. Williams is an 88-year-old woman who has been in good health. She was living independently and able to drive her car prior to a fall this week. She had surgery to repair her broken hip. Part of her rehabilitation includes getting her up walking. Mrs. Williams has been in pain and is afraid to allow you to get her up.

What Is Your Response/Action?

You could talk to Mrs. Williams and tell her that you will coordinate with the RN to have her walk when she is feeling the best after her pain medication. You could also tell Mrs. Williams that you will go slowly to move her out of bed and that walking will ultimately help her feel better.

Answers to Workbook Exercises

33

The following exercises will assist you to apply what you have read in Chapter 33, "Rehabilitation and Return to Self-Care." For each exercise, read the objective and use information you have read in Chapter 33 to answer the questions, complete the sentences, or label the diagrams.

EXERCISE 33-1

Objective: To recognize and correctly spell words related to rehabilitative care.

Directions: Unscramble the words in the Word List at the left. Then circle the same words in the Word Search grid at the right.

Word List

1. CATIVE ___*ACTIVE*___
2. AVITONIMOT ___*MOTIVATION*___
3. GENRA FO NOITOM ___*RANGE OF MOTION*___
4. SICOTROHT ___*ORTHOTICS*___
5. BIMOZLTAOINI ___*MOBILIZATION*___
6. SPASVIE ___*PASSIVE*___
7. CITSILOH ___*HOLISTIC*___
8. IHERIABLTOATNI ___*REHABILITATION*___

Word Search

A	L	E	R	T	U	Y	A	Z	C	M	H	C	F	O	H	B	C
I	C	Q	Z	K	S	D	T	D	I	T	G	K	P	W	S	R	I
M	O	T	I	V	A	T	I	O	N	S	I	Z	S	O	C	E	D
J	P	A	I	C	Z	X	H	V	A	X	B	R	Z	W	A	H	S
K	G	Z	W	V	O	B	Z	V	H	Z	V	L	Z	A	P	A	K
C	Z	D	D	F	E	I	Z	S	D	Z	K	Z	R	O	V	B	R
B	O	F	S	F	U	G	R	O	P	C	Y	B	E	C	T	I	B
H	P	J	C	T	M	K	F	M	D	Q	S	D	I	Z	I	L	G
R	A	N	G	E	O	F	M	O	T	I	O	N	X	E	Y	I	S
K	S	T	Q	H	B	G	T	R	R	L	R	G	B	A	Z	T	L
L	S	A	M	X	I	A	Y	J	Z	F	T	Y	Z	F	C	A	J
D	I	J	D	U	L	Q	B	X	F	O	H	I	P	Z	O	T	B
M	V	O	S	S	I	M	B	W	B	H	O	L	I	S	T	I	C
F	E	C	G	Y	Z	O	L	B	H	D	T	K	O	D	V	O	Z
I	Q	T	A	I	A	T	G	K	O	D	I	O	I	J	M	N	D
E	P	B	H	X	T	C	P	Z	V	E	C	M	Z	C	Q	I	M
J	K	T	Y	D	I	J	Q	E	T	W	S	H	X	R	T	F	B
G	R	W	Z	Y	O	Z	C	D	Z	G	X	Y	K	S	P	K	O
B	L	X	L	Z	N	S	F	Z	K	C	O	I	D	E	O	A	J

EXERCISE 33-2

Objective: To apply what you have learned about rehabilitation and return to self-care.

Directions: Read the following riddles carefully before writing the correct answer on the blank line.

1. If your patient expresses frequent feelings of excessive tiredness and weariness, he may be showing this common symptom of depression. *Hint:* If you were in the military you would wear this item.

   fatigue

2. A stroke or trauma can cause this function of the hand to become weak. *Hint:* This can also be a stagehand in a movie production.

   grip

3. Before beginning bladder or bowel training, keep track of the current excretory pattern for 2–3 days by writing it in this item. *Hint:* This is also a fallen tree without branches.

   log

EXERCISE 33-3

Objective: To recognize important aspects of holistic care and appropriate actions to be taken.

Directions: Place the correct letters next to the holistic need described in each situation. Then circle the best response to meet that need. More than one letter can be selected for each situation.

PH = physical needs	SOC = social needs
EC = economic needs	SP = spiritual needs
PSY = psychological needs	M = mental needs
EM = emotional needs	

1. Your patient has been incontinent of urine since coming home from the hospital.

   LETTERS: PH, PSY, EM **What would you do?**

   A. You complain of the increasing amount of work this is for you.
   B. You encourage him to stay positive.
   C. You start a log to establish a voiding or evacuation pattern.
   (D.) You do both B and C.

2. Your stroke patient takes a very long time to dress herself.

   LETTERS: PH, PSY, EM **What would you do?**

   A. You notify the nurse.
   B. You help her so that it only takes a few minutes.
   C. You keep her in her pajamas until all other work is completed.
   (D.) No matter how long it takes, you let her select her own clothing and do as much of the dressing as she can.

3. Although the patient appears to receive comfort from it, you find that on days when the minister comes to see the patient, you are forced to reorganize your patient care duties to accommodate his visit.

LETTERS: SP, SOC **What would you do?**

(A.) You speak positively of the visit both before and after it occurs.
B. You report the minister to the nurse.
C. You continue with your schedule while he is there.
D. You encourage the minister to come only on days when you are not there.

4. During range-of-motion exercises, the patient mentions that he can't sleep at night because he is worried about his increasing health care bill.

LETTERS: EC, PSY, EM **What would you do?**

(A.) You notify the nurse, who can make a referral to the financial counselor.
B. You tell him not to worry so much, and to just concentrate on the exercises.
C. You tell him about your financial difficulties.
D. You tell your family about his problem.

5. The child you are working with watches television all day. He will complete his rehabilitation program soon and will go back to school.

LETTERS: M **What would you do?**

(A.) You encourage him to do the homework left by the teacher.
B. You do nothing because it is not related to patient care.
C. You call the minister to speak to the child.
D. You do the homework for him.

6. The elderly patient you care for has diminished speaking ability. He is understandable, but it takes him a long time to get his thoughts communicated. Today he wants to talk about his deceased wife, since this would have been their 50th wedding anniversary.

LETTERS: EM, PSY, SOC **What would you do?**

(A.) Encourage him to talk about his wife, and spend as much time listening to him as you can spare.
B. Remind him that he shouldn't live in the past.
C. Refer him to the speech therapist.
D. Continue working and hope that he will take his nap soon.

7. Mrs. Green is in rehabilitation for hand and arm injuries she received in an automobile accident. Her family lives far away, and she cannot afford to telephone them regularly.

LETTERS: SOC, EC **What would you do?**

A. Tell her not to think about them.
B. Give her crafts such as basket-weaving to occupy her mind.
(C.) Offer to write short letters to her family for her, encouraging them to write.
D. Do nothing, this is not related to her well-being.

8. Your patient spends quite a long time in bed each day and is unable to move or change position without help.

   LETTERS: PH **What would you do?**

   A. Make sure she assists you as much as possible when repositioning her in bed.
   B. Take the time to give her backrubs twice a day.
   C. Put her body in good alignment when positioning her with pillows.
   (D.) All of the above.

EXERCISE 33-4

Objective: To recognize the definitions of words used in patient rehabilitation activities.

Directions: Place the letters of the correct definition next to the matching word(s) from the Word List.

Word List

J 1. incontinence
D 2. prosthetics
E 3. mobilization
P 4. apathy
H 5. suppository
N 6. occupational therapist
K 7. range-of-motion exercises
I 8. holistic
R 9. physical therapist
Q 10. rehabilitation nurse
S 11. abduction
M 12. orthotics
A 13. passive
O 14. psychosocial
F 15. active
G 16. motivation
C 17. depression
B 18. fatigue
L 19. psychological

Definitions

A. Not active, but acted upon
B. A feeling of tiredness or weariness
C. Low spirits that may or may not cause a change in activity
D. Artificial limbs or substitutes for missing body parts
E. Making movable; putting into action
F. Producing, involving, or participating in activity or movement
G. The reason, desire, or purpose that causes one to do something
H. A semisolid preparation (sometimes medicated) that is inserted into the vagina or rectum
I. An approach to meeting the needs of the whole patient that comes from the belief that human beings function as complete units and cannot be treated part by part

J. The inability to control the bowels or the bladder

K. These exercises move each muscle and joint through its full range of motion and assist the patient who is confined to exercise his muscles and joints

L. All aspects of the mind, such as feelings and thoughts

M. The science concerned with making and fitting prosthetic devices

N. Trained person who assists the patient with performing activities of daily living(ADLs)

O. All aspects of living together in a group with other human beings

P. A lack of feeling or interest in things

Q. A nurse with special training in the causes and treatment of disabilities, who is sometimes certified in his area of specialty, having the title of certified rehabilitation registered nurse (CRRN)

R. Person trained to assist the patient with activities related to motion

S. Moving a body part away from the body midline

EXERCISE 33-5

Objective: To apply what you have learned about rehabilitation and return to self-care.

Directions: Circle the letter next to the statement that best completes the sentence or describes the sentence as true or false. If the sentence is false, draw a line through the incorrect part of the sentence and write the correction on the blank line.

1. Rehabilitation takes time and patience, and it often may not
- A. do any good.
- (B.) bring about a complete return to normal.
- C. challenge the patient.
- D. involve the patient.

2. The nursing assistant helps the patient gain skill in
- A. becoming dependent.
- B. feeding only.
- C. dressing only.
- (D.) dressing, personal hygiene tasks, and feeding.

3. The child's natural curiosity can be very helpful in the rehabilitation process by
- A. keeping him uninformed.
- B. providing fear of the unknown.
- C. stopping his involvement in the process.
- (D.) getting him interested in his treatment.

4. Observations of the patient that should be reported to the occupational therapist are all of the following *except*
   A. signs of being tired.
   B. signs of pain.
   C. tolerance of each procedure.
   (D.) the nursing assistant's level of curiosity.

5. The nursing assistant's role in rehabilitation is to assist other team members by all of the following *except*
   A. listening to the patient.
   B. maintaining a safe environment.
   (C.) medicating the patient.
   D. observing the patient.

6. An example of the nursing assistant developing a helping relationship with the patient is to ~~discourage~~ him ~~from participating~~ in his plan of care.
   A. True
   (B.) False
   Correct Answer: *encourage, to participate*

7. The nursing assistant should encourage the patient to do as many personal care tasks as she is capable of performing.
   (A.) True
   B. False
   Correct Answer: ______

8. Patients should be encouraged to dress in
   A. a hospital gown.
   B. the middle of the night, if they are awake.
   C. the bathroom.
   (D.) street clothes to enhance their feelings of self-esteem.

9. Cultural and religious beliefs may play an important role in the rehabilitative process.
   (A.) True
   B. False
   Correct Answer: ______

10. When dressing the patient, dress the weakest or most involved ______ first.
    A. nursing assistant
    B. family member
    (C.) extremity
    D. visitor

11. Transitional subacute care patients receive care that is a substitute for continued hospital stay.
    (A.) True
    B. False
    Correct Answer: ______

12. Chronic subacute care patients may be classified as having ~~a high~~ hope of ultimate recovery and functional independence.

A. True

(B.) False

Correct Answer: *little*

COMPETENCY CHECKLIST 33-1: REHABILITATION AND RETURN TO SELF-CARE

ACTIVITY	S	U	COMMENTS
1. Student will demonstrate the correct method of bathing the patient with a disability.			
2. Student will demonstrate the correct method of dressing and grooming the patient.			
3. Student will demonstrate the correct method of feeding the patient with a disability.			
4. Student will demonstrate the correct method of assisting the patient with a disability with bowel and bladder training.			
5. Student will demonstrate the correct method of inserting a rectal suppository.			
6. Student will demonstrate the correct method of performing range-of-motion exercises.			

34

The Terminally Ill Patient and Postmortem Care

CHAPTER OVERVIEW

Instructor Notes

I. **Care of Dying Patients**

II. **Organ and Tissue Donation**

III. **Psychological/Psychosocial Aspects of Caring for a Terminally Ill Patient**
   A. Stages of Dying

IV. **The Patient's Family or Significant Other**

V. **Hospice Care**
   A. Principles of Hospice Care
   B. Characteristics of Hospice Programs

VI. **Making the Patient Comfortable**

VII. **Signs of Approaching Death**

VIII. **Postmortem Care (PMC)**

Instructor Notes

OBJECTIVES

When the students have completed this chapter, they will be able to:

- Cite an advantage of organ donation.
- Assist in meeting the psychological, spiritual, or psychosocial needs of the terminally ill patient.
- List common feelings of a patient who is dying.
- Assist in meeting the special care needs of the elderly patient's family or significant other.
- Describe hospice care.
- Identify comfort measures for the terminally ill patient.
- Describe *palliative care*, care designed to comfort, instead of cure, the patient.
- Identify the signs of approaching death.
- Explain *DNR* (do not resuscitate) status.
- Give postmortem care gently and respectfully.
- Explain how to protect the patient's valuables.

KEY TERMS

Acceptance: Admitting, understanding, or facing the truth or reality of the situation, for example, one's death

Advance Directive: Prewritten instructions on withholding resuscitation and life-prolonging measures and equipment

Anger: A strong emotional response of displeasure, irritation, and resentment

Bargaining: Trying to make a deal to change the situation

Denial: Refusal to admit the truth or face reality

Depression: A state of sadness, grief, or low spirits that may or may not cause change of activity

Expired: Deceased, dead

Hospice: Program that allows a dying patient to remain at home or in a non-hospital environment and die there while receiving professionally supervised care

Morgue: A place for temporarily keeping dead bodies for identification, autopsy, retrieval by funeral home staff, and burial

Palliative Care: Care designed to comfort, instead of cure, the patient

Postmortem: After death

Rigor Mortis: The natural stiffening of a body and limbs shortly after death

Terminally Ill: Having an illness that can be expected to cause death, usually within a predictable time

CORE STUDENT ASSIGNMENTS

Instructor Notes

Students should:

- Read this chapter in their textbook, *Being a Nursing Assistant*.
- Underline any words or sentences they do not understand. Write down any questions they have.
- Complete the Chapter Review in their textbook.
- Read the Time Management Tip for this chapter and think about how they might use this tip in their work.
- Complete the Nursing Assistant in Action exercise.

OPTIONAL STUDENT ASSIGNMENTS

Students should:

- Complete all workbook assignments for this chapter in their copy of *Workbook for Being a Nursing Assistant*.
- Use the CD/CD-Rom disk enclosed with their textbook to hear the pronunciation of the key terms in the chapter.
- Watch the "Communication" portion of the "Age-Specific Competency" video and the "Patient's Right to Refuse Care" portion of the "Patient's Rights" video from the Care Provider Skills series.
- Use the Website address **(www.prenhall.com/wolgin)** to access the free, interactive Companion Website created for this textbook. Get hints, instant feedback, and textbook references to chapter-related multiple-choice questions. Read and react to the Nursing Assistant in Action exercise. Link to other interesting sites.

METHODOLOGY AND SUGGESTED ACTIVITIES

I. Lecture/Discussion

- Answer any questions the students may have.
- Discuss the key terms and related abbreviations. Repeat them out loud and practice using them in sentences.
- Discuss the Time Management Tip for this chapter.
- Discuss the Nursing Assistant in Action exercise.
- Discuss the Critical Thinking points for this chapter.
- Discuss personal safety and protection. Emphasize the importance of following Universal Precautions. Stress the need to wear protective equipment.
- Discuss the importance of Advance Directives for people of all ages.
- Discuss scenarios of people's reactions to terminal diagnoses.
- Discuss ways that families can be involved with care.
- Review the stages of dying.
- Invite a hospice nurse to talk to the students.
- Discuss signs and symptoms of approaching death.
- Have a mortician talk with the students.

Instructor Notes

II. Role Play/Lab

- Show the videos for this chapter. Role play situations where the patient refuses care. Have the students respond.
- Have the students share experiences they've had with death and dying.
- Have the students practice postmortem care. Emphasize the importance of respect for the dead and cultural and religious differences.

III. Evaluation

- Review the answers to the Chapter Review with students.
- Review the answer to the workbook exercises with students.
- Review the students' understanding of the Time Management Tip.
- To evaluate student comprehension, give a quiz.
- To evaluate student skills, administer the competency checklist.
- Have the students visit the interactive Companion Website and take the quiz.

ANSWERS TO CHAPTER REVIEW

FILL IN THE BLANK

Read each sentence and fill in the blank line(s) with the word or words that complete the sentence. (Note: Hyphenated words get one line.)

1. When a patient is ___*terminally*___ ill, they have an illness that is expected to cause death usually within a predicted time.
2. When a patient is dying, respect the patient and family's need for ___*privacy*___ as much as possible.
3. A program that allows a dying patient to remain at home or in a nonhospital facility is called ___*hospice*___.
4. Care designed to comfort rather than cure is called ___*palliative*___ care.
5. Rigor mortis is the natural ___*stiffening*___ of the body after death.

MULTIPLE CHOICE

Choose the best answer for each question or statement.

1. People have different ideas about death and dying. As a nursing assistant, it is important that you
   A. impose your ideas and religious beliefs on patients.
   (B.) respect the cultures and religious beliefs of others.
   C. say "no" or "you must follow policy" when patient or family requests pose a problem or inconvience to you.
   D. All of the above.

Instructor Notes

2. Some common stages of dying are
   A. denial, anger, depression, bargaining, and acceptance.
   B. denial, depression, anger, bargaining, and acceptance.
   C. anger, denial, depression, repression, and acceptance.
   D. anger, repression, denial, bargaining, and acceptance.
3. All of the following are signs of approaching death *except*
   A. the hands and feet become cold to the touch.
   B. the patient's face may become pale.
   C. the arms and legs become stiff.
   D. the patient may perspire heavily even though his body is cold.
4. A physician's order that states that emergency care must be given to a patient is
   A. DNR.
   B. Advanced Directive.
   C. slow code.
   D. None of the above.
5. Postmortem care should be completed
   A. after rigor mortis has set in.
   B. only in the morgue.
   C. by a funeral attendant.
   D. before rigor mortis has set in.

CRITICAL THINKING

CUSTOMER SERVICE

Encourage students to reflect and share their thoughts and experiences. Respect their privacy and confidentiality. Share your own viewpoints with the students.

CULTURAL CARE

Encourage students to reflect and share their thoughts and experiences. Respect their privacy and confidentiality. Share your own viewpoints with the students.

COOPERATION WITHIN THE TEAM

Encourage students to reflect and share their thoughts and experiences. Respect their privacy and confidentiality. Share your own viewpoints with the students.

Instructor Notes

NURSING ASSISTANT IN ACTION

Mr. Justice is a patient on your unit who is terminally ill with an Advance Directive in place. His son who lives in another town has arrived to visit and just learned his father is dying. The Advance Directive states you are not to give fluids or nutrition to Mr. Justice. His son is upset and tells you he will have you fired from your job if you do not start giving his father some water immediately.

What Is Your Response/Action?

You should not argue or become angry at the son. He is most likely upset about his father's approaching death. You should immediately contact the nurse so she can talk with the son and Mr. Justice. You can express your care and concern about Mr. Justice and your desire to fulfill his wishes.

34

Answers to Workbook Exercises

The following exercises will assist you to apply what you have read in Chapter 34, "The Terminally Ill Patient and Postmortem Care." For each exercise, read the objective and use information you have read in Chapter 34 to answer the questions, complete the sentences, or label the diagrams.

EXERCISE 34-1

Objective: To recognize and correctly spell words related to the care of terminally ill patients and providing postmortem care.

Directions: Unscramble the words in the Word List at the left. Then circle the same words in the Word Search grid at the right.

Word List

1. SHPOCIE *HOSPICE*
2. LILPAAVTIE *PALLIATIVE*
3. DINLEA *DENIAL*
4. GNINIAGRAB *BARGAINING*
5. PRDEEISNSO *DEPRESSION*
6. CEPCAATCNE *ACCEPTANCE*
7. TIRIPSAUL NEDE *SPIRITUAL NEED*

Word Search

V	D	S	P	G	A	B	K	U	X	Q	V	I	L
F	T	D	W	X	Y	U	Y	O	M	C	T	O	T
E	H	N	O	I	S	S	E	R	P	E	D	L	Y
A	Z	O	Y	D	F	R	A	M	D	I	E	Q	R
C	Y	X	S	T	Z	I	G	Q	X	L	N	P	D
C	L	N	Q	P	A	L	L	I	A	T	I	V	E
E	U	A	O	B	I	W	F	X	S	K	A	F	F
P	D	G	Y	K	X	C	U	O	M	W	L	U	D
T	B	H	M	B	O	T	E	H	A	C	A	C	I
A	I	C	L	R	D	G	Q	L	U	E	E	M	V
N	B	A	R	G	A	I	N	I	N	G	I	O	F
C	S	P	I	R	I	T	U	A	L	N	E	E	D
E	N	V	J	V	N	E	P	D	J	C	P	K	I
A	H	D	Z	B	F	H	E	Q	N	I	G	X	M
T	Z	I	W	K	R	A	P	Z	U	B	V	A	K

EXERCISE 34-2

Objective: To apply what you have learned about care of the terminally ill patient.

Directions: Read the following riddles carefully before writing the correct answer on the blank line.

1. If you ask me I will tell you that I get more from the patients than I give. Who am I? *Hint:* Rhymes with "very dear."
   volunteer
2. I can provide cleanliness, moisture, and lubrication, and I taste good too. Who am I? *Hint:* I'm not made of only cotton like my cousin, "Q."
   glycerine/lemon swab
3. If the patient can feel clean, comfortable, and cared for she will die with this important characteristic. *Hint:* Important aspect of being human.
   dignity

EXERCISE 34-3

Objective: To recognize the needs of terminally ill patients.

Directions: Place the correct letters with the matching phrases. More than one set of letters may be selected for each phrase.

PN = personal need	VN = visual need
CN = communication need	EN = elimination need
OHN = oral hygiene need	SN = spiritual need
PON = positioning need	NN = nutrition need
OXN = oxygen therapy need	

OXN, PN 1. Check nostrils for dryness and behind the ears for redness of the skin, where the tubing may cause irritation.

SN 2. Learn your institution's policy concerning religious observances and requirements at the time of death.

PN, OHN 3. Use a glycerine applicator for the mouth.

PN, EN 4. As the patient becomes weaker, he may require more of your help with bathing or toileting.

PN, EN 5. Change the bedding whenever necessary to keep the skin dry.

PON, PN 6. Change the patient's position at least every 2 hours.

CN, PN 7. Speak to the patient, even though she may appear unconscious.

NN, PN 8. Semisoft foods may be easier to swallow than liquids.

VN, PN 9. Adjust the light in the room to suit the patient.

PN 10. Members of the nursing staff should stay calm and sympathetic when working with the patient, his family, and significant others.

EXERCISE 34-4

Objective: To recognize the five stages of death and dying.

Directions: Place the correct letters with the matching phrases.

D = denial A = anger B = bargaining
DP = depression AC = acceptance

DP 1. "I know now that I won't last long. Life is too short! There are so many things I wish I had done with my life. Do you have time to listen to me if I tell you a little story right now?"

D 2. "This can't be happening! The tests must be wrong. . . . I never smoked or drank in my life!"

A 3. "Well, you sure are slow today! If you take much longer with this bath I'll be dead before you finish!"

B 4. "I have prayed every day since I found out about this problem I have. I have told God that if I get through this I will devote the rest of my life to the poor and unfortunate."

AC 5. "I guess this is really going to happen to me. I don't feel like talking today. I would just like to listen to the music on the radio and rest. Please close the door and pull the window shades down for me."

EXERCISE 34-5

Objective: To apply what you have learned about the importance of the patient's family or significant other(s).

Directions: Circle the letter next to the statement that best completes the sentence or describes the sentence as true or false. If the sentence is false, draw a line through the incorrect part of the sentence and write the correction on the blank line.

1. Members of the family should be ________ if they wish to spend increased amounts of time with the terminally ill patient.
   A. discouraged
   (B.) encouraged
   C. denied
   D. rescheduled

2. You can demonstrate to members of the family that the patient is well cared for by ~~leaving the room as soon as~~ they arrive for a visit.
   A. True
   (B.) False
   Correct Answer: completing the patient care even though

3. The family may want to stay with the patient, even if he
   A. is unconscious.
   B. is receiving care from the nursing assistant.
   C. has died.
   (D.) all of the above.

4. It is important that the family realize that the patient's needs are being met even though she is near death.
   (A.) True
   B. False
   Correct Answer: ______________________

5. The patient's family may ask many questions; therefore, it is important that the nursing assistant
   A. know all the answers.
   B. only answer five questions per day.
   C. tell them to ask the nurse.
   (D.) understand what kind of questions he is allowed to answer and which questions should be referred to the nurse.

6. When the patient is visited by the pastor, rabbi, minister, or other religious leader, make sure you
   A. include the visitors.
   B. provide suitable music.
   C. provide patient care.
   (D.) provide privacy for them.

7. Unconscious patients require more time
   A. and less thorough care.
   (B.) and as thorough care as conscious patients.
   C. and less work for the nursing assistant.
   D. but are more responsive than conscious patients.

8. You can help the patient's family most by maintaining a concerned and efficient approach to your work.
   (A.) True
   B. False
   Correct Answer: ______________________

9. An Advance Directive describes the type and extent of care the patient wants at the end of life.
   (A.) True
   B. False
   Correct Answer: ______________________

10. The patient's family should be directed to the ________ so that they do not neglect their nutritional needs if they have spent long periods of time at the hospital.
   A. chapel
   B. lounge
   C. nurse's station
   (D.) cafeteria

EXERCISE 34-6

Objective: To recognize the definitions of words related to the care of the terminally ill patient and postmortem care.

Directions: Place the letter of the correct definition next to the matching word(s) from the Word List.

Word List

__E__ **1.** terminally ill

__D__ **2.** expired

__H__ **3.** denial

__F__ **4.** postmortem

__I__ **5.** hospice

__J__ **6.** bargaining

__C__ **7.** anger

__K__ **8.** morgue

__B__ **9.** rigor mortis

__A__ **10.** acceptance

__L__ **11.** depression

__G__ **12.** significant other

__M__ **13.** Advance Directive

Definitions

A. Accepting, understanding, or facing the truth or reality of the situation
B. Natural stiffening of a body and limbs shortly after death
C. A strong emotional response of displeasure, irritation, and resentment
D. Deceased, dead
E. Having an illness that can be expected to lead to death, usually within a predictable time
F. After death
G. A key person having important meaning to the patient, and who provides key emotional and physical support
H. Refusal to admit the truth or face reality
I. Program that allows a dying patient to remain at home or in a nonhospital environment and die there while receiving professionally supervised care
J. Trying to make a deal to change the situation
K. A place for temporarily keeping dead bodies for identification, autopsy, retrieval by funeral home staff, and burial
L. State of sadness, grief, or low spirits that may or may not cause change of activity
M. Prewritten instructions on withholding resuscitation and life-prolonging measures and equipment.

EXERCISE 34-7

Objective: To recognize the body system changes that produce the signs of approaching death.

Directions: Place the correct letters with the matching phrases. More than one set of letters may be selected for each phrase.

CC = circulatory changes
RSC = respiratory system changes
MSC = muscular system changes
NSC = nervous system changes
PYC = psychological changes
EXC = excretory system changes

CC **1.** The patient's hands and feet feel cold to the touch.

PYC **2.** The patient may speak to persons who have died.

EXC **3.** Urine output will decrease and eventually stop.

CC **4.** The face will become pale.

PYC **5.** The eyes may appear to stare blankly.

CC, NSC **6.** The patient may perspire heavily but feel cold.

NSC, CC **7.** The dying patient may feel little or no pain.

MSC **8.** Swallowing ability decreases.

MSC **9.** The body becomes limp.

CC **10.** The pulse will be irregular, weak, or very rapid.

RSC **11.** The breathing pattern will become irregular, slower, or more difficult.

NSC, PYC **12.** The patient may be confused or disoriented.

EXERCISE 34-8

Objective: To apply what you have learned about postmortem care.

Directions: Circle the letter of the correct answer for each question.

1. The body of the deceased person must be
A. treated quickly before the family arrives.
B. removed immediately and taken to the morgue.
C. pronounced dead by the nurse.
(D.) treated with respect.

2. After the patient has expired, ________ care is given.
A. catheter
B. postoperative
C. postpartum
(D.) postmortem

3. The dentures must be

(A.) placed in the mouth immediately after death.
B. discarded.
C. placed in a bag and labeled with the patient's time of death.
D. cleaned and stored.

4. The body should be placed in a flat, ________ position.

A. posterior
B. standing
(C.) dignified
D. sitting

5. At the direction of the ________ , turn off the oxygen and IV.

A. family
B. clergy
C. significant other
(D.) nurse or doctor

6. Follow the ________ policy on care of the patient's belongings.

A. finders keepers
B. family
C. sticky finger
(D.) institution's specific

7. In most instances, jewelry, especially wedding rings,

A. is removed immediately.
B. is given to any relative present at the death.
C. is removed by relatives as soon as death occurs.
(D.) should be taped in place instead of being removed, until the surviving spouse or family makes the decision to remove it.

8. Postmortem care should be done before ________ occurs.

A. procrastination
B. nursing assistant resistance
C. corpus delecti
(D.) rigor mortis

9. ________ must be worn by the nursing assistant when providing postmortem care.

A. A bath blanket
B. Disposable shoe covers
(C.) Disposable gloves
D. A face mask

10. Signs of approaching death include all of the following *except*

A. face becomes pale.
B. loss of muscle tone.
(C.) pulse gets stronger.
D. urine output decreases.

11. Straighten up the room and remove any ________ before the family comes to view the body.
    A. valuables
    B. furniture
    (C.) emergency equipment
    D. all of the above

12. Turn off any ________ over the bed when finished with postmortem care.
    A. call lights
    B. electric blankets
    (C.) bright lights
    D. fans

COMPETENCY CHECKLIST 34-1: POSTMORTEM CARE

ACTIVITY	S	U	COMMENTS
Student will correctly demonstrate postmortem care.			

35

Beginning Your Career as a Nursing Assistant

CHAPTER OVERVIEW

Instructor Notes

I. Preparing for the Competency Evaluation Exam
- A. Clinical Skills Examination
- B. Written/Oral Examination
- C. Test Fees and Time Requirements
- D. Nurse Aide Registry
- E. Sample Test

II. Pursuing Employment Opportunities
- A. Where to Look for Jobs
  1. Personal Contacts
  2. Want Ads/Classifieds
  3. Employment Agencies
  4. Local Hospitals/Nursing Homes/Facilities
- B. Application Process
- C. Preparing a Résumé
- D. The Job Interview
- E. Job Offer
- F. Orientation
- G. Continuing to Learn
- H. Planning Your Career Path

III. Positioning Yourself for Promotion
- A. Changing Jobs
- B. Resignation Letters

Instructor Notes

OBJECTIVES

When the students have completed this chapter, they will be able to:

- List the steps to be taken in completing competency evaluation and testing.
- Describe the function of the state Nurse Aide Registry.
- Select a method of preparing for competency testing.
- Successfully complete a model test.
- Identify job opportunities and be prepared for an interview.
- Write one or two possible career plans using the career options chart provided.
- Describe how their competencies can be assessed in an employment setting.

KEY TERMS

Competency: A demonstrable skill or ability

Continuing Education: Formal classes, courses, or training programs to develop new knowledge or qualify one for career advancement

Evaluation: Assessment of one's ability or skill to perform a given task

Staff Development: On-the-job training or classes provided to enhance or expand an employee's skills or abilities

CORE STUDENT ASSIGNMENTS

Students should:

- Read this chapter in their textbook, *Being a Nursing Assistant.*
- Underline any words or sentences they do not understand. Write down any questions they have.
- Complete the Chapter Review in their textbook.
- Read the Time Management Tip for this chapter and think about how they might use this tip in their work.
- Complete the Nursing Assistant in Action exercise.

OPTIONAL STUDENT ASSIGNMENTS

Students should:

- Complete all workbook assignments for this chapter in their copy of *Workbook for Being a Nursing Assistant.*
- Use the CD/CD-Rom disk enclosed with their textbook to hear the pronunciation of the key terms in the chapter.
- Watch the "Focus on Professionalism" video from the Care Provider Skills series.
- Use the Website address **(www.prenhall.com/wolgin)** to access the free, interactive Companion Website created for this textbook. Get hints, instant feedback, and textbook references to chapter-related multiple-choice questions. Read and react to the Nursing Assistant in Action exercise. Link to other interesting sites.

METHODOLOGY AND SUGGESTED ACTIVITIES

Instructor Notes

I. Lecture/Discussion

- Answer any questions the students may have.
- Discuss the key terms and related abbreviations. Repeat them out loud and practice using them in sentences.
- Discuss the Time Management Tip for this chapter.
- Discuss the Nursing Assistant in Action exercise.
- Discuss the Critical Thinking points for this chapter.
- Invite a few former students to return as an informal panel to describe their jobs. Have your students prepare questions in advance.
- Discuss nursing assistant requirements in your state and career options.
- Discuss test-taking strategies.
- Discuss anxiety-reducing strategies.
- Discuss job possibilities in your area or institution.
- Discuss possible next steps for a career. Have the student set 1-year and 5-year goals.
- Review any institution tuition reimbursement or scholarship programs.

II. Role Play/Lab

- Show the video for this chapter. Discuss what characteristics make a good professional. Have the students recall experiences with health care workers that made them feel well cared for.
- Have the students practice by taking the sample test.
- Pair the students and have them role play interviewing each other.
- Display different résumé styles and discuss their strengths and weaknesses.
- Display orientation and continuing education materials, flyers, and catalogs.

III. Evaluation

- Review the answers to the Chapter Review with students.
- Review the answer to the workbook exercises with students.
- Review the students' understanding of the Time Management Tip.
- To evaluate student comprehension, give a quiz.
- Have the students visit the interactive Companion Website and take the quiz.

ANSWERS TO CHAPTER REVIEW

FILL IN THE BLANK

Read each sentence and fill in the blank line(s) with the word or words that complete the sentence. (Note: Hyphenated words get one line.)

1. A demonstratable skill or ability is called a ___*competency*___.
2. The ___*Nurse*___ ___*Aide*___ ___*Registry*___ is a list kept by each state to show who is certified in that state.

Instructor Notes

3. A(n) ___résumé___ is a one-page description of who you are and what kind of skills you have.

4. The period of time that the institution teaches you about your new job is called ___orientation___.

5. On the job training of classes to enhance or expand an employee's skills or abilities is called ___staff___ ___development___.

MULTIPLE CHOICE

Choose the best answer for each question or statement.

1. When taking the clinical examination portion of the *Nurse Aide State Examination*
   A. you may ask questions of the observer.
   (B.) you may *not* ask questions of the observer.
   C. say you "must always follow policy" anytime you do not know the correct steps.
   D. request prompting only on the skills that are confusing to you.

2. All of the following except one are good places to look for employment.
   A. Want ads
   B. Personal contacts
   C. Local hospitals, nursing homes, and facilities
   (D.) Library

3. Include all of the following on your résumé *except*
   A. your name.
   B. your address.
   (C.) your health history.
   D. your work history.

4. After a job interview you should:
   A. tell the interviewers you will not believe anything they tell you if it is not in writing.
   B. demand to be told immediately if the job will be offered to you.
   C. wait to hear from the interviewer before you contact the agency.
   (D.) smile and thank the interviewers for their time.

5. Which of the following is *not* considered in a promotion?
   A. Your attendance including tardiness
   B. Your willingness and ability to learn new skills
   (C.) The reason you were off sick for 2 days last year
   D. Your most recent performance evaluation or references

CRITICAL THINKING

Instructor Notes

CUSTOMER SERVICE

Encourage students to reflect and share their thoughts and experiences. Respect their privacy and confidentiality. Share your own viewpoints with the students.

CULTURAL CARE

Encourage students to reflect and share their thoughts and experiences. Respect their privacy and confidentiality. Share your own viewpoints with the students.

COOPERATION WITHIN THE TEAM

Encourage students to reflect and share their thoughts and experiences. Respect their privacy and confidentiality. Share your own viewpoints with the students.

NURSING ASSISTANT IN ACTION

You are scheduled to work the night shift and are attending a birthday party prior to going to work. Your host is passing out shots of tequila to toast the guest of honor. Everyone else at the party accepts a glass for the toast. You decline telling your host you are going to work shortly and should not be drinking now. Your friend says, "Don't be such a jerk. Call in sick or chew some breath mints. No one at your job will know the difference."

What Is Your Response/Action?

You should respond that your job is very important so asking in at the last minute is not a good idea. Drinking alcohol could decrease your ability to make good decisions and take good care of patients. Be proud of your job and the responsible position you will have—lives depend on you.

Instructor Notes

35

Answers to Workbook Exercises

The following exercises will assist you to apply what you have read in Chapter 35, "Beginning Your Career as a Nursing Assistant." For each exercise, read the objective and use information you have read in Chapter 35 to answer the questions, complete the sentences, or label the diagrams.

EXERCISE 35-1

Objective: To demonstrate the use of a career plan for a nursing assistant.

Directions: Label the career path drawn in Figure 35-1 with the careers in the Word List below. Next, starting with the year you will begin working as a nursing assistant, label each new job with an additional 5 years until you have completed the career path.

Word List

Food Service Worker	Radiologist, MD
Laboratory Director/Manager	Registered Nurse
Advanced Nursing Assistant	Patient Care Technician
Medical Assistant	EKG Technician
Laboratory Aide	

FIGURE 35-1

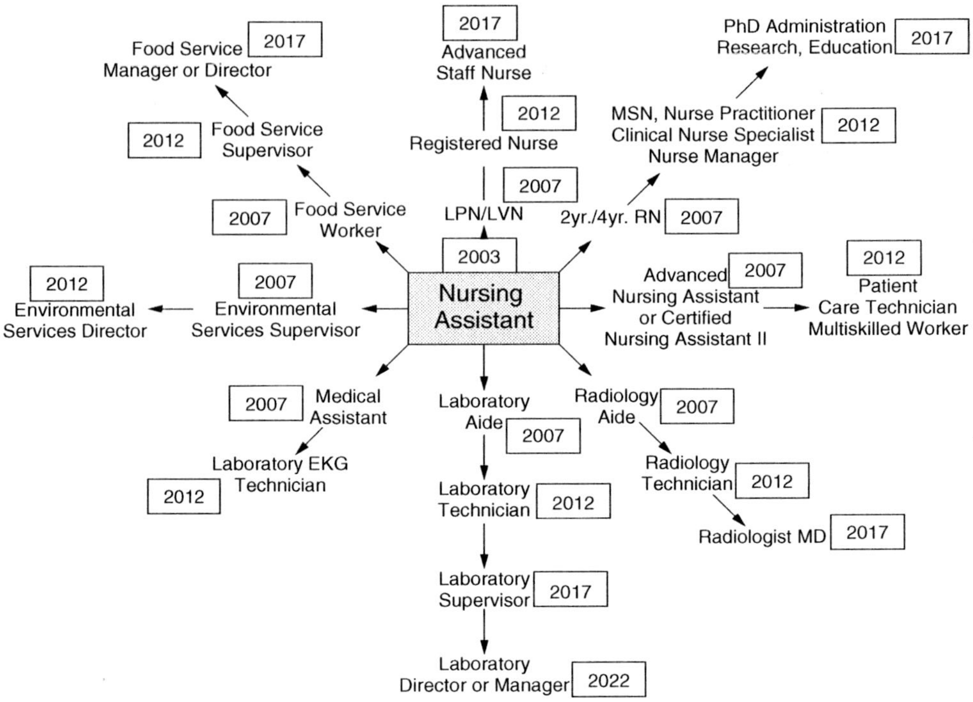

EXERCISE 35-2

Objective: To recognize the definitions of words used in beginning your career as a nursing assistant.

Directions: Draw a line from the correct word(s) in the Word List to the matching Definitions.

Word List	Definitions
staff development	Assessment of one's ability or skill to perform a given task
evaluation	Formal classes or training programs to develop new knowledge or qualify one for career advancement
continuing education	A demonstrable skill or ability
competency	On-the-job training or classes provided to enhance or expand an employee's skills or abilities

EXERCISE 35-3

Objective: To apply what you have learned about beginning your career as a nursing assistant.

Directions: Circle the letter next to the statement that best completes the sentence or describes the sentence as true or false. If the sentence is false, draw a line through the incorrect part of the sentence and write the correction on the blank line.

1. The Omnibus Budget Reconciliation Act of 1987 (OBRA) requires health care facilities to hire nursing assistants
   A. who hold certificates.
   B. who study hard.
   (C.) who hold certificates or licenses from state-approved training programs and have completed the Nursing Assistant Competency Evaluation examination.
   D. who hold up well under stress.

2. Candidates for the competency examination must have completed a state-approved training course consisting of
   A. a maximum of 75 hours of hard labor.
   B. a minimum of 25 hours of classroom time.
   C. a minimum laboratory experience of 45 hours.
   (D.) a minimum of 75 hours of theory, lab practice, and supervised patient care.

3. The Clinical Skills Examination requires the involvement of
   (A.) an actor.
   B. a director.
   C. a producer.
   D. an agent.

4. Some of the tasks you may be asked to demonstrate are
   A. cooking, cleaning, and shopping.
   B. fishing, hunting, and gathering.
   (C.) toileting, applying a safety device, and personal care.
   D. occupying a made bed.

5. This is an important time for you to
   A. ask questions of the actor.
   B. draw conclusions about patient diagnoses.
   C. offer examples of how excellent you are.
   (D.) demonstrate competencies you have acquired during training.

6. After the Clinical Skills Examination, you will be asked to take a written (oral in some situations) examination consisting of
   A. 100 true or false questions.
   (B.) 50 or more multiple-choice questions.
   C. 75 hours of written testimony.
   D. 50 open-book questions.

7. An important part of the multiple-choice examination will include the use of
   A. oral responses of the patient.
   (B.) medical terms and abbreviations.
   C. multiplication tables.
   D. study groups.

8. Upon completing your training course, you have a ________ within which you must complete the testing process and register with the Nurse Aide Registry.
   A. "doorway to disaster"
   B. "hallway to success"
   (C.) "window of opportunity"
   D. "house of cards"

9. The Nurse Aide Registry keeps an official list of
   (A.) registered nursing assistants.
   B. missed "windows of opportunity."
   C. examination appointments.
   D. examination fees.

10. The best contacts for possible employment are
   A. local health care facilities.
   B. family and friends.
   C. Help Wanted classified advertisements in the newspaper.
   (D.) all of the above.

11. Most prospective employers will require that you
   (A.) fill out an application.
   B. work the first pay period for free.
   C. pay for an application.
   D. bring a friend to be with you during the interview.

12. You should be sure to include your ________ skills on the résumé.
   A. animal
   B. dancing
   C. singing
   (D.) people

13. Be sure that your stated objective on the résumé
   A. relates to the job for which you are applying.
   B. is clearly written.
   C. relates to the training you have received.
   (D.) all of the above.

14. In health care, the ability to be flexible with the hours you are willing and able to work is important to getting hired.
   (A.) True
   B. False
   Correct Answer: ______________________________

15. It is important to ________ and shake the interviewer's hand when the interview is over.

(A.) smile
B. look very serious
C. frown
D. avoid eye contact during the interview

16. If a job is offered to you, get a written statement of what the conditions of employment are.

(A.) True
B. False

Correct Answer: ______________________________

17. It is preferred that you accept in writing because this gives you a chance to

A. write a thank you note.
(B.) restate the salary, hours, or shifts you will work and the date you will start the job.
C. give a verbal reply.
D. change the agreement to better suit your expectations.

18. After you have been hired, you can expect

A. to relax and quit learning.
(B.) an orientation to the new job provided by the employer.
C. to take a vacation immediately.
D. to know everything about how to do your new job.

19. To make the most of your years of work in the future, you should

A. consult a psychic.
(B.) create a career path to use as a guide.
C. avoid further training.
D. avoid change whenever possible.

20. Education or career counselors at local colleges can provide you with free information on

A. how to advance your training.
B. how to get funding for school.
C. how to develop a career path.
(D.) all of the above.

21. Gaining experience as a nursing assistant will open many opportunities for employment if you decide to change your career in the future.

(A.) True
B. False

Correct Answer: ______________________________

22. Guidelines for keeping a job include ________ and ________.

A. tardiness, not coming to work
B. using alcohol, drugs before coming to work
C. violating confidentiality rules, abusing patients
(D.) none of the above

APPENDIX A Medical Terms, Abbreviations, and Specialities

OVERVIEW

I. Abbreviations and Their Meanings

II. Word Elements: Roots, Prefixes, and Suffixes

III. Medical Specialties

Instructor Notes

Instructor Notes

OBJECTIVES

When the students have completed Appendix A, "Medical Terms, Abbreviations, and Specialties," they will be able to:

- Define the list of abbreviations commonly used in health care institutions.
- Identify different physicians' titles and describe their meanings.
- Name and describe medical specialties.

KEY TERMS

Abbreviation: A shortened form of a word or phrase used to represent the complete form

Medical Terminology: The special vocabulary of words used in the health care professions

Prefix: A word element added to the beginning of a root

Roman Numerals: The letters used to represent numbers in the ancient Roman system

Root: The body or main part of a word

Suffix: A word element used to change or add to the meaning of a root; it is always added to the end of a root

CORE STUDENT ASSIGNMENTS

Students should:

- Read this chapter in their textbook, *Being a Nursing Assistant*.
- Underline any words or sentences they do not understand. Write down any questions they have.

OPTIONAL STUDENT ASSIGNMENTS

Students should:

- Complete all workbook assignments for this chapter in their copy of *Workbook for Being a Nursing Assistant*.
- Use the CD/CD-Rom disk enclosed with their textbook to hear the pronunciation of the key terms in the chapter.
- Use the Website address **(www.prenhall.com/wolgin)** to access the free, interactive Companion Website created for this textbook. Get hints, instant feedback, and textbook references to chapter-related multiple-choice questions. Read and react to the Nursing Assistant in Action exercise. Link to other interesting sites.

METHODOLOGY AND SUGGESTED ACTIVITIES

Instructor Notes

I. Lecture/Discussion

- Answer any questions the students may have.
- Discuss the key terms and related abbreviations. Repeat them out loud and practice using them in sentences.
- Offer additional examples and/or case studies of new forms in medicine.
- Create a list of common medical and surgical procedures.
- Utilize flash card exercises as a class project. Write each specialty on an individual card. Assign one card per student for group discussion of the definition of the specialty.
- Review and discuss institution-specific abbreviations.

II. Evaluation

- Review the answer to the workbook exercises with students.
- To evaluate student comprehension, give a quiz.
- Have the students visit the interactive Companion Website and take the quiz.

Instructor Notes

Answers to Workbook Exercises

The following exercises will assist you to apply what you have read in Appendix A, "Medical Terms, Abbreviations, and Specialties." For each exercise, read the objective and use information you have read in Appendix A, to answer the questions or complete the sentences.

EXERCISE A-1

Objective: To recognize and correctly spell commonly used abbreviations.

Directions: Define the following commonly used abbreviations:

1. w/c *wheelchair*
2. IV *intravenous line*
3. CVA *cerebrovascular accident*
4. Q.I.D *4 times/day*
5. pre *before*
6. per *by, through*
7. O_2 *oxygen*
8. hypo *below*
9. hr *hour*
10. $\bar{c}$ *with*
11. @ *at*
12. B.I.D. *2 times/day*
13. Ca *cancer*
14. C.C.U. *Coronary Care Unit*
15. amb. *ambulatory*
16. C.V.A. *cerebrovascular accident*
17. DX *diagnosis*
18. ASAP *as soon as possible*
19. po *by mouth*

EXERCISE A-2

Objective: To recognize the correct physician title by its definition.

Directions: Draw a line matching each physician's title with the correct definition.

allergist	a doctor who treats patients with diseases of the heart and circulatory system
cardiologist	a doctor who treats diseases and disorders of the muscular and skeletal systems
gynecologist	a doctor who treats patients with allergies
orthopedist	a doctor who treats patients with mental disorders
psychiatrist	a doctor who treats patients with diseases of the female reproductive organs

EXERCISE A-3

Objective: To recognize the definitions of frequently used terms.

Directions: Use the words listed below to correctly fill in the blanks in the following sentences.

Word List

abbreviation	prefix	Roman numerals
medical terminology	root	suffix

1. A shortened word or phrase used to represent the complete form is a(n). ___*abbreviation*___.
2. The special vocabulary used in the health care professions is referred to as ___*medical*___ ___*terminology*___.
3. The word element that is always added to the end of a root to change or add meaning is the ___*suffix*___.
4. The body or main part of a word is the ___*root*___.
5. ___*Roman*___ ___*numerals*___ are the letters used to represent numbers in the ancient Roman system.
6. A(n) ___*prefix*___ is a word element added to the beginning of a root.

EXERCISE A-4

Objective: To recognize and label Roman numerals.

Directions: Write the Roman numerals for 1 to 5.

1. I
2. II
3. III
4. IV
5. V

EXERCISE A-5

Objective: To recognize similarity between medical terms.

Directions: Draw a line matching word elements to their related terminology and meaning.

1. ante	macroscopy	A. seen **large,** as with naked eye
2. cyto	hypotension	B. **before** onset of fever
3. macro	cytogenesis	C. **low** blood pressure
4. a	intracranial	D. **within** the skull
5. hypo	antefebrile	E. production (origin) **of the cell**
6. intra	afebrile	F. **without** fever

EXERCISE A-6

Objective: To recognize and correctly label abbreviations of terms and the meaning of abbreviations.

Directions: Write the abbreviations for the following terms:

1. nothing by mouth NPO
2. oxygen O_2
3. intravenous IV
4. before surgery preop
5. head of bed HoB

Write the meaning of the following abbreviations:

6. R.N. registered nurse
7. Spec. specimen
8. ADL activities of daily living
9. TPR temperature, pulse, respiration
10. C.S.R. Central supply room

EXERCISE A-7

Objective: To learn the list of abbreviations and their meanings. This is a big list, and there is a lot of important information here. It will be easier to remember what all the different abbreviations are if you try to learn them one at a time. One easy way to learn the list is to study from flash cards. You can create your own set of flash cards by using 3 × 5 index cards. Write the abbreviation on one side and the meaning on the other side. Now you can test yourself.

Directions:

1. Arrange all the cards so the name of the abbreviation is facing up and the meaning is facing down.
2. Read the name of the first abbreviation in your stack.
3. Try to remember the meaning from studying your textbook.
4. Say the meaning out loud.
5. Turn the card over and read the meaning to see if you were right.
6. If you were correct, put the card in a pile on the left, and you are finished studying this card.
7. If you were wrong, put the card in a pile on the right, so you can study it later.
8. Repeat this for all the cards.
9. Now go back to the pile of cards on the right and study these.
10. Read each card front and back five times.
11. Close your eyes and try to say the name of the abbreviation and its meaning.
12. Open your eyes and see if you were correct.
13. Repeat this for all the cards that you originally put on the right side.
14. When you feel that you have learned them all, test yourself again.
15. Ask a friend or relative to test you by holding the first card up so you can see the abbreviation. Read the abbreviation and recite the meaning.
16. Your friend can read the meaning to determine if you are correct.
17. Repeat this for all the cards.
18. Turn the stack upside down.
19. Now go through the cards and read the meaning and tell the name of the abbreviation.
20. Continue in this way over and over again, until you have learned all the abbreviations and their meanings.